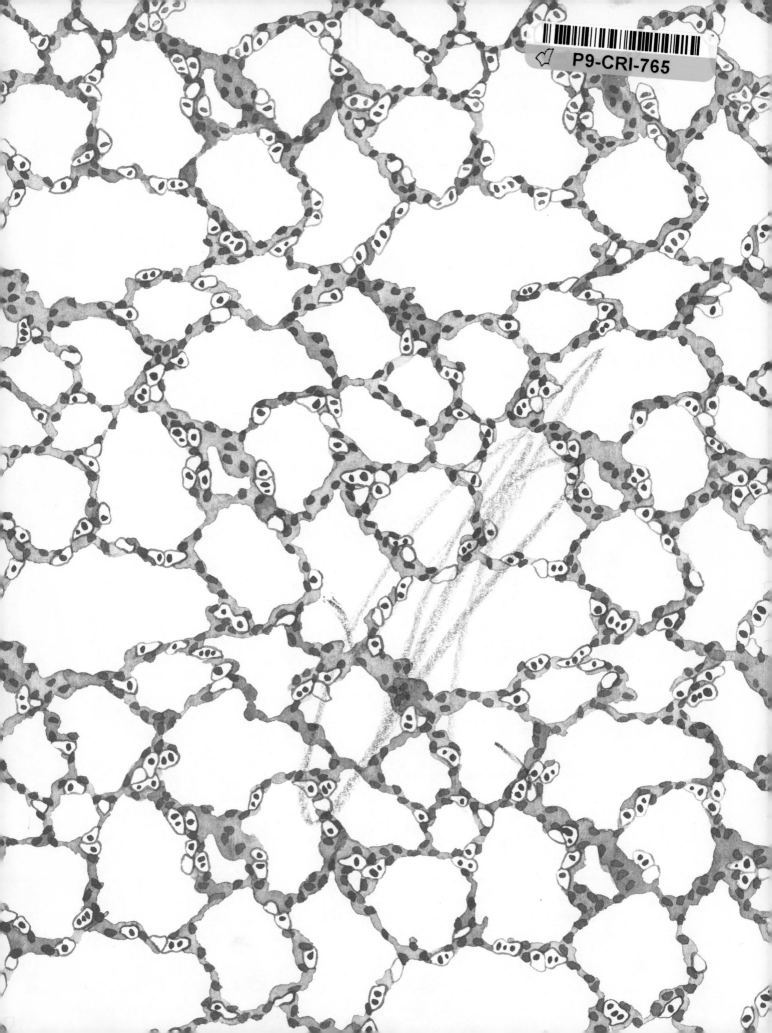

P9-CRI-765

NURSING84 BOOKS™

Nurse's Clinical Library™
Other volumes in this series:
Cardiovascular Disorders
Endocrine Disorders
Neurologic Disorders
Renal and Urologic Disorders

Nurse's Reference Library®
Diseases
Diagnostics
Drugs
Assessment
Procedures
Definitions
Practices

New Nursing Skillbook™
series
Giving Emergency Care
    Competently
Monitoring Fluid and
    Electrolytes Precisely
Assessing Vital Functions
    Accurately
Coping with Neurologic
    Problems Proficiently
Reading EKGs Correctly
Combatting Cardiovascular
    Diseases Skillfully
Nursing Critically Ill Patients

Nursing Photobook™
series
Providing Respiratory Care
Managing I.V. Therapy
Dealing with Emergencies
Giving Medications
Assessing Your Patients
Using Monitors
Providing Early Mobility
Giving Cardiac Care
Performing GI Procedures
Implementing Urologic
    Procedures
Controlling Infection
Ensuring Intensive Care
Coping with Neurologic
    Disorders
Caring for Surgical Patients
Working with Orthopedic
    Patients
Nursing Pediatric Patients
Helping Geriatric Patients
Attending Ob/Gyn Patients
Aiding Ambulatory Patients
Carrying Out Special
    Procedures

Nursing Now™
Shock
Hypertension
Drug Interactions
Cardiac Crises
Respiratory Emergencies

***Nursing84* Drug Handbook**™

Cover: color-enhanced
pulmonary X-ray.
Photograph by Howard Sochurek.

Inside front and back covers:
cross section of alveoli.

NURSE'S CLINICAL LIBRARY™
RESPIRATORY DISORDERS

NURSING84 BOOKS™
SPRINGHOUSE CORPORATION
Springhouse, Pennsylvania

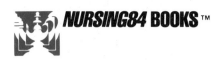

NURSING84 BOOKS™

The clinical procedures described and recommended in this publication are based on research and consultation with medical and nursing authorities. To the best of our knowledge, these procedures reflect currently accepted clinical practice; nevertheless, they can't be considered absolute and universal recommendations. For individual application, treatment recommendations must be considered in light of the patient's clinical condition and, before administration of new or infrequently used drugs, in light of latest package-insert information. The authors and the publisher disclaim responsibility for any adverse effects resulting directly or indirectly from the suggested procedures, from any undetected errors, or from the reader's misunderstanding of the text.

© 1984 by Springhouse Corporation, 1111 Bethlehem Pike, Springhouse, Pa. 19477

All rights reserved. Reproduction in whole or part by any means whatsoever without written permission of the publisher is prohibited by law. Patient-teaching aids in this book may be reproduced by office copier for distribution to patients. Written permission is required for any other use or to copy any other material in this book. Printed in the United States of America.

NCL2-010384

Library of Congress Cataloging in Publication Data
Main entry under title:
Respiratory disorders.

(Nurse's clinical library)
"Nursing84 Books."
Includes bibliographies and index.
1. Respiratory disease nursing—Addresses, essays, lectures. I. Series.
[DNLM: 1. Lung diseases—Nursing.
2. Respiratory tract disease—Nursing. WY 163 R4335]
RC735.5.R466   1984
616.2'0024613   83-20354
ISBN 0-916730-58-1

Nurse's Clinical Library™

Editorial Director
Helen Klusek Hamilton

Clinical Director
Minnie Bowen Rose, RN, BSN, MEd

Art Director
Sonja E. Douglas

Clinical staff

Senior Clinical Editor
Regina Daley Ford, RN, BSN, MA

Acquisitions Editors
Elizabeth J. Cobbs; Patricia A. Devine, RN, BSN

Clinical Editors
Joanne Patzek DaCunha, RN; Diane Cochet, RN, BSN; Carole Arlene Pyle, RN, BSN, MA, CCRN

Contributing Clinical Editors
Mary Chapman Gyetvan, RN, BSEd; Jo-Ann Hopkins Olmstead, RN, BS; Patricia Dwyer Schull, RN, BS, MSN; Nina Poorman Welsh, RN

Drug Information Manager
Larry N. Gever, RPh, PharmD

Editorial staff

Editorial Manager
Matthew Cahill

Associate Editors
Lisa Z. Cohen, Martin DiCarlantonio, Nancy Holmes, June Norris, Patricia Minard Shinehouse

Contributing Editors
Elaine Schott-Jones, Joan Twisdom

Copy Supervisor
David R. Moreau

Copy Editors
Diane M. Labus, Jo Lennon

Contributing Copy Editors
Susan L. Baumann, Reni Fetterolf, Max A. Fogel, David D. Jones, Doris Weinstock

Production Coordinator
Sally Johnson

Editorial Assistants
Mary Ann Bowes, Maree DeRosa, Bernadette Glenn

Indexer
Barbara Hodgson

Researchers
Vonda Heller, Elaine Shelly

Design staff

Senior Designer
Linda Jovinelly Franklin

Contributing Designers
Maryanne Buschini, Anthony Gasparich, Donna Monturo, Mary Wise

Illustrators
Michael Adams, Dimitrios Bastas, Maryanne Buschini, David Christiana, Design Management, Jean Gardner, Anthony Gasparich, Tom Herbert, Robert Jackson, Robert Jones, David Noyes, Robert Phillips, George Retseck, Eileen Rudnick, Dennis Schofield, Daniel F. Sneberger

Production staff

Art Production Manager
Robert Perry

Art Assistants
Diane Fox, Donald Knauss, Sandy Sanders, Craig T. Siman, Louise Stamper, Thom Staudenmayer

Typography Manager
David C. Kosten

Typography Assistants
Janice Haber, Ethel Halle, Debra Judy, Diane Paluba, Nancy Wirs

Senior Production Manager
Deborah C. Meiris

Production Manager
Wilbur D. Davidson

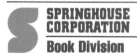

SPRINGHOUSE CORPORATION
Book Division

Chairman
Eugene W. Jackson

President
Daniel L. Cheney

Vice-President and Director
Timothy King

Vice-President, Book Operations
Thomas A. Temple

Vice-President, Production and Purchasing
Bacil Guiley

Research Director
Elizabeth O'Brien

Advisory Board

At the time of publication, the advisors held the following positions:

Charold Baer, RN, PhD, Professor and Chairperson, Department of Medical-Surgical Nursing, University of Oregon Health Sciences Center, Portland

Lillian Brunner, RN, MSN, ScD, FAAN, Consultant in Nursing, Presbyterian–University of Pennsylvania Medical Center, Philadelphia

Bruce Clayton, PharmD, Associate Professor and Vice-Chairman, Department of Pharmacy Practice, College of Pharmacy, University of Nebraska Medical Center, Omaha

Leonard Crowley, MD, Clinical Assistant Professor, Department of Laboratory Medicine and Pathology, and Department of Family Practice, University of Minnesota, Minneapolis; Pathologist, St. Mary's Hospital, Minneapolis

Judith Donlen, RNC, MSN, Assistant Director of Nursing Education, Department of Nursing, Children's Hospital of Philadelphia

Kathleen Dracup, RN, DNS, CCRN, FAAN, Assistant Professor, School of Nursing, Center for Health Sciences, University of California, Los Angeles

DeAnn Englert, RN, MSN, Assistant Professor, School of Nursing, Louisiana State University Medical Center, New Orleans

Sr. Rebecca Fidler, MT(ASCP), PhD, Chairperson of Health Sciences and Professor of Medical Technology, Salem College, Salem, West Virginia

Mitchell Jacobsen, MD, Coordinator of Continuing Education, Mt. Sinai Medical Center, Milwaukee

John Laszlo, MD, Director, Clinical Programs, Duke Comprehensive Cancer Center, Duke University Medical Center, Durham, N.C.

Evan McLeod, MD, Director, Pulmonary Rehabilitation Program, Michael Reese Hospital, Chicago

Madeline Wake, RN, MSN, Director of Continuing Education in Nursing, Marquette University, Milwaukee

Connie Walleck, RN, MS, CNRN, Nurse Clinician II/Research Assistant, University of Maryland Hospital, Baltimore

Johnsie W. Woody, RN, Respiratory Nurse Clinician, Duke University Medical Center, Durham, N.C.

CONTENTS

CONTRIBUTORS AND CLINICAL CONSULTANTS

Contributors

At the time of publication, the contributors held the following positions:

Virginia Barrett, RN, CCRN, Student, LaSalle College, Philadelphia, Pa.

Deborah L. Dalrymple, RN, BSN, Clinical Instructor, Montgomery County Community College, Blue Bell, Pa.; Staff Nurse, I.V. Therapy, Doylestown Hospital, Doylestown, Pa.

Kathleen Viall Gallagher, RN, MSN, Former Instructor, Associate Degree Program, School of Nursing, Hahnemann University, Philadelphia, Pa.

Shirley Given, HT(ASCP), Supervisor, Histology, Crozer-Chester Medical Center, Upland, Pa.

Sheila A. Glennon, RN, MA, CCRN, Chief, Division of Critical Care Nursing, Norwalk Hospital, Norwalk, Conn.

Tobie V. Hittle, RN, BSN, CCRN, Head Nurse, Intensive Care Unit, Genesee Hospital, Rochester, N.Y.

Sr. Eileen Marie Hollen, RN, BSN, CCRN, Special Care Unit Supervisor, Nazareth Hospital, Philadelphia, Pa.

Anita Johnston-Early, RN, Oncology Nurse Investigator and Protocol Coordinator, Veterans Administration Medical Center, Washington, D.C.

Susan A. Kayes, BS, SM(ASCP), Supervisor, Microbiology Department, Putnam Memorial Hospital, Bennington, Vt.

Ruth S. Kitson, RN, BAA, Clinical Coordinator, ICU, CCU, CVS Cardiology, Toronto Western Hospital, Toronto, Ont.

Marcella Majors, RN, MSN, Pulmonary Nurse Clinical Specialist, Providence Hospital, Cincinnati, Ohio; Assistant Professor, Field Service Faculty, College of Nursing and Health, University of Cincinnati.

Barbara A. Mlynczak, RN, CCRN, Coordinator, Division of Clinical Nursing Education, Anne Arundel General Hospital, Annapolis, Md.

Marilee Warner Mohr, RN, MSN, Clinical Supervisor, Ob/Gyn Division, Lankenau Hospital, Philadelphia, Pa.; Faculty, College of Nursing, Pennsylvania State University, Delaware County Campus, Media, Pa.

Mae E. Paulfrey, RN, MN, Assistant Professor, University of San Francisco, School of Nursing, San Francisco, Calif.

Janice G. Stewart, RN, MSN, Special Projects Coordinator, Thomas Jefferson University Hospital, Philadelphia, Pa.

Irene Vernaglia Toomey, RN, CCRN, School Nurse, Halifax Elementary School, Halifax, Mass.

Bertha Warren, RN, MSN, Pulmonary Clinical Nurse Specialist, Sepulveda Veterans Administration Medical Center, Sepulveda, Calif.

Terri E. Weaver, RN, MSN, Pulmonary Clinical Nurse Specialist, Hospital of the University of Pennsylvania; Clinical Instructor, Adult Health and Illness Section, School of Nursing, University of Pennsylvania, Philadelphia.

Linda M. Woodin, RN, BSN, Unit Instructor, Department of Nursing, Medical-Surgical Division, Lehigh Valley Hospital Center, Allentown, Pa.

Clinical Consultants

At the time of publication, the clinical consultants held the following positions:

Joan P. Chalikian, RN, MSN, CCRN, Clinical Specialist, Pulmonary Nursing, Crozer-Chester Medical Center, Upland, Pa.

Alan M. Chausow, MD, ABIM, Pulmonary Medicine Boards, Attending Physician, Michael Reese Hospital and Medical Center, Chicago; Assistant Professor of Medicine, University of Chicago.

Elizabeth R. Cox, RN, BS, Infection Control Practitioner, Bryn Mawr Hospital, Bryn Mawr, Pa.

Patricia Turk Horvath, RN, MSN, Assistant Professor, Graduate Program, School of Nursing, Kent State University, Kent, Ohio.

Edward E. Landis, Jr., MD, Medical Director, Respiratory Therapy, Pulmonary Consultant, Charlotte Memorial Hospital and the Nalle Clinic, Charlotte, N.C.

Neil R. McIntyre, MD, Assistant Professor of Medicine, Duke University Medical Center, Durham, N.C.

Carlene R. Peat, RN, BSN, Supervisor, Respiratory Care Department, Kaiser Foundation Hospital, Walnut Creek, Calif.

Mack A. Thomas, MD, FACS, Chief, Anesthesiology Service, Veterans Administration Medical Center and Director of Education, Charity Hospital Department of Anesthesia, New Orleans, La.

Peter G. Tuteur, MD, Coursemaster, Department of Internal Medicine, Washington University School of Medicine, St. Louis, Mo.

Terri E. Weaver, RN, MSN, Pulmonary Clinical Nurse Specialist, Hospital of the University of Pennsylvania; Clinical Instructor, School of Nursing, University of Pennsylvania, Philadelphia.

William Weiss, MD, Professor of Medicine, Hahnemann University School of Medicine, Philadelphia, Pa.

Johnsie Whitt Woody, RN, Respiratory Nurse Clinician, Duke University Medical Center, Durham, N.C.

FOREWORD

Competent respiratory nursing can improve the quality of life and function for the 2 million people who continue to seek treatment for respiratory disorders each year. Nurses are now assuming a central role in respiratory care and are involved in all phases from prevention to acute and rehabilitative care. In fact, they're being recognized as coordinators of the new respiratory care team, scheduling the delivery and monitoring the effects of a host of constellatory treatments and services.

No longer primarily supportive, nursing care of respiratory disease requires a ready grasp of respiratory mechanics and the implications of their dysfunction for interacting vital systems. Nurses must know how to distinguish between CO_2 narcosis and simple fatigue, and know when best to schedule chest physiotherapy, IPPB, and other treatments. Their accurate interventions—suction, turning, mobility, coughing and deep breathing exercises—are crucial to the patient's ventilatory status. Careful nursing attention can prevent the need for intubation and can determine whether the patient improves or proceeds into respiratory failure.

Nurses are pivotal figures in helping the patient gain and maintain independence. They must evaluate self-care, teach relaxation techniques and energy conservation, and be able to spot problems and rally the proper medical, social, and psychological resources. In the community, nurses are advocates for disease prevention, warning about the risk of smoking, and educating about occupational and environmental respiratory carcinogens.

As educators, primary care-givers, and coordinators of respiratory care, nurses need a thorough grounding in respiratory fundamentals and up-to-date knowledge of available treatments. RESPIRATORY DISORDERS, the second volume in a new reference series for nurses, supplies both theoretical and practical information about respiratory nursing today.

An introductory chapter reviews the principles of normal respiratory anatomy and physiology, the mechanisms of respiratory dysfunction, and its direct effect on acid-base balance and major body systems. A second chapter explains respiratory assessment techniques, and supplies guidelines for developing nursing diagnoses based on assessment findings. The third chapter outlines the diagnostic tests that verify respiratory disorders, and the nurse's role in the diagnostic process.

Successive chapters in this volume discuss specific respiratory disorders. Each chapter contains three major sections. *Pathophysiology* covers the origins of each disorder, distinguishing signs and symptoms, deviant physiology, and its impact on the body. *Medical management* summarizes appropriate diagnostic tests and findings, current treatment, and prognosis. *Nursing management* focuses on the steps of the nursing process. For each disorder, this section relates pertinent items to include in the nursing history, and significant assessment findings and their implications. It details the type of nursing diagnoses that may flow from the assessment findings, and expands on the goals of nursing care, nursing interventions for attaining those goals, tips for recognizing life-threatening complications such as tension pneumothorax and pulmonary embolism, and guidelines for evaluating the success of nursing interventions.

Interspersed throughout the text are numerous color diagrams, anatomic drawings, charts, graphs, teaching aids, and supplementary material. The appendix adds information about the drugs most often used to treat respiratory disorders, along with possible side effects and important nursing considerations.

With respiratory disorders the most rapidly increasing of the 10 leading causes of death and disability, and a fast-growing population over age 55, nurses are challenged to hone their knowledge of current respiratory care. This volume will help you meet that challenge confidently.

TERRI E. WEAVER, RN, MSN
Pulmonary Clinical Nurse Specialist
Hospital of the University of Pennsylvania
Clinical Instructor/Lecturer, School of Nursing
University of Pennsylvania

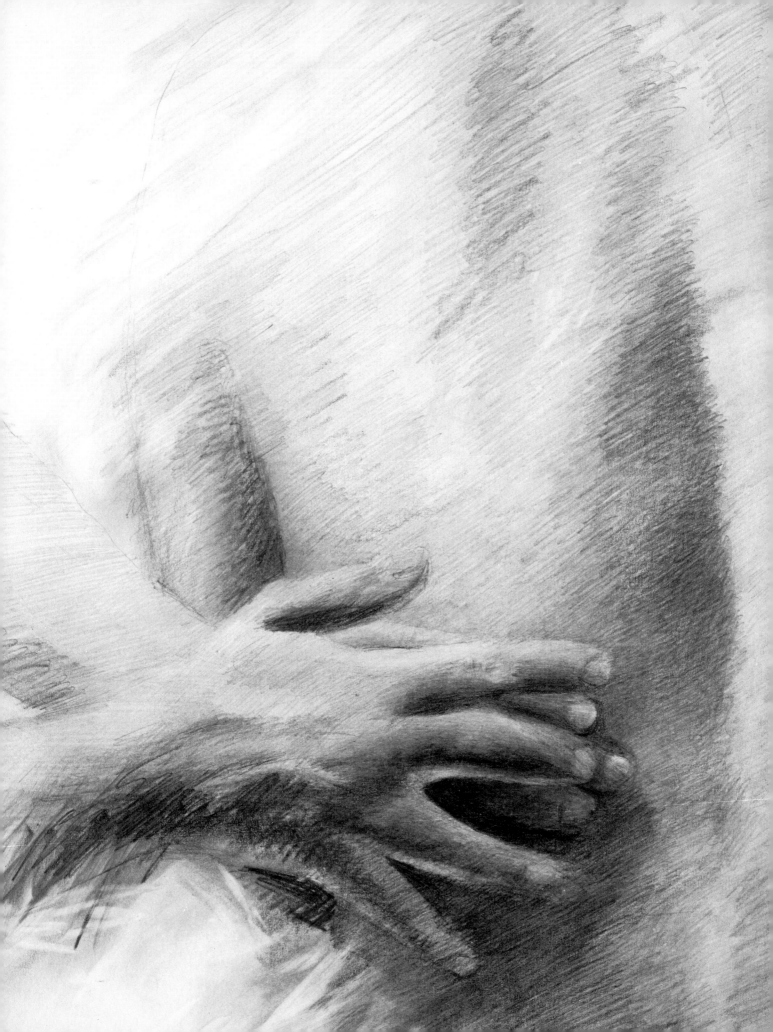

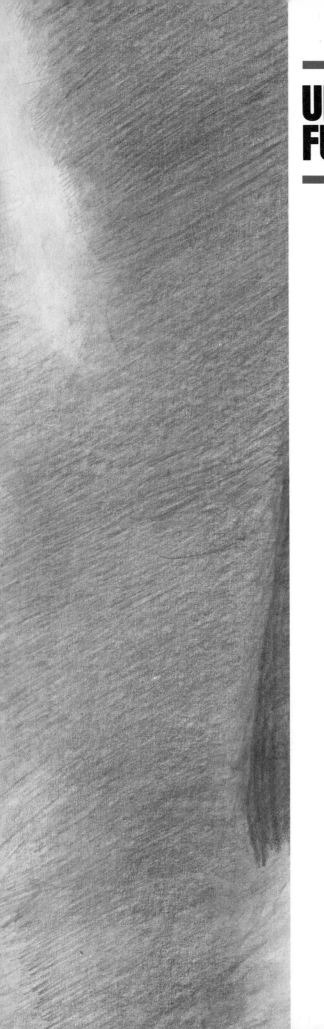

UNDERSTANDING FUNDAMENTALS

1 REVIEWING BASIC PRINCIPLES

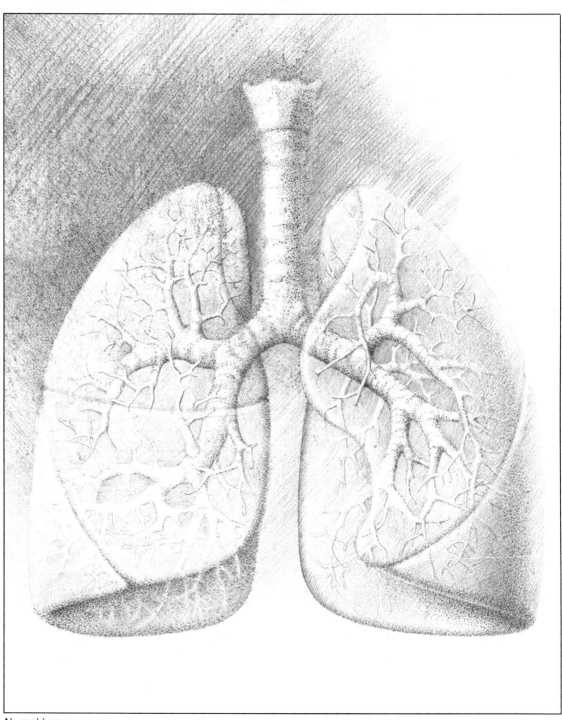

Normal lungs

One in every five Americans suffers from some form of respiratory disease, ranging from chronic sinusitis to severe chronic obstructive pulmonary disease. And the numbers are increasing.

While drugs now control many diseases of the past, such as tuberculosis, respiratory disease currently ranks as the second leading cause of disability and the sixth leading cause of death. Mortality rates are rising steadily at 1.4% per year. The most dramatic increase has been for women—40% in the last 10 years, compared with a 9% increase for men—related primarily to an increase in smoking among women.

In your practice, you'll be seeing more patients with severe chronic respiratory diseases. You'll also be seeing patients who are living longer with their chronic conditions, because of recent technologic advances in medicine. Such advances now permit direct measurement of alveolar oxygenation and carbon dioxide exchange for more effective monitoring of respiratory and metabolic status. They include ventilator refinements, which offer new flexibility in gas-flow delivery to compensate for specific pulmonary disorders. And they include improved tracheostomy and endotracheal tube design, meaning fewer complications and a greater survival rate for patients requiring long-term acute respiratory management. In addition, advances in treating other body system disorders have increased the number of patients with residual severe impairment of respiratory function after survival of critical illness.

Technologic advances have also helped develop respiratory care as a distinct nursing specialty. As an integral member of the new respiratory care team, you're now expected to identify and help solve problems, formulate nursing diagnoses and plans of care, and provide treatment based on current thinking and sophisticated equipment. You're called on to educate the patient and his family about respiratory disorder and its management, and to prepare them to handle long-term care at home. You may also be involved in home visits to ensure that the patient maintains an adequate standard of self-care.

The expanded responsibilities of respiratory care require proficiency in all nursing skills—from assessment to evaluation. To meet these responsibilities, you must first understand fully the function, physiology, and pathophysiology of the respiratory system.

RESPIRATORY FUNCTION

The respiratory system is the body's life-support mechanism in more ways than the obvious. To be sure, its primary function is to bring together roughly equal flows of air and blood, and to effect the crucial exchange of carbon dioxide and oxygen in the lungs. This exchange supports a subordinate but no less critical function—helping to maintain acid-base balance. One way or another, this complex system supports *all* vital functions. Effective respiratory function can compensate for severe physiologic deficits in other body systems; its dysfunction provokes widespread systemic dysfunction. Beyond this, the lungs themselves have several minor functions:
• storing small amounts of blood
• acting as a minor excretion route for certain drugs and metabolites, such as anesthetic vapors and gases, through the action of catecholomethyltransferase and dimethylating enzymes
• helping to inactivate serotonin by taking it up into endothelial cells
• producing angiotensin II, the most potent vasoconstrictor known, from its inactive precursor, angiotensin I. (Even though angiotensin I is present in other cells, the pulmonary capillaries provide the most efficient site for its conversion to angiotensin II.)

Pulmonary circulation

The respiratory system's primary purpose, of course, is the exchange of carbon dioxide and oxygen. To achieve this exchange, the airways of the tracheobronchial tree are shadowed by a similar network of blood vessels. Oxygen-depleted blood being routed to the lungs for replenishment is pumped from the right ventricle to the pulmonary trunk. This trunk then branches laterally into the right and left pulmonary arteries, which further divide into smaller arteries and closely follow the bronchial airways throughout the lungs. Eventually, pulmonary arteries branch into arterioles and venules that form capillary beds around and protruding into the alveoli, the site of gas exchange. After oxygen diffusion, oxygenated blood travels to the left atrium to be pumped throughout systemic circulation.

The tissues of the lung and pleura receive blood from the bronchial arteries, which arise from the aorta and its branches. The bronchial arteries are part of systemic circulation and play no part in the oxygenation of blood.

An extensive network of lymph vessels drains the pulmonary pleura and the dense

Frontal sinus

Inferior nasal concha

Superior nasal concha

Middle nasal concha

Naris

Sphenoid sinus

Choana

Nasopharynx

Oropharynx

Laryngopharynx

Esophagus

Soft palate

Oral cavity

Epiglottis

Thyroid cartilage

Trachea

Carina

Left primary bronchus

Hilum

Left secondary
(segmental) bronchus

Mediastinum

Bronchiole

Alveolus

Reviewing respiratory basics

The respiratory system exchanges carbon dioxide produced by cellular metabolism for atmospheric oxygen. Divided into upper and lower tracts, it includes the organs responsible for external respiration.

Upper tract
The upper respiratory tract consists of the nose, mouth, nasopharynx, oropharynx, laryngopharynx, and larynx. Air enters the body through the nostrils (nares), where small hairs (vibrissae) filter out dust and large foreign particles. It then passes into the two nasal passages, separated by the septum. Cartilage forms the anterior walls, and bony structures (conchae or turbinates) form the posterior walls. The conchae warm and humidify air before it passes into the nasopharynx. Their mucous layer also traps finer foreign particles, which the cilia carry to the pharynx to be swallowed. The four paranasal sinuses, which provide speech resonance, drain through the meatuses near the conchae.

Air passes from the nasal cavity into the muscular nasopharynx through the choanae, which remain constantly open.

The oropharynx, the posterior wall of the mouth, connects nasopharynx and laryngopharynx. The laryngopharynx extends to the esophagus and larynx.

The larynx, which contains the vocal cords, connects the pharynx with the trachea by means of cartilaginous and muscular walls. It includes the large, shield-shaped thyroid cartilage situated just under the jawline. The larynx is protected during swallowing by the epiglottis, a flexible cartilage that bends reflexively to close the larynx to swallowed substances.

Lower tract
The lower respiratory tract is subdivided into the conducting airways (trachea, primary bronchi, lobar and segmental bronchi) and the acinus, which is

Laminar flow

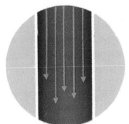

This linear pattern occurs at low flow rates, with minimal airflow resistance in the small peripheral airways.

Turbulent flow

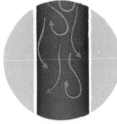

This eddying pattern occurs at high flow rates, with much airflow resistance, in the trachea and large central bronchi.

Transitional flow

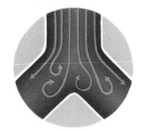

This mixed pattern occurs at lower flow rates in the larger airways, especially where they branch, converge, or narrow because of obstruction.

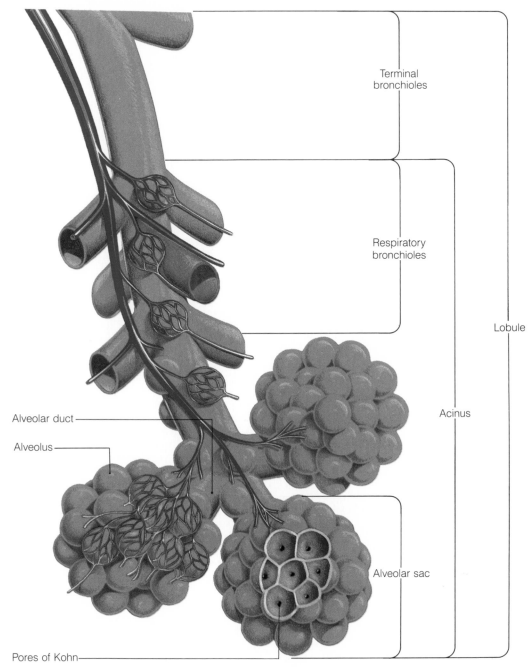

the area of gas exchange (respiratory bronchioles, alveolar ducts, and alveoli). Mucous membrane lines the respiratory tract, and constant movement of mucus by ciliary action cleanses the tract and carries foreign matter upward for swallowing or expectoration.

The tubular trachea, half in the neck and half in the thorax, extends about 5″ (12 cm) from the only complete tracheal ring, the cricoid cartilage, to the carina at the level of the sixth or seventh thoracic vertebra. C-shaped cartilage rings reinforce and protect the trachea, preventing its collapse.

The right and left primary (mainstem) bronchi begin at the carina, or tracheal bifurcation. The right primary bronchus is shorter, wider, and more vertical than the left. The primary bronchi divide into the five secondary (lobar) bronchi and—accompanied by blood vessels, nerves, and lymphatics—enter the lungs at the hilum. Each lobar bronchus enters a lobe.

Within its lobe, each of the secondary bronchi branches into segmental and smaller bronchi and finally into bronchioles. Each bronchiole, in turn, branches into a lobule. The lobule includes the terminal bronchioles, which conclude the conducting airways; and the acinus, the chief respiratory unit for gas exchange. Within the acinus, terminal bronchioles branch into respiratory bronchioles, which structurally resemble bronchioles but also feed directly into alveoli at sites along their walls. These respiratory bronchioles end in alveolar sacs, clusters of capillary-swathed alveoli, and it's through their thin walls that two-way gas diffusion takes place.

Respiratory membrane
The thin alveolar walls contain two basic epithelial cell types. Type I cells, the most abundant, are thin, flat, squamous cells across which gas exchange occurs. Type II cells secrete a surfactant that coats *(continued)*

Terminal bronchioles

Respiratory bronchioles

Lobule

Acinus

Alveolar duct

Alveolus

Alveolar sac

Pores of Kohn

Normal

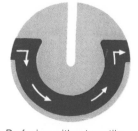

Ventilation matches perfusion.

Shunt

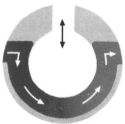

Perfusion without ventilation usually results from airway obstruction, particularly caused by acute diseases, such as atelectasis, pneumonia.

Dead-space ventilation

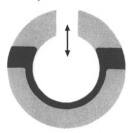

Normal ventilation without perfusion usually results from a perfusion defect, such as pulmonary embolism.

Silent unit

Absence of ventilation and perfusion usually stems from multiple causes, such as pulmonary embolism with resultant ARDS.

the alveolus and facilitates gas exchange by lowering surface tension. These alveolar cells, along with a minute interstitial space, capillary basement membrane, and endothelial cell in the capillary wall, collectively make up the "respiratory membrane" separating the alveolus and capillary.

The entire structure is less than 1 micron thick. Any increase in thickness or decrease in surfactant production decreases the rate of gas diffusion across the membrane.

Lungs and accessory structures

Straddling the heart, the cone-shaped lungs fill the thoracic cavity, the right lung shorter and broader than the left. Each lung's concave base rests on the diaphragm, and the apex extends about ½" (1 cm) above the first rib. Above and behind the heart lies the hilum, the opening through which pass the lung's root structures—primary bronchus, pulmonary and bronchial blood vessels, lymphatics, and nerves. Except at the hilum, where root and pulmonary ligaments anchor them, the lungs are freely movable.

Pleura. Composed of a visceral layer and a parietal layer, the pleura totally encloses the lung. The visceral pleura hugs the contours of the lung surface, including the fissures between lobes. The parietal pleura lines the inner surface of the chest wall and the upper surface of the diaphragm, doubles back around the mediastinum, and joins the visceral layer at the lung root. The space between the pleural layers, the pleural cavity, is only a potential space. A thin film of serous fluid fills this cavity, lubricating the pleural surfaces to slide smoothly against each other while creating a cohesive force between the layers, which compels the lungs to move synchronously with the chest wall during breathing.

Thoracic cavity. The area within the chest wall—the thoracic cavity—is bounded below by the diaphragm; above by the scalene muscles and the fascia of the neck; and circumferentially by the ribs, intercostal muscles, vertebrae, sternum, and ligaments.

Mediastinum. The space between the lungs—the mediastinum—includes the heart and pericardium; the thoracic aorta; the pulmonary artery and veins; the vena cavae and azygos veins; the thymus, lymph nodes, and vessels; the trachea, esophagus, and thoracic duct; and the vagus, cardiac, and phrenic nerves.

Gas diffusion and the law of partial pressures

The concept of diffusion draws on Dalton's law of partial pressures. This law states that in a mixture of gases, the pressure (tension) exerted by each gas is independent of the other gases present and directly corresponds to the percentage it represents of the total mixture.

Here's how Dalton's law works. Atmospheric air inspired at sea level exerts a pressure of 760 mm Hg against all parts of the body. Oxygen represents 21% of air, and therefore exerts a partial pressure (Po_2) of 158 mm Hg, or 21% of 760 mm Hg. Carbon dioxide, a trace element of atmospheric air, has a partial pressure (Pco_2) of 0.3 mm Hg. Nitrogen, making up 78% of air, has a partial pressure of 596 mm Hg. Lastly, water vapor has a partial pressure (PH_2O) of 5.7 mm Hg.

During inspiration, the upper respiratory tract warms and humidifies atmospheric air, increasing the partial pressure of water vapor to 47 mm Hg. Partial pressures of the other gases decline since total pressure must remain at 760 mm Hg. Before entering the alveoli, inspired air mixes with gas that wasn't exhaled on the previous expiration. Since this gas contains more carbon dioxide and less oxygen than inspired air, partial pressures must change again.

Gas that finally enters the alveoli for diffusion across the respiratory membrane registers still further partial pressure changes but remains high in oxygen pressure and low in carbon dioxide pressure. It's met by deoxygenated blood from the right ventricle with low oxygen and high carbon dioxide pressure. The differential in partial pressures of oxygen and carbon dioxide causes the two gases to cross the respiratory membrane toward the lower side of their respective pressure gradients. Oxygen diffuses into the blood and carbon dioxide diffuses outward, equalizing the gas pressures on both sides of the respiratory membrane.

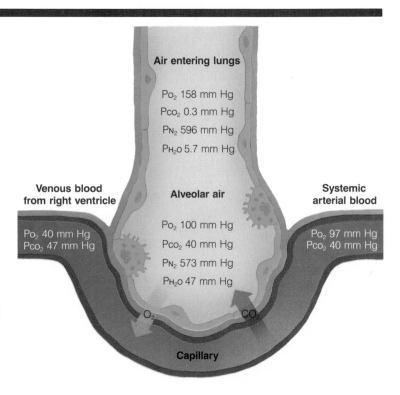

Air entering lungs

Po_2 158 mm Hg
Pco_2 0.3 mm Hg
PN_2 596 mm Hg
PH_2O 5.7 mm Hg

Venous blood from right ventricle

Alveolar air

Po_2 100 mm Hg
Pco_2 40 mm Hg
PN_2 573 mm Hg
PH_2O 47 mm Hg

Systemic arterial blood

Po_2 40 mm Hg
Pco_2 47 mm Hg

Po_2 97 mm Hg
Pco_2 40 mm Hg

O_2

CO_2

Capillary

connective tissue around the bronchi, respiratory bronchioles, pulmonary arteries, and veins. Circulating freely, lymph flows into collecting trunks, which empty into the bronchopulmonary lymph nodes at the hilum.

RESPIRATORY PHYSIOLOGY

Breathing involves two actions: inspiration, an active process, and expiration, a relatively passive one. Breathing is regulated by both mechanical and chemical factors, and is influenced by lung expansibility (compliance), and the size of airways and the resistance to flow that they impart.

Neurologic control of breathing

For the most part, breathing is automatic and usually involuntary. It's neurologically regulated, with the help of chemoreceptors and certain physiologic factors.

Neurologic regulators. These regulators for the mechanical aspects of breathing reside in the medulla oblongata and the pons. Called respiratory centers, they are really groups of scattered neurons that function as a unit to regulate breathing. The primary location in the medulla is called the medullary respiratory center. Here, neurons associated with inspiration and neurons associated with expiration apparently interact to regulate respiratory rate and depth. They react to impulses from other areas, particularly the pons. In the pons, two neuron groups, or centers, regulate respiratory rhythm by interacting with the medullary respiratory center to smooth the transitions from inspiration to expiration and back. The apneustic center of the pons stimulates inspiratory neurons in the medulla to precipitate inspiration. In turn, these inspiratory neurons stimulate the pneumotaxic center of the pons to precipitate expiration. They do this in two ways: by inhibiting the apneustic center and by stimulating the expiratory neurons in the medulla. Thus, the pons, as pacemaker, regulates rhythm, while the medulla regulates rate and depth.

Conscious control of breathing through nerve impulses from the motor areas of the cerebral cortex can override the involuntary respiratory centers. This permits voluntary breath control for such activities as speaking, singing, and swimming. But this conscious control is only temporary, and the respiratory centers, in turn, override cortical impulses to meet ventilatory needs.

Central and peripheral chemoreceptors. Responding to changes in blood CO_2, O_2, and pH, these chemoreceptors monitor the body's ventilatory status and signal the respiratory centers to adjust respiratory rate and depth. The central chemoreceptors, located in the anterior medulla, are particularly sensitive to alterations in PCO_2 and acid-base balance. For example, physical exertion raises the level of carbon dioxide in the blood; the gas diffuses easily from cerebral capillaries into the cerebrospinal fluid bathing the central nervous system, where it reacts with water to form carbonic acid and yield hydrogen ions. Chemoreceptors detect this rising acidity and stimulate the respiratory centers to increase respiratory rate and depth. As expiration of carbon dioxide lowers carbonic acid levels, the chemoreceptors stimulate the respiratory centers to reduce respiratory rate and depth. Conversely, if blood levels of carbon dioxide fall below normal, the central chemoreceptors initiate a cessation of breathing (apnea) until ongoing cellular metabolism produces sufficient carbon dioxide to stimulate the respiratory centers again.

Peripheral chemoreceptors, located in the aortic and carotid bodies, primarily monitor blood-oxygen level. When the blood level of oxygen falls, the oxygen content of interstitial fluid around the peripheral chemoreceptors also falls, and the receptors stimulate the respiratory centers to increase respiratory rate and/or depth to introduce additional oxygen.

Physiologic factors. Along with the important chemical and neurologic factors, several physiologic factors significantly affect breathing: lung inflation, changes in blood pressure and temperature, airway irritation, and sensory stimulation.

Lung inflation. This stimulates stretch receptors in the alveolar ducts, which send a stream of impulses along the vagus nerves to the central nervous system. These afferent impulses inhibit the inspiratory center, which then stops sending expansion impulses to the diaphragm and external intercostal muscles. Consequently, these muscles stop expanding, and passive expiration follows. This reflex, the Hering-Breuer reflex, is an important regulator of normal respiration; but a secondary mechanism independent of the vagus is also operative and becomes apparent when the normal pathway is blocked. For example, cutting the vagus nerves prolongs and deepens inspiration, but eventually the inspiratory center stops sending expansion messages and allows expiration to occur.

Blood pressure changes. Sudden, sharp

Mechanics of normal, quiet breathing

Inspiration
• Central nervous system (CNS) stimulates diaphragm contraction.
• Diaphragm descends as it contracts, vertically enlarging thorax; external intercostal muscles also contract (especially during deep or forced inspiration), raising and rotating ribs and sternum and horizontally enlarging thorax.
• Thorax expansion lowers intrapleural pressure; pleural cohesion causes lungs to expand with thorax; lung expansion lowers intrapulmonic (bronchoalveolar) pressure below atmospheric pressure.
• Intrapulmonic/atmospheric pressure gradient pulls air into lungs until the two pressures equalize.

Expiration
• CNS impulses to diaphragm cease; diaphragm slowly relaxes, and lungs and thorax recoil to resting size and position.
• This recoil (usually passive, but aided during deep or forced expiration by CNS-stimulated contraction of internal intercostal muscles) reduces thorax to resting size.
• Compression of lungs and thorax causes intrapulmonic pressure to rise above atmospheric pressure.
• Intrapulmonic/atmospheric pressure gradient forces air out of lungs until the two pressures equalize.

Innervation of respiratory structures

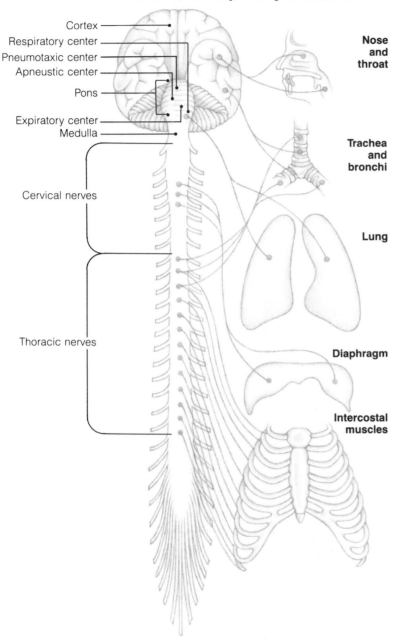

Cortex
Respiratory center
Pneumotaxic center
Apneustic center
Pons
Expiratory center
Medulla

Cervical nerves

Thoracic nerves

Nose and throat

Trachea and bronchi

Lung

Diaphragm

Intercostal muscles

Stimulation from external sources and from higher brain centers acts on respiratory centers in the pons and medulla. These centers in turn send impulses to the various parts of the respiratory apparatus to alter respiration patterns.

changes stimulate pressoreceptors in the aortic and carotid sinuses. With a sudden rise in blood pressure, the receptors send impulses along vagus and glossopharyngeal nerves to the respiratory centers. These impulses depress respiratory activity and temporarily make respiration slower and shallower. With a sudden blood pressure drop, as occurs with severe hemorrhage, pressoreceptor impulses slow down and the respiratory center activity quickens correspondingly, increasing respiratory rate and depth.

Temperature changes. Changes in the temperature of the blood passing through the respiratory centers may also trigger changes in respiration. A temperature increase during fever or exertion quickens the respiratory rate; and a temperature drop, as in hypothermia, initiates a drop in respiratory rate.

Airway irritation. Foreign particles stimulate the protective "irritant" receptors in the mucous membrane that lines the respiratory tract. In the nose, this causes a sneeze to expel the irritant. In the larynx or trachea, such invasion induces a cough.

Sensory stimulation. Stimulation of various receptors may cause a temporary reflex reaction. Sudden heat or cold, or alarming sounds or sights may provoke a gasp, accelerated respiratory rate, or momentary apnea.

Working together, these various control mechanisms regulate ventilation to provide continuous airflow to the lungs. However, the amount of air that actually reaches the lungs with oxygen and then departs carrying carbon dioxide depends on lung volume and capacity (see *Measuring lung volumes* on page 17), resistance to airflow, and compliance.

Physical forces

Effective gas exchange is opposed by three forces of resistance that can restrict respiration and add to the work of breathing: elastic resistance, nonelastic (viscous) resistance, and airflow resistance.

Elastic resistance. This refers to the lung's natural tendency to contract because of the elasticity of its tissue. This elasticity derives partly from elastic fibers throughout the lung, which stretch during inspiration and then spring back during expiration. But it derives primarily from surface tension of the fluid lining the individual alveoli, which constantly promotes alveolar collapse. Two forces counter lung elasticity: chest-wall rigidity combined with pleural fluid tension, and secretion of surfactant in the alveoli to reduce alveolar surface tension.

During inspiration, the cohesive force of the fluid between the visceral and parietal pleurae combined with negative intrapleural pressure causes the lung to expand with the chest wall and, during expiration, halts lung deflation at the chest wall's point of maximum contraction. The lung and chest wall function smoothly as a counterbalanced unit, as long as the pleurae remain intact. When the pleurae are interrupted, such as by external puncture or by rupture of a bleb, this pleural force of attraction is broken and lung collapse results, as in pneumothorax.

In the alveoli, epithelial cells secrete surfactant, a lipoprotein, which coats the fluid lining the alveoli and prevents fluid contact with alveolar air. This creates a surface tension 2 to 14 times less than the fluid/air tension and reduces alveolar tendency to collapse. Thus, any disease process that interferes with surfactant production promotes lung collapse.

Nonelastic (viscous) resistance. This results from the force exerted on the thorax by the diaphragm and the abdominal contents, which inhibits the thorax from expanding downward. Not usually sufficient to compromise inspiration, such resistance becomes a problem under conditions of obesity, abdominal distention, ascites, and late-term pregnancy.

Airflow resistance. This derives from a change in airway radius or pattern of airflow. Airway radius, a critical factor, decreases as large bronchi branch out through the lung, and also when accumulated secretions narrow the bronchi or condensation narrows ventilator tubing. A 50% reduction in airway radius causes a sixteenfold increase in resistance to gas flow. For the patient on a ventilator, airway length is also a factor. The ventilator tubing becomes an extension of the tracheobronchial tree, and this change in airway length directly affects airway resistance; doubling the length doubles the resistance. Understanding this helps you remember the strict limitations on the length of ventilator tubing.

The pattern of gas flow—whether laminar, turbulent, or transitional (see *Reviewing respiratory basics* on page 10)—also affects resistance. Laminar flow offers minimal resistance to gas flow. The smooth angles in the small airways of the bronchial tree produce this desirable flow pattern. Turbulent flow creates added friction and raises resistance to flow. Normal in the trachea and larger bronchi, turbulent flow can occur in the smaller airways as a result of bronchoconstriction or excessive secretions. For the patient on a ventilator, condensation in the tubing can also change the flow pattern. Keep in mind that high gas-flow rates also induce turbulence and thus require higher pressures to deliver a normal tidal volume. A mix of patterns, called transitional flow, occurs around obstructions and at transitional points in the larger airways, such as branches.

Compliance. The reciprocal of elasticity,

compliance is the lung's ability to expand, to yield to intraalveolar pressure during inspiration. Compliance has two influencing factors: lung expansibility; and expansibility of the chest wall, including the thorax and diaphragm. Chest-wall compliance isn't routinely measured, since it's affected by skeletal muscle contraction and valid measurement demands total muscle relaxation. Lung compliance, however, doesn't depend on physical relaxation for valid measurement. Lung compliance may be static or dynamic. The most common measurement, static compliance, is made under static conditions. It's a product of the tidal volume divided by the pressure required to deliver that volume; this determines the change in volume for every centimeter of water-pressure increase. Normal static compliance is 100 cc/cm water. Dynamic compliance is measured under nonstatic conditions, usually during inspiration. It's the volume above which an increase in pressure will not increase the volume of gas delivered. Normal dynamic compliance is 50 cc/cm water.

Understanding diffusion

Gas moves from an area of greater pressure to one of lesser pressure. During ventilation, the action of chest wall, pleurae, and lungs produces changes in intrapulmonic and intrapleural pressure necessary to move air into and out of the lungs. The next step in gas exchange, diffusion of oxygen into the blood and carbon dioxide out, occurs because the partial pressures of those gases on each side of the respiratory membrane create steep pressure gradients that promote gas transfer in opposite directions.

Rapid gas exchange. Normally, gas exchange takes place in half the time allowed for it. Exposure of blood to the respiratory membrane lasts about 0.8 second at rest. Almost full oxygen saturation of the blood occurs in half that time, and carbon dioxide exchange occurs 20 times faster than oxygen exchange. So, if a specific lung area receives an adequate volume of blood flow, flow rate will not compromise gas exchange.

The speed at which gas exchange occurs and the specific pressure needed to effect the exchange depend on the degree to which a gas is soluble in blood. Since carbon dioxide is much more soluble than oxygen, it diffuses more rapidly than oxygen and requires a much lower pressure gradient to do so, even when resistance to diffusion increases. In the

Pulmonary innervation

Vagal and sympathetic efferents and vagal afferents innervate the lungs, forming networks around the bronchial and arterial trees. Stimulation via the vagal efferents causes bronchoconstriction, and via the sympathetic efferents, vasoconstriction.

The three main vagal afferents have varied responses: *Irritant* receptors lie just under the surface of the airways and seem to respond to irritant gases, smoke, dust, and histamine by causing coughing and bronchoconstriction. *J (juxtacapillary) receptors* are believed to lie in the alveolar walls and to respond to exercise, emboli, edema, and irritant gases by causing hyperventilation. *Stretch receptors* lie in the smooth muscle of the smaller airways and respond to lung distention by signaling the central nervous system to halt inspiration (Hering-Breuer reflex).

Oxyhemoglobin dissociation curve

The oxyhemoglobin dissociation curve shows hemoglobin saturation (affinity for oxygen) at any PO_2, and thus the efficiency of oxygen transport and delivery. Note that the curve flattens out at a PO_2 of about 75 mm Hg; at this level, most of the hemoglobin is saturated, and an increase in PO_2 won't greatly improve saturation. Note, too, that when PO_2 falls below 60 mm Hg, rapid and extensive desaturation can occur, resulting in hypoxia.

Factors that alter hemoglobin affinity and shift the curve include pH, PCO_2, and temperature. A rise in pH, or a drop in PCO_2 or temperature, induces hemoglobin to bond with oxygen, producing higher saturation at a given PO_2 and shifting the curve to the left. But these same factors inhibit oxygen release at the cellular level. Conversely, a drop in pH, or a rise in PCO_2 or temperature, induces hemoglobin to release oxygen, producing lower saturations at a given PO_2 and shifting the curve to the right. But these factors also inhibit hemoglobin bonding in the lungs.

Key:

Normal _____

↑ pH
↓ Temp _____
↓ PCO_2

↓ pH
↑ Temp _____
↑ PCO_2

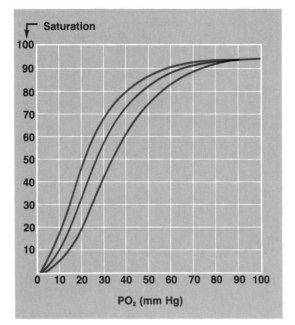

case of added resistance from a thickened respiratory membrane, as occurs with pulmonary fibrosis, carbon dioxide may still diffuse outward with its partial pressure in systemic blood remaining normal, while oxygen diffusion and PO_2 decrease.

Oxygen transport. Once diffusion takes place, arterial blood transports oxygen to the tissues in two ways: physically dissolved in plasma, and chemically bound to hemoglobin. Plasma carries comparatively little oxygen. Henry's law governs this relationship: the amount of a gas dissolved in a liquid is directly proportional to the pressure of the gas against the liquid. As gas pressure rises, the amount of gas that dissolves into the liquid to equalize that pressure differential also rises, depending on the solubility of the gas. Because oxygen resists dissolving in plasma, only about 3% is transported in this manner.

Hemoglobin carries about 97% of the oxygen in the blood, depending on the PO_2 level. High PO_2, as in pulmonary capillaries, causes oxygen to bind to the protein's ferrous iron (heme, or Fe^{++}) molecules to form oxyhemoglobin (HbO_2). Low PO_2, as at the cellular level, reverses the bond, so oxygen is released. Barriers to this process include certain chemicals, such as nitrites, that convert hemoglobin to a ferric state (Fe^{+++}), called methemoglobin, and annul its ability to combine with oxygen; and carbon monoxide, which has an attraction to hemoglobin hundreds of times greater than oxygen and easily displaces oxygen in the bonding process.

Hemoglobin bound to oxygen to its fullest ex-

tent (normally about 1.34 ml oxygen per gram of hemoglobin) is considered 100% saturated. Less complete combinations are expressed in lower percentages. Saturation near 100% turns hemoglobin bright red, as in normal arterial blood. Desaturated (reduced) hemoglobin is purple and imparts the bluish tone of cyanosis to the skin. Cyanosis, however, is unreliable as an indicator of hypoxemia (decreased blood oxygen), since it doesn't show up until at least 5 g of hemoglobin is desaturated—a situation more serious clinically for the anemic patient with total hemoglobin of only 8 g than for the polycythemic patient with a hemoglobin total of 20 g.

Once oxygen-laden arterial blood reaches body tissues, internal respiration, or gas exchange between systemic capillaries and interstitial fluid, takes place along pressure gradients. Oxygen moves into the interstitial fluid to nourish the cells, and carbon dioxide leaves the fluid to travel in the blood. At this point, blood moves across the capillaries from the arterial to the venous system to begin its journey to the lungs where the waste CO_2 is exchanged for oxygen.

Carbon dioxide transport. The blood carries carbon dioxide to the lungs in three ways: dissolved in plasma, coupled with hemoglobin as carbaminohemoglobin, and combined with water as carbonic acid and its component ions. (See *Carbon dioxide transport* on page 18.) Only 7% is carried in blood plasma, and the reaction requires many long seconds to complete. Some of this 7% has a measurable partial pressure; the rest reacts very slowly with water to form carbonic acid (H_2CO_3), which may further break down into hydrogen ions (H^+) and bicarbonate ions (HCO_3^-); both of these processes are reversible.

About 23% of the carbon dioxide reacts somewhat faster with hemoglobin in the red blood cells and forms the compound carbaminohemoglobin.

About 70% of the carbon dioxide converts to carbonic acid in the red blood cells, a process that occurs in a fraction of a second because of the presence of the catalyzing enzyme carbonic anhydrase. Equally fast, the carbonic acid breaks down into hydrogen ions and bicarbonate ions; the hydrogen ions remain cell-bound, neutralized by the hemoglobin, while the bicarbonate ions trade places with chloride ions in the surrounding plasma. In this process, called chloride shift, the red blood cells expel excess bicarbonate yet remain electrically neutral.

When venous blood enters the lung for gas

Measuring lung volumes

You can measure certain of your patient's lung volumes using a spirometer, and calculate others from the results. Typically, you'll measure tidal volume and vital capacity.

• *Tidal volume (V_T):* the amount of air that enters or leaves the lungs during normal quiet breathing. Average inspiratory and expiratory tidal volumes each equal 500 ml.

• *Inspiratory reserve volume (IRV):* the amount of air that can be forcibly inhaled in excess of the tidal volume. Average inspiratory reserve volume is 3,000 ml.

• *Expiratory reserve volume (ERV):* the amount of air that can be forcibly exhaled beyond the tidal volume. Average expiratory reserve volume is 1,200 ml.

Certain lung volumes can't be measured with a spirometer:

• *Residual volume (RV):* the amount of air remaining in the lungs after the deepest possible expiration. Unresponsive to voluntary effort, it can be removed only by collapse of the lungs. Average residual volume is 1,200 ml.

• *Dead-space air:* air filling respiratory airways that conduct air to the alveoli but play no part in gas exchange. These airways include the nose, mouth, pharynx, larynx, trachea, and bronchial tree, but not the alveoli. Average dead-space air is 150 ml for an adult male and 110 ml for an adult female.

• *Physiologic dead-space air:* the sum of anatomic dead-space air and air in any non-functioning or partly functioning alveoli. Such defective alveoli, no longer active in gas exchange, may be adequately ventilated but lack a blood supply because of disease, or may receive enough blood but lack ventilation.

Adding various lung volumes allows evaluation of several lung capacities:

• *Vital capacity (VC):* the amount of air exhaled by the deepest possible expiration after the deepest possible inspiration. The sum of tidal, inspiratory reserve, and expiratory reserve volumes, it's usually about 4,700 ml.

• *Functional residual capacity (FRC):* the amount of air remaining in the lungs after normal (tidal) expiration. The sum of the expiratory reserve and residual volumes, it ensures a steady supply of air in the lungs so that gas exchange can occur continuously, even between breaths. Without it, resulting fluctuations in blood gas values would produce constant oxygen shortage.

• *Inspiratory capacity (IC):* the maximum amount of air inhaled after normal (tidal) expiration. It's the sum of the tidal and inspiratory reserve volumes.

• *Total lung capacity (TLC):* the amount of air in the lungs after the fullest possible inspiration. The sum of functional vital capacity and residual volume, it's usually about 5,900 ml.

• *Minute volume* or *minute ventilation (VE):* the product of the tidal volume multiplied by the number of respirations per minute. For example, a person with a tidal volume of 500 ml breathing 12 times per minute has a minute volume of 6,000 ml.

• *Maximal breathing capacity:* the amount of air moved in and out of the lungs in 1 minute of forced breathing. It's calculated by having a person breathe as rapidly and deeply as possible for a given number of seconds, usually 15, and then multiplying that number, in this case by 4, to arrive at a figure for a minute's respiration. The resulting figure may be as high as 100 liters/minute during strenuous exercise.

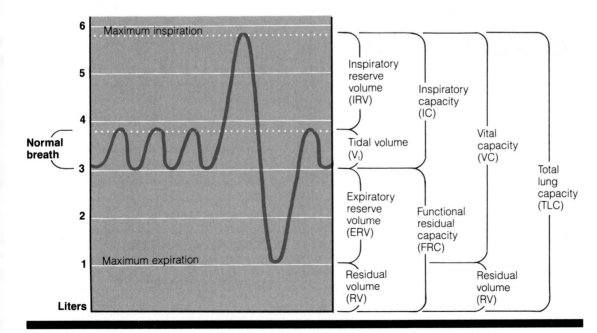

Carbon dioxide transport

The tissues release carbon dioxide into the bloodstream where it travels to the lungs in three forms: as a gas dissolved in plasma, combined with hemoglobin, and combined with water as carbonic acid.

Transport of carbon dioxide in the blood

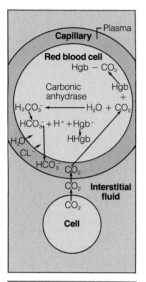

exchange, all reversible chemical processes reverse, reforming carbon dioxide. The gas diffuses into the alveoli and is expired.

The degree to which oxygen in the alveoli trades places with carbon dioxide in the blood depends largely on the amount of oxygen the lungs can draw in and the amount of blood available in the lungs to oppose it. This ratio of ventilation to perfusion determines the effectiveness of gas exchange.

Ventilation/perfusion ratio

In the ideal model for gas exchange, the amount of air in the alveoli (ventilation) matches the amount of blood in the capillaries (perfusion), and gas exchange takes place easily along complementary pressure gradients. In fact, the match is unequal. The alveoli receive air at a rate of about 4 liters/minute, while the capillaries supply blood at a rate of about 5 liters/minute, creating a ventilation/perfusion (V/Q) mismatch of 4:5 or 0.8. But even this ratio is average and does not hold constant throughout the lung. Gravitational force makes ventilation relatively greater at the apex of the lung, and blood flow greater at the base, widening the V/Q gap further. Alveoli at the apex are underperfused in relation to ventilation, resulting in a V/Q ratio of about 3.0. This ratio gradually reverses down through the lung, so that alveoli at the base are overperfused in relation to ventilation, for a V/Q ratio of about 0.6.

Since the quality of the V/Q match affects the quality of gas exchange, the result is an unequal exchange pattern throughout the lung. Because of reduced blood flow, the PO_2 at the apex is over 40 mm Hg lower than the PO_2 at the base, although exercise increases apical oxygen uptake as it increases apical perfusion. The difference in PCO_2 from apex to base, reflected by pH change, is much less. However, only areas with a low V/Q ratio, rather than a high V/Q ratio as at the apex, lead to impaired gas exchange.

RESPIRATORY PATHOPHYSIOLOGY

Understanding respiratory anatomy and physiology is the fundamental first step in identifying respiratory pathophysiology and understanding its implications and the ramifications of treatment—increasingly important today, given the nurse's expanding role in health assessment. The ability to interpret clinical findings for specific respiratory disorders rests on an understanding of the overall mechanisms of respiratory dysfunction.

Ineffective gas exchange

A central problem in respiratory disorders is ineffective gas exchange between the alveoli and the pulmonary capillaries, a problem that can affect all body systems. For gas exchange to be effective, ventilation and perfusion must match as closely as possible. V/Q mismatch accounts for most of the defective gas exchange in respiratory disorder. Such mismatching may result from a ventilation/perfusion dysfunction or a change in lung mechanics.

V/Q dysfunction. When ineffective exchange results from a physiologic abnormality, the effect may be reduced ventilation to a unit (shunt), reduced perfusion to a unit (dead-space ventilation), or both (silent unit). (See *Reviewing respiratory basics* on page 11.) Note that shunting is the term applied whenever unoxygenated blood returns to the left heart. An abnormal shunt may occur because an actual physical defect allows unoxygenated blood to bypass fully functioning alveoli, or because an airway obstruction prevents oxygen from reaching an adequately perfused area of the lung. But keep in mind that a physical shunt occurs in the normal lung: the pulmonary veins collect oxygen-depleted blood from the bronchial artery, which perfuses the bronchi; and from the thebesian veins, which drain the heart muscle. Shunting of this poorly oxygenated blood into arterial blood depresses arterial PO_2, but not significantly for the normal person. However, the person with heart disease may also have a physical defect between the right and left heart, which diverts greater amounts of unoxygenated blood directly into arterial blood flow and seriously depresses arterial PO_2. Most abnormal shunting, though, results from airway obstruction.

Variations of the three ventilation/perfusion abnormalities exist, depending on the overall lung V/Q ratio. Respiratory disorders are often physiologically categorized as shunt-producing, if the V/Q ratio falls below 0.8, or dead space-producing, if the V/Q exceeds 0.8.

Changes in mechanics. Ineffective gas exchange can also occur because changes in lung mechanics demand higher internal pressures to produce adequate breath volumes. This increases the work of breathing and reduces the effectiveness of diffusion. Changes in mechanics fall into two classes: changes in compliance and changes in resistance.

Changes in compliance. These changes in ability to expand can occur in either the lung or the chest wall. Lung compliance increases when the elastic fibers of the lung are destroyed, as in emphysema. The lung expands easily during inspiration but contracts with difficulty, thus adding to the work of breathing during expiration. Lung compliance usually remains normal in chronic bronchitis and bronchial asthma, since airway spasm, rather than a change in the lung's cellular structure, creates the obstruction to gas flow. Lung compliance decreases in interstitial and alveolar pulmonary diseases—such as pulmonary edema, pulmonary fibrosis, and sarcoidosis—because characteristic cellular changes make inspiration more difficult.

Chest-wall compliance is affected by thoracic deformity, muscle spasm, and abdominal distention. Compliance may decrease in ankylosing spondylitis, kyphosis, marked obesity, extreme pectus excavatum, scoliosis, and disorders causing muscle spasticity.

Changes in resistance. These changes in the pressure needed to produce airflow may occur in the lung tissue itself, as with sarcoidosis and other interstitial lung diseases; in the chest wall, as with pleurisy and other pleural disorders; or in the airways. However, airway resistance alone accounts for 80% of all respiratory system resistance. Airway resistance typically mounts with obstructive diseases such as asthma, chronic bronchitis, and emphysema. Consequently, the work of breathing increases, particularly during expiration, to compensate for narrowed airways and diminished gas exchange.

Signs of ineffective gas exchange. When gas exchange is ineffective, the end result is hypoxia (tissue-oxygen deficiency), although this deficiency may be evident only on exertion when oxygen demand intensifies. This deficiency may occur at any point from ventilation to transport to cell metabolism, but the end result is oxygen deficiency at the cellular level. Such a decrease in cellular oxygen concentration means the cell must resort to anaerobic metabolism to supply its energy needs, a situation that leads to lactic acidosis.

The mechanisms of hypoxia vary because oxygen delivery to the cells depends on the blood's oxygen-carrying capacity, cardiac output, and peripheral blood flow. For example, insufficient hemoglobin, as in anemia, reduces the blood's ability to transport adequate oxygen. Low blood volume, as from severe hemorrhage or an embolus or other vascular impedance, also reduces the amount of blood available to carry oxygen to the cells. The various physiologic pathways suggest these classifications of hypoxia:

• *Hypoxic (anoxic or arterial) hypoxia.* Deficient oxygenation of arterial blood despite its normal oxygen-carrying capacity, possibly resulting from airway obstruction.

• *Anemic hypoxia.* Reduced blood oxygen-carrying capacity because of hemoglobin deficiency.

• *Stagnant (circulatory) hypoxia.* Normal blood oxygen-carrying capacity but inadequate tissue oxygenation because of vascular obstruction and reduced capillary blood flow.

• *Histotoxic (metabolic) hypoxia.* Normal blood PO_2, but inadequate tissue oxygenation because of impaired oxidative-enzyme cellular mechanisms that prevent cells from metabolizing oxygen. Such hypoxia is particularly acute if the cell's demand for oxygen is excessively high.

Other signs of ineffective gas exchange include hypoxemia, which refers solely to a decrease in the oxygen concentration of the blood and is often used incorrectly as a synonym for hypoxia. Hypocapnia is a decrease in the carbon dioxide concentration of the blood; and, conversely, hypercapnia is an increase in blood retention of carbon dioxide. (See Chapter 2 for additional signs.)

Ineffective gas exchange has an additional implication beyond poor tissue oxygenation; it promotes retention of carbon dioxide and threatens homeostasis by tipping the systemic acid-base balance. But the body has three normal regulatory mechanisms for dulling this toxic effect before it can tax other body systems.

Compensatory mechanisms. Normally, the body's acid-base balance hovers at 7.4 or remains within a very narrow pH range of 7.35 to 7.45. This is crucial, since an acute drop to 7.1 (acidosis) or a rise to 7.5 (alkalosis) may be life-threatening. Anything that tips the balance to the acid side, by producing hydrogen ions, lowers the pH; conversely, anything that tips the balance toward the basic side, by producing bicarbonate ions, decreases acidity and raises the pH. Body fluids fluctuate constantly, their composition altered by acids, carbon dioxide, and water from cellular metabolism of carbohydrates, proteins, and fats. Carbon dioxide and water unite to form carbonic acid, which dissociates into hydrogen ions and bicarbonate ions. Three regulatory mechanisms neutralize or eliminate an excess of either hydrogen or bicarbonate ions and maintain the body's normal pH: acid-

Effects of chronic ineffective gas exchange

Renal
Release of
  erythropoietin
Increased retention
  of bicarbonate ion,
  sodium, and water
Fluid overload

Neurologic
Dulling of medullary
  respiratory center
Respiration stimulated
  by aortic and
  carotid bodies

**Prolonged
hypoxia and
hypercapnia**

Musculoskeletal
Pulmonary osteo-
  arthropathy
  (arthralgia, digital
  clubbing,
  subperiosteal
  proliferation
  of long bones)
Increased myoglobin
  in muscles

Cardiovascular
Pulmonary capillary
  vasoconstriction
Increased
  pulmonary vascular
  resistance
Pulmonary
  hypertension
Shunting of
  oxygenated blood
Cor pulmonale

Hematopoietic
Polycythemia
Increased risk
  of embolism and
  thrombosis

Prolonged hypoxia and hypercapnia, as seen in patients with chronic respiratory disorders, eventually take their toll on other vital systems:

Neurologic
With progressive hypercapnia, the regulatory mechanisms of respiration may adjust to tolerate higher Pco_2 levels. But severe hypercapnia dulls the medullary respiratory center, forcing peripheral chemoreceptors in the aortic and carotid bodies to direct respiration. Since these receptors respond to low Po_2, and any treatment involving high concentrations of oxygen will suppress this hypoxic drive and thus suppress respiration, oxygen therapy must be strictly controlled in accordance with blood gas analysis.

Cardiovascular
Respiratory neuromuscular disorder or lung or pulmonary vascular disease can produce cor pulmonale (CP), acute or chronic enlargement of the right ventricle. Usually, CP is chronic, secondary to chronic obstructive disease, such as pulmonary emphysema or chronic bronchitis. In acute form, CP may develop from massive pulmonary embolism, with or without heart failure, or from acute pulmonary infection or other condition that sharply increases hypoxemia.

CP may result from widespread destruction of lung tissue or pulmonary capillaries that reduces the pulmonary vascular bed, from increased pulmonary vascular resistance, shunting of unoxygenated blood, or from pulmonary vasoconstriction and pulmonary artery hypertension because of decreased Po_2. Pulmonary hypertension, the most common cause, may occur sporadically at first under conditions of increased pulmonary blood flow, as with exertion or fever. Eventually a constant, it leads to right ventricular muscle dilation and hypertrophy, followed by right-heart failure, reduced cardiac output, and cardiovascular collapse.

Musculoskeletal
A compensatory increase in muscle content of the oxygen-binding heme protein myoglobin improves oxygen transport to contracting muscles when Po_2 is low. In addition, an increase in pulmonary vasculature in response to chronic hypoxia may be the cause of pulmonary osteoarthropathy, also called

secondary hypertrophic osteoarthropathy. This condition—which shows up as bone and tissue changes in the extremities (arthralgia, clubbing, proliferation of subperiosteal tissues in long bones)—may accompany bronchial carcinoma, bronchiectasis, or pulmonary abscess.

Renal
Sustained hypercapnia causes renal retention of bicarbonate ions, sodium, and water to dilute the effects of excess hydrogen ions, a compensatory action that can lead to fluid overload. Sustained hypoxia stimulates the kidneys to release erythropoietic factor into the blood. This factor causes a plasma transport protein to yield erythropoietin, the compound that spurs red blood cell production and raises hematocrit.

Hematopoietic
Chronic hypoxemia often causes polycythemia, a compensatory attempt to increase the blood's oxygen-carrying capacity by increasing the number of red blood cells. However, such an increase thickens the blood, which makes embolism and thrombosis more likely, and increases the heart's work load—dangers that outweigh the advantage of improved oxygen capacity, especially for the patient with cor pulmonale.

base buffers, the respiratory system itself, and the renal system.

Buffer systems. These pairs of weak acids and related bases operate in seconds to reduce the danger of stronger incoming acids and bases. By combining with a strong acid, which would dissociate to yield many hydrogen ions and thus sharply lower the pH, these buffers create a weaker acid that dissociates into fewer hydrogen ions and has a gentler effect on pH. They react similarly to neutralize a strong base, thereby keeping pH fluctuations to a minimum. Chief buffers of body fluids are bicarbonates, phosphates, and proteins, such as hemoglobin. The bicarbonate buffers, however, are mainly responsible for monitoring blood and interstitial fluid. Among the buffer systems, the bicarbonates alone have a limitless outlet in the respiratory system to reduce acidity and renew themselves by increased expiration of carbon dioxide.

Respiratory system. The second acid-base regulator is the respiratory system, which normally can restore homeostasis within minutes. Since the amount of carbon dioxide in plasma determines the amount of carbonic acid and hydrogen ions produced, any rise in PCO_2 means a rise in acidity; and any drop in PCO_2 means a rise in alkalinity. Working together to sense and correct pH changes, the medullary respiratory centers and the lungs strive to keep PCO_2 at 40 mm Hg, a level that makes it possible for the lungs to excrete carbon dioxide at the same rate the cells produce it. They succeed by altering respiration rate and depth to eliminate more or less carbon dioxide, and therefore acid, as necessary to control pH. But when the respiratory disorder itself causes prolonged hyperventilation or hypoventilation beyond the limits needed to adjust pH, or otherwise prevent effective carbon dioxide exchange, respiratory alkalosis or acidosis results.

Renal system. The body's third and long-term regulator, the renal system, intervenes when the first two compensatory mechanisms fail to correct pH imbalance. Within several hours or over several days, the kidneys adjust pH by excreting nonvolatile (fixed) acids—those that the lungs can't excrete—and by either excreting hydrogen ions and reabsorbing bicarbonate ions to correct excess acidity, or reversing this action to correct alkalosis. In cases of metabolic acidosis or metabolic alkalosis, which stem from altered metabolic rather than respiratory patterns, renal and respiratory compensatory mechanisms work together. The kidneys adjust the levels of appropriate ions, while the lungs change respiration rate and depth to reduce or conserve carbon dioxide.

Thus, coping mechanisms exist to offset the effects of inefficient gas exchange. Compensation for acid-base imbalance involves a systemic shift in the opposite direction that moves pH back within normal limits. A primary respiratory imbalance produces an opposing compensatory metabolic response; the reverse also holds true. For example, respiratory acidosis provokes conservation of bicarbonate ions and excretion of hydrogen ions (compensatory metabolic alkalosis).

But when disease or disorder keeps compensatory systems from operating effectively, the result may be multiple systemic dysfunction requiring outside intervention. For example, the patient with COPD who develops diabetic ketoacidosis can't compensate by increasing expiration of carbon dioxide. Remember, too, that the patient with chronic respiratory disease will show an elevated bicarbonate level as his kidneys compensate for carbon dioxide retention to maintain a normal pH; correcting the elevated bicarbonate level only aggravates acidosis. Thus, in treating systemic dysfunction, it's crucial for you to treat the primary problem, not the compensatory response.

The years ahead

With incidence and mortality rates for respiratory disorders rising steadily each year, you'll find your role as a teacher and your involvement in the community also increasing. As always, your enduring responsibility to the general population centers on advocating health promotion and disease prevention, and includes educating about environmental pollutants, such as tobacco, the chief culprit of self-imposed heart and lung damage. With your patients and their families, who must deal with the fact of advanced respiratory disease, you'll be relaying information about short- and long-term management, the importance and technique of proper home care, and the availability of support services to help them cope with changes in life-style. To teach effectively, you must first have a thorough understanding of normal respiratory physiology and the pathophysiology of respiratory disorders. Such understanding will help you convey complex biologic and technical information in a way that's comprehensive and comprehensible to patients and their families.

Points to remember

• Poor gas exchange lies at the root of all respiratory disorders.
• Respiratory disorders can result from a defect in ventilation, perfusion, or both.
• Changes in the body's acid-base balance accompany respiratory disorders, and the respiratory system can compensate for these changes to a limited degree.

2 ASSESSING RESPIRATORY DYNAMICS

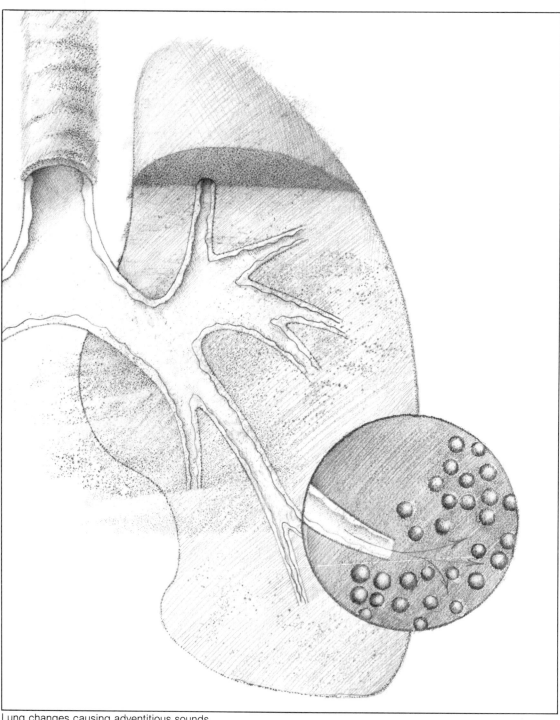

Lung changes causing adventitious sounds

Respiratory assessment is a vital part of patient care, and it pays to do it well. Obviously, doing it well requires practice and polished skills of history taking, observation, inspection, palpation, percussion, and auscultation. But that's not all. Doing it well requires understanding when and what kind of assessment is needed and knowing what respiratory changes tell about the patient's condition.

When is respiratory assessment needed? It's essential on hospital admission, at regular intervals during illness, and during routine health evaluation and screening. When caring for hospitalized patients, you should perform respiratory assessment at least once daily for patients who are ambulatory; more frequently for patients who are acutely ill or particularly susceptible to disease, like children and the elderly.

And why is respiratory assessment so important? It may uncover changes in function that threaten the patient's life or hinder daily activities. As you remember, the two functions of the respiratory system are maintenance of oxygen and carbon dioxide exchange in the lungs and tissues and regulation of acid-base balance. Consequently, changes in respiratory function can result in acid-base disturbances, tissue hypoxia, and even sudden death. Using correct assessment, you can detect such changes early and intervene quickly, perhaps preventing complications. You can also determine how respiratory dysfunction disrupts activities of daily living and design a care plan that addresses the patient's special needs.

Check first for respiratory distress

Your first priority in respiratory assessment is to make sure the patient isn't suffering severe hypoxia or other acute respiratory difficulty. Observe the patient for these signs of respiratory distress:
- decreased level of consciousness
- shortness of breath when speaking
- rapid, very deep or very shallow, or depressed respirations
- use of accessory muscles when breathing
- intercostal and sternal retractions
- cyanosis
- external sounds (such as crowing, wheezing, or stridor)
- diaphoresis
- nasal flaring
- extreme apprehension or agitation.

If the patient shows most or all of these signs and symptoms, you'll have to postpone a detailed respiratory assessment. But you may do a quick check of lung sounds to help determine the patient's problem. Decreased or absent sounds may point to airway obstruction or pneumothorax, both of which require immediate intervention. Carry out necessary emergency procedures and contact the doctor promptly.

Prepare for detailed assessment

Before performing a detailed respiratory assessment:

Check the environment. Be sure the examining area is quiet so you can take the patient's history without interference and accurately auscultate his lungs. Have the area well lit to detect variations of skin color. (If possible, use natural light, because fluorescent light doesn't show true skin color.)

Gather the equipment. You'll need a nasal speculum, a tongue depressor, a penlight, a hand mirror, a cotton-tipped applicator or swabstick, and a stethoscope. You may also wish to use a marking pen and a centimeter ruler to mark points of reference on the patient's body.

Prepare the patient. First, encourage him to relax. Introduce yourself, and explain to the patient what you're about to do and why. Encourage him to ask questions. Provide privacy to minimize any embarrassment. Next, ask him to undress to the waist and put on an examining gown. (If the patient's wearing a bra, ask her to remove it.) Drape the patient for privacy and warmth.

Place the patient in a comfortable position that allows you access to his posterior, anterior, and lateral chest. If his condition permits, have him sit on the edge of the bed or examining table, or in a chair, leaning slightly forward with his hands on his thighs. If this isn't possible, place him in semi-Fowler's position for the interview and anterior chest examination. Later, it may be necessary to reposition him laterally for the posterior examination. After you carry out these preparatory steps, you're ready to begin a detailed assessment.

THE NURSING HISTORY

Begin detailed assessment with the nursing history. You may wish to take the history over several meetings to avoid tiring acutely ill patients. Include the following steps for a complete history.

Record biographical data

Remember that the patient's age and sex can affect his thoracic configuration. And, when asking about the patient's life-style and occupation, be alert to possible environmental or occupational hazards that can affect his lungs and breathing.

Determine the chief complaint

Record the patient's description of his chief complaint. The most common chief complaints in patients with respiratory disorders are cough—with or without sputum production or hemoptysis—dyspnea, and chest pain.

Explore the history of present illness

When you have identified the patient's chief complaint, define his illness in greater detail by asking the following types of questions:

About cough. *Does your cough usually occur at a specific time of day? How does it sound—dry, hacking, barking, congested?* Try to determine whether the patient's cough is related to cigarette smoking or other irritants. (The most common causes of coughing are smoking and chronic bronchitis.)

Are you taking any drug or receiving treatment to clear the cough? If so, how often? Have you recently been exposed to anyone with a similar cough? Was that person's cough caused by a cold or flu?

About sputum production. *How much sputum are you coughing up per day?* Remember, the tracheobronchial tree can produce up to 3 oz (90 ml) of sputum per day.

What time of day do you cough up the most sputum? Smokers cough the most in the morning; nonsmokers generally don't. Coughing from an irritant occurs most often during exposure to it—for example, at work.

Is sputum production increasing? This may result from external stimuli or from such internal causes as chronic bronchial infection or a lung abscess. Excess production of sputum that separates into layers may indicate bronchiectasis.

Does the sputum contain mucus or look frothy? What color is it? Has its color changed? Does it smell bad? Foul-smelling sputum may result from an anaerobic infection, such as an abscess. Blood-tinged or rust-colored sputum may result from trauma caused by coughing or from such underlying conditions as bronchitis, pulmonary infarction or infections, tuberculosis, and tumors. A color change from white to yellow or green indicates infection.

About dyspnea. *Are you always short of breath, or do you have intermittent attacks of breathlessness?* Onset of dyspnea may be slow or abrupt. For example, a patient with asthma may experience acute dyspnea intermittently.

What relieves the attacks—repositioning yourself, relaxing, taking medication? Do the attacks cause your lips and nail beds to turn blue? Does body position, time of day, or any activity affect your breathing? Paroxysmal nocturnal dyspnea and orthopnea are commonly associated with chronic lung disease but may be related to cardiac dysfunction.

How many stairs can you climb, or how many blocks can you walk, before you begin to feel short of breath? Do such activities as taking a shower or shopping make you feel that way? Dyspnea that follows activity suggests poor ventilation or perfusion, or inefficient breathing mechanisms.

Do you experience any associated discomfort, such as cough, unusual sweating, or chest pain? Does the breathlessness seem to be stable or getting worse? Is it accompanied by external sounds, such as wheezing or stridor? Wheezing results from small-airway obstruction (for example, from an aspirated foreign body, from a tumor, from asthma, or from congestive heart failure). Stridor results from tracheal compression or laryngeal edema.

About chest pain. *Is the pain localized? Is it constant, or do you experience attacks? Have you ever had a chest injury? Does a specific activity (such as movement of the upper body or exercise) produce pain?* Respiratory disorders usually cause musculoskeletal chest pain; that is, pain related to motion. (Remember, the lungs have no pain-sensitive nerves; however, the parietal pleura and the tracheobronchial tree do.) Of course, chest pain is also commonly associated with cardiovascular disorders.

Is the pain accompanied by other discomfort, such as coughing, sneezing, or shortness of breath? Does the pain occur when you breathe normally, or only when you breathe deeply? Pain on deep breathing is often pleuritic. *Does splinting relieve the pain?*

After you have elicited a detailed description of the chief complaint and the present illness, you can begin to formulate nursing diagnoses, as shown in the chart on page 25.

Review past history

Next, focus on the past history. Be sure to consider the following body systems, procedures, and conditions:

Respiratory system. Ask the patient if he's

Using the chief complaint in nursing diagnoses

Chief complaint	Effect of sign or symptom	Nursing diagnosis
Dyspnea	*Acute:* • Diaphoresis, restlessness *Chronic:* • Barrel chest, accessory muscle change *Acute and chronic:* • Fatigue, exhaustion • Emotional distress • Hypoventilation/hyperventilation (may lead to respiratory acidosis/alkalosis)	• Alteration in comfort • Ineffective breathing pattern • Fear of breathlessness, ineffective breathing pattern, impaired gas exchange, impaired physical mobility
Chest pain	• Decreased ventilation (may lead to infection or pneumonia) • Increased CO_2 retention and respiratory acidosis • Discomfort • Pain	• Impaired gas exchange, ineffective breathing pattern • Fear of chest pain, alteration in comfort
Cough	*Chronic and short term (less than 1 month):* • Hazardous elevation in intrathoracic pressure, intracranial pressure, and blood pressure (may lead to congestive heart failure, ruptured aneurysm) • Cough syncope • Musculoskeletal pain • Fractured ribs *Chronic and long term (more than 1 month):* • Fatigue • Weight loss, anorexia *Forced cough:* • Collapsed airways (atelectasis) • Rupture of thin-walled alveoli (may lead to pneumothorax) • Hemoptysis, second-degree irritation of tracheobronchial tree	• Alteration in CO_2 level • Alteration in comfort • Alteration in nutrition (less than body requirements) • Impaired gas exchange • Fear of seeing blood
Increased and abnormal secretions	*Increased sputum:* • Mucous plugs (may lead to airway obstruction, atelectasis, prevention of alveolar gas exchange, hypoxia, respiratory acidosis) • Increased secretions and/or abnormal fluids retained in lung (may lead to infection, tracheobronchitis, bronchopneumonia) *Hemoptysis:* • Obstruction with blood (may lead to asphyxiation, atelectasis, pneumonia) • Blood-streaked sputum; severe blood loss may lead to shock	• Ineffective airway clearance, impaired gas exchange • Ineffective airway clearance, impaired gas exchange, alteration in tissue perfusion • Fear of seeing blood

ever had pneumonia, pleurisy, asthma, bronchitis, emphysema, or tuberculosis. Also ask how often he gets colds. Note that congenital or trauma-related deformities may distort cardiac and pulmonary structures.

Cardiovascular system. Ask the patient if he's ever had hypertension, myocardial infarction, or congestive heart failure. A history of such disorders is particularly significant because of the close relationship between the cardiovascular and respiratory systems.

Chest surgery and procedures. Find out if the patient has had any thoracic surgery or undergone any chest- or lung-related procedures, such as bronchoscopy or thoracentesis. Remember that such procedures as thoracoplasty or pneumonectomy change the findings at the physical examination.

Laboratory tests. Ask if the patient has recently had a chest X-ray, pulmonary function test, electrocardiogram, arterial blood gas analysis, sputum culture, or skin test for tuberculosis. If so, find out where these tests were performed, and obtain the results.

Allergies. Ask about hypersensitivity to drugs, foods, pets, dust, or pollen. Also ask if the patient has any allergic signs and symptoms, such as coughing, sneezing, sinusitis, or dyspnea, and if he's ever been treated for allergy. Chronic allergies may lead to other respiratory disorders.

Drugs and vaccines. Ask the patient if he takes any drugs for cough control, expectoration, nasal congestion, chest pain, or dyspnea. Also note any drugs the patient is taking for other conditions. Ask the patient if he's ever been vaccinated against pneumonia or flu.

Review family history
Ask the patient if anyone in his family has had asthma, cystic fibrosis, or emphysema, all of which may be genetically transmitted. Similarly, ask about lung cancer, infectious diseases (such as tuberculosis), chronic allergies, cardiovascular and respiratory disorders, kyphosis, scoliosis, obesity, and neuromuscular dysfunction.

Review psychosocial history
Next, direct your questions to the following aspects of the patient's life-style, which can have great impact on respiratory function.

Home and work conditions. Persons living near a constant source of air pollution, such as a chemical factory, may develop respiratory disorders. Exposure to cigarette smoke at home or at work may aggravate respiratory symptoms. Crowded living conditions facilitate transmission of communicable respiratory disease. Exposure to animals may precipitate allergic or asthmatic attacks.

Hobbies. Such seemingly innocent pastimes as building model airplanes or refinishing furniture may expose the patient to harsh chemical irritants.

Stress. Some respiratory conditions, especially asthma, can be aggravated by stress.

Smoking. Knowing the patient's smoking habits is essential for any comprehensive respiratory assessment. Ask the patient if he smokes cigarettes, cigars, pipe tobacco, or marijuana. If he smokes cigarettes, find out how many packs per day and how long he's been smoking at this rate. Note the number of pack years (packs smoked per day multiplied by years). If he doesn't smoke now, ask if he used to smoke, how much, and when he stopped. Smoking is often associated with pulmonary disease, especially lung cancer, chronic bronchitis, and emphysema. The risk of lung disease is higher among smokers exposed to environmental respiratory irritants. So when asking the patient about his daily activities, be especially alert to conditions that suggest exposure to chemicals, noxious fumes, chromium, and dust containing nickel, uranium, or asbestos.

Daily routine. Respiratory signs and symptoms can interfere with such activities as climbing stairs or traveling to work.

Fill in missing data
Complete the history by asking about the following signs and symptoms that are commonly associated with respiratory disorders.
• *General.* Fever, chills, and fatigue may accompany respiratory symptoms.
• *Cutaneous.* Nocturnal diaphoresis may be associated with tuberculosis.
• *Hematologic.* Anemia decreases the blood's oxygen-carrying capacity; polycythemia may occur in response to chronic hypoxemia.
• *Oral and nasal.* Halitosis may result from a pulmonary infection, such as an abscess or bronchiectasis. Nasal discharge, sinus pain or infection, or postnasal drip may result from seasonal allergies or chronic sinus problems.
• *Cardiovascular.* Ankle edema, paroxysmal nocturnal dyspnea, orthopnea, or chest pain that worsens with exercise, eating, or stress may reflect a cardiovascular disorder.
• *Gastrointestinal.* Unexplained weight loss suggests possible deterioration from disease, such as from lung cancer. Loss of appetite resulting from breathing difficulty is associated with chronic obstructive pulmonary disease.
• *Neurologic.* Confusion, syncope, and restlessness may be associated with cerebral hypoxia.
• *Musculoskeletal.* Chronic hypoxia may cause fatigue and weakness.
• *Psychological.* Some respiratory signs and symptoms (for example, wheezing and hyperventilation) may be associated with emotional problems.

THE PHYSICAL EXAMINATION
If the patient's condition permits, follow the history with a detailed physical examination. But if the patient shows signs of acute respiratory distress, proceed differently. Above all, don't waste time. Focus your examination on areas that will help identify the cause of respiratory distress and guide emergency intervention. For example, auscultate lung sounds in the dyspneic, cyanotic patient to identify areas of decreased or absent sounds that characterize pneumothorax or airway obstruction. Later, after the airway has been restored and the patient's more comfortable, you can complete your detailed examination.

Inspect the patient's skin

Begin the detailed physical examination by inspecting the patient's skin color. Central cyanosis, which affects all body organs, results from prolonged hypoxia. Its presence helps you gauge the severity of the patient's illness. Look for central cyanosis in highly vascular areas: lips, nail beds, tip of the nose, ear helices, and underside of the tongue. To detect cyanosis in a patient with dark brown or black skin, inspect the nose, cheeks, and mucosa inside the lips. Facial skin may be pale gray in a cyanotic dark-skinned patient. (Remember, though, that severely anemic patients with respiratory difficulty don't appear cyanotic.) Be sure you know how to distinguish central cyanosis from peripheral cyanosis. The latter results from local vasoconstriction and is apparent only in the nail beds and sometimes the lips. Also examine the skin for dryness— a possible sign of dehydration—or for diaphoresis, which may be associated with fever and infection. Bright cherry-red mucous membranes may result from carbon monoxide poisoning. While inspecting the skin, observe the fingers for clubbing, a sign of chronic respiratory dysfunction and of certain cardiovascular and gastrointestinal disorders. Use the quick assessment technique in the illustration to detect clubbing.

Examine the nose

Inspect the patient's nose for symmetry and for tumors or other external deformities. Look for narrowing of the nose associated with chronic nasal obstruction and note dependence on mouth breathing. Also check for nasal flaring, in which the nostrils alternately dilate with inspiration and contract with expiration, to detect increased respiratory effort.

Palpate the nose to detect any swelling, pain, fractures, or loss of structure. Test nostril patency by occluding one nostril with digital compression while having the patient inhale through the open nostril with his mouth closed. Repeat for the other nostril.

Tip the patient's head back slightly to examine the interior nose. Using a nasal speculum, check the nostrils for discharge, swelling, obstructions, and bleeding. Note the condition and color of the nasal mucosa (it should be slightly redder than oral mucosa). To confirm your observations, examine the nose with a penlight. Place one palm on the patient's forehead, and gently lift the bulbous portion of the nose with your thumb. Shine the penlight into the nostrils with your other hand. Check

Assessing the fingers for clubbing

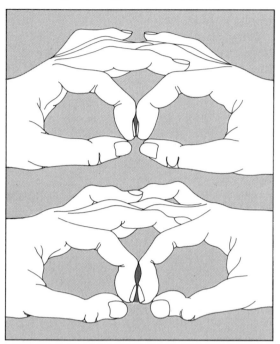

To quickly assess the fingers for clubbing, have the patient place the first phalanges of the forefingers together. Normally, the bases of the nails are concave and create a small, diamond-shaped space when the first phalanges are opposed (as shown in the illustration at top). When clubbed fingers are opposed, the now convex bases of the nails can touch without leaving a space (as shown in the illustration at bottom).

the nasal septum for perforation by shining the penlight into one nostril and inspecting the illuminated septum.

Clearly document all your observations and consider the possible causes of nasal abnormalities. Nasal obstruction may involve one or both nostrils. A foreign body, neoplasm, or significant deviation of the septum (it's rarely perfectly straight) may cause unilateral obstruction. An S-shaped deviation of the septum may cause bilateral obstruction. Most commonly, bilateral obstruction results from rhinitis and, less commonly, nasal polyps. Perforation of the nasal septum often follows frequent sniffing of cocaine. A watery nasal discharge with sneezing and stuffiness accompanies nasal allergy. A discharge of clear, watery mucus marks the viral start of the common cold; discharge that thickens and becomes purulent marks superimposed bacterial infection. Epistaxis may follow repeated nose picking or other trauma or may be a sign of serious disease. Notify the doctor of recurring epistaxis. Keep in mind that a neoplasm usually produces a bloody discharge, not the brisk bleeding of epistaxis. Inflammation of the nasal turbinates—the three projec-

Assessing the paranasal sinuses

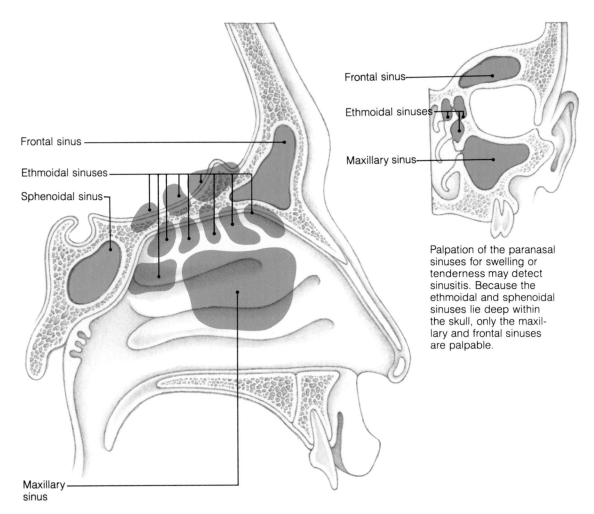

Frontal sinus

Ethmoidal sinuses

Sphenoidal sinus

Maxillary sinus

Frontal sinus

Ethmoidal sinuses

Maxillary sinus

Palpation of the paranasal sinuses for swelling or tenderness may detect sinusitis. Because the ethmoidal and sphenoidal sinuses lie deep within the skull, only the maxillary and frontal sinuses are palpable.

tions on the lateral wall of the nasal chamber—may cause swelling and reddening of the mucosa. Allergy, however, turns the mucosa pale and bluish.

Next, palpate the paranasal sinuses. Palpate the maxillary sinuses for tenderness and swelling by pressing the patient's cheeks over the maxillary areas. Palpate his frontal sinuses by placing your thumbs just below the eyebrows and pressing upward. Palpate both sides simultaneously to elicit unilateral tenderness. Also check the eyelids for swelling that may accompany sinus disease. While checking these facial structures, listen for external sounds of moisture or mucus and for stridor or wheezing.

Examine the mouth and trachea

If the patient wears dentures, ask him to remove them. Using a tongue depressor, a cotton-tipped applicator, and a penlight, examine the oropharynx for color changes, inflammation, white patches, ulcerations,

bleeding, exudate, and lesions. Check the soft palate, anterior and posterior pillars of fauces, uvula, tonsils, posterior pharynx, teeth, gums, tongue, floor of the mouth, mucous membranes, and lips. Remember, a dark-skinned patient normally has dark patches on the mucous membranes.

To examine the lingual tonsils, gently pull the tongue forward with a piece of gauze, and observe the tonsils with the hand mirror. Keep in mind that large tonsils don't always imply disease, but they can make respiration or swallowing difficult. Reddened, edematous tonsils with white or yellow dots or streaks of exudate characterize acute tonsillitis. Abscess formation may complicate infection, producing a large grayish patch on the tonsils. Using a tongue depressor, bring the patient's pharynx into view and ask him to say "eh." Observe for symmetrical rise and fall of the soft palate. Next, check for mucopurulent discharge (postnasal drip) on the posterior pharyngeal wall, which may result from rhinitis or sinus infection. Touch both sides of the posterior pharynx with the applicator to check the patient's gag reflex. (This test is particularly helpful when you're assessing an older patient with decreased sensitivity to touch or one who has suffered a cerebrovascular accident, or CVA; it helps you determine such a patient's ability to swallow oral secretions and food.) To determine the patient's ability to clear his respiratory tract of accumulated secretions, ask him to cough. If he's unresponsive to verbal commands because of CVA or other cerebral trauma, or because of drug or alcohol ingestion, elicit a cough by gently touching the posterior oropharynx with a swabstick.

Inspect the patient's trachea for midline position, and observe again for any use of accessory neck muscles in breathing. If you can't see the trachea, palpate for it at the midline position, using the fingertips of one hand. Starting at the middle of the patient's chin, gently slide your fingertips down the center of the neck. After locating the larynx, you should be able to feel the trachea in the area of the sternal notch. Deviation of the trachea to either side indicates deformity and requires further investigation. Also, observe and palpate the neck over the trachea for swelling, bruises, tenderness, and masses that might obstruct breathing.

Locate thoracic landmarks
Before examining the thorax, become familiar with surface landmarks. These landmarks are imaginary lines or anatomic guides like bony prominences, such as ribs, and intercostal spaces. When you know thoracic landmarks (see *Locating thoracic landmarks*), you'll be able to locate the underlying respiratory structures and describe the site of any abnormalities more precisely.

Inspect the posterior chest
Begin examination of the thorax by inspecting the posterior chest. Instruct the patient to sit and lean forward slightly, with shoulders rounded and arms crossed on the chest. If the patient can't lean forward, place him on his side. When you use the lateral position, examine the uppermost side of the chest first; then roll the patient onto his other side and repeat the examination for comparison. (Always note the patient's tolerance of position changes; observe for such signs as shortness of breath, holding of breath because of pain, color change, and use of accessory muscles.) After checking the posterior chest for wounds, le-

Locating thoracic landmarks
Use the landmarks in these illustrations as guides when assessing the patient's respiratory status:

Posterior view

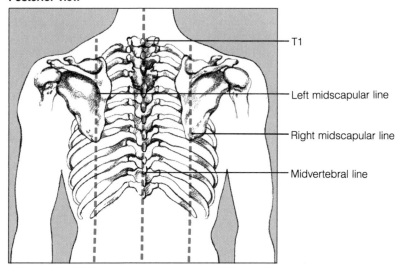

- T1
- Left midscapular line
- Right midscapular line
- Midvertebral line

Right lateral view   **Left lateral view**

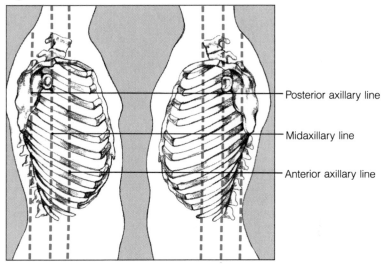

- Posterior axillary line
- Midaxillary line
- Anterior axillary line

Anterior view

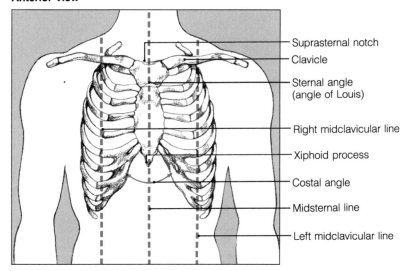

- Suprasternal notch
- Clavicle
- Sternal angle (angle of Louis)
- Right midclavicular line
- Xiphoid process
- Costal angle
- Midsternal line
- Left midclavicular line

Identifying lung lobes

To locate lung lobes, use the common chest wall landmarks shown here. In the posterior view, the oblique fissures divide the upper lobes from the lower lobes of both lungs. Externally, you can approximate the location of these fissures by imagining bilateral lines drawn laterally and inferiorly from the third thoracic spinous process to the inferior border of the scapula.

In the left lateral view, the left oblique fissure divides the left upper lobe (LUL) from the left lower lobe (LLL). Externally, you can approximate the location of this fissure by imagining a line drawn anteriorly and inferiorly from the third thoracic spinous process to the sixth rib, midclavicular line.

In the right lateral view, you can determine the location of the right oblique fissure as you did for the left oblique fissure. To approximate the division of the right upper lobe (RUL) and the right middle lobe (RML), imagine a line drawn medially from the fifth rib, midaxillary line, to the fourth rib, midclavicular line.

In the anterior view, you can locate the apices and the inferior borders of both lungs. The apices lie ¾″ to 1½″ (2 to 4 cm) above the clavicle. The inferior borders run from the sixth rib, midclavicular line, to the eighth rib, midaxillary line.

The horizontal fissure divides the right upper lobe from the right middle lobe. Externally, you can approximate the location of this fissure by imagining a line drawn anteriorly and superiorly from the fifth rib, midaxillary line, to the fourth rib, midclavicular line.

The oblique fissures divide the lower lobes from the upper and middle lobes. Externally, you can approximate the location of these fissures by imagining bilateral lines drawn medially and inferiorly from the fifth rib, midaxillary line, to the sixth rib, midclavicular line.

Posterior view

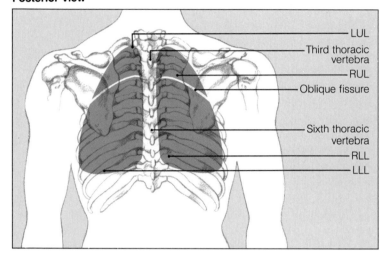

Right lateral view   **Left lateral view**

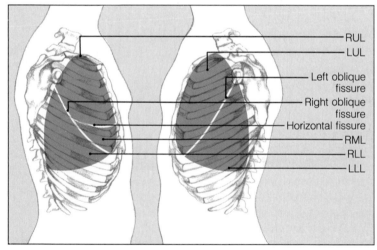

Anterior view

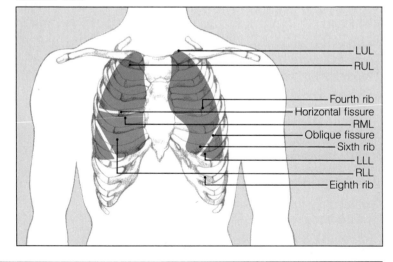

sions, masses, or scars, observe the rate, rhythm, and depth of respirations. The normal respiratory rate for an adult is 12 to 20 breaths/minute. Respirations should be regular and inaudible, with the sides of the chest expanding equally. Unequal expansion may result from massive pleural effusion, atelectasis, pneumothorax, or chest pain. To avoid missing unequal expansion, inspect the chest during both quiet and deep breathing. Normal respirations consist of inspiration, a slight pause, and slightly longer expiration. Prolonged expiratory time suggests air outflow impedance.

Next, observe the patient's chest for local lag or impaired movement. Normally, the chest moves upward and outward symmetrically on inspiration. Impairment may result from pain, exertion from poor positioning, or obstruction from abdominal distention. Paradoxical movement of the chest wall may result from fractured ribs or flail chest. Note the slope of the patient's ribs. Check for retraction of intercostal spaces during inspiration and for abnormal bulging of intercostal spaces during expiration. Intercostal retractions usually indicate obstruction to the free inflow of air, which increases inspiratory effort. Intercostal bulging usually results from forced, prolonged expiration as in asthma or emphysema. Then observe for such spinal deformities as lordosis, kyphosis, and scoliosis.

Palpate the posterior chest

Palpate the patient's posterior chest to assess the thorax, to identify thoracic structures, and to check chest expansion and vocal or tactile fremitus. Begin by feeling for muscle mass with your fingers and palms (use a grasping action of the fingers to assess position and consistency). Normally, it feels firm, smooth, and symmetrical. As you palpate muscle mass, also check skin temperature and turgor. Be sure to note the presence of crepitus (especially around a wound site). Crepitus, or subcutaneous emphysema, is a crackling sensation beneath the fingertips that indicates trapped air within the tissues. Then, palpate the thoracic spine, noting tenderness, swelling, or such deformities as lordosis, kyphosis, and scoliosis. Next, using your metacarpophalangeal joints and finger pads, gently palpate the intercostal spaces and ribs for abnormal retractions, bulging, and tenderness. Normally, the intercostal spaces delineate the downward slope of the ribs. In a patient with an increased anteroposterior diameter caused by

obstructive lung disease, you'll feel ribs that are abnormally horizontal.

Palpate the thoracic landmarks. To help you identify the division between the patient's upper and lower lobes, instruct him to raise his arms above his head; then, palpate the borders of the scapulae. The lower borders of the scapulae should line up with the divisions between the upper and lower lobes. The inferior border of the lower lobes is usually located at the 10th thoracic spinous process and may descend, on full inspiration, to the 12th thoracic spinous process.

To locate the lower lung borders in a patient lying on his side, palpate the visible free-floating ribs or costal margins; then, count four intercostal spaces upward for the general location of the lower lung fields.

Palpate for symmetrical expansion of the thorax. Place your palms—fingers together and thumbs abducted toward the spine—flat on the bilateral sections of the patient's lower posterior chest wall. Position your thumbs at the 10th rib, and grasp the lateral rib cage with your hands. As the patient inhales, the posterior chest should move upward and outward and your thumbs should move apart; when he exhales, your thumbs should return to midline and touch each other again. Repeat this technique on the upper posterior chest.

Palpate for vocal or tactile fremitus. Use the top portion of each palm and follow the palpation sequences (see *Sequences for palpation*, page 31). To check for vocal fremitus, ask the patient to repeat "99" as you proceed. Palpable vibrations will be transmitted from the bronchopulmonary system, along the solid surface of the chest wall, to your palms and fingers. Expect fremitus to be most intense in thin persons. In muscular or obese persons, the additional subcutaneous tissue tends to dampen vibrations. Note the symmetry of the vibrations and the areas of enhanced, diminished, or absent fremitus. (Remember, fremitus should be most distinct in the patient's upper chest, where the trachea branches into the right and left mainstem bronchi, and less so in the lower regions of the thorax.) Anything that lies between the vibrations traveling down the tracheobronchial tree and your hand on the chest wall can decrease or mask fremitus. Air or fluid in the pleural space has this dampening effect. Consolidation of the lungs enhances vocal fremitus because vibrations travel better through solid or semisolid material than through normally porous lung tissue. But to increase fremitus, the consoli-

Sequences for palpation

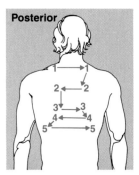

Posterior

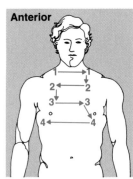

Anterior

Follow the sequences illustrated here to palpate the posterior and anterior chest.

dated area must connect to a patent bronchus and extend to the lung's surface so that vibrations are palpable.

Other palpable vibrations include tussive fremitus, pleural friction fremitus, and rhonchal fremitus. Tussive fremitus is the vibration that results from coughing; pleural friction fremitus, the vibration of inflamed pleural surfaces rubbing together. Rhonchal fremitus is the vibration of air moving through secretions in the trachea or bronchi. Unlike pleural friction fremitus, rhonchal fremitus clears with coughing.

You can estimate the level of the patient's diaphragm on both sides of his posterior chest by placing the ulnar side of your extended hand parallel to the anticipated diaphragm level. Instruct the patient to repeat "99" as you move your hand downward. The level where you no longer feel fremitus corresponds approximately to the diaphragm level.

Percuss the posterior chest
To learn the density and location of such anatomic structures as the lungs and diaphragm, you must identify five percussion sounds: flat, dull, resonant, hyperresonant, and tympanic (see *Identifying percussion sounds*). Start by percussing across the top of each shoulder. The area overlying the lung apices—approximately 2″ (5 cm)—should be resonant. Then, percuss downward toward the diaphragm, at 2″ intervals, comparing right and left sides as you proceed (see *Sequences for percussion and auscultation*, page 36). The thoracic area (except over the scapulae) should produce resonance when you percuss. At the level of the diaphragm, resonance should change to dullness. A dull sound over the lungs indicates fluid or solid tissue. Hyperresonance or tympany over the lungs suggests pneumothorax or large emphysematous blebs. A marked difference in diaphragm level from one side to the other is an abnormal finding.

Next, measure diaphragmatic excursion. Instruct the patient to take a deep breath and hold it while you percuss downward until dullness identifies the lower border of the lung field. Mark this point. Now ask him to exhale and again hold his breath as you percuss upward to the area of dullness. Mark this point, too. Repeat the procedure on the opposite side. Now measure the distances between the two marks on each side. Normal diaphragmatic excursion is about 1¼″ to 2¼″ (3 to 6 cm). (The diaphragm is usually slightly higher on the right side.)

Auscultate the posterior chest
To assess airflow through the respiratory system, auscultate the lungs and identify normal and abnormal (adventitious) breath sounds (see *Assessing breath sounds*). Lung auscultation helps detect abnormal fluid or mucus, as well as obstructed passages. It also helps evaluate the condition of the alveoli and surrounding pleura.

Before auscultating the posterior chest, remove clothing and bed linen from the body area to be examined. If the patient has a lot of hair on his posterior chest, wet and mat the hair with a damp washcloth to prevent it from causing rubbing sounds that can be confused with rales. Then, warm the stethoscope's diaphragm with your hands to avoid startling the patient.

When auscultating the patient's chest, instruct him to take full, slow breaths through his mouth. (Breath sounds intensify with deep breathing, but nose breathing changes the pitch of the sounds.) Listen for one full inspiration and expiration before moving the stethoscope. Remember, a patient may try to accommodate you by breathing quickly and deeply with every movement of the stethoscope, which can cause hyperventilation. If the patient becomes light-headed or dizzy, stop auscultating and allow him to breathe normally for a few minutes. Using the diaphragm of the stethoscope, begin auscultating above the patient's scapulae. Move to the area between the scapulae and the vertebral column. Then, move laterally beneath the scapulae, to the right and left lower lobes. Move the stethoscope's diaphragm methodically, and compare the sounds you hear on both sides of the chest before moving to the next area.

Normally, you'll hear vesicular breath sounds—soft, low-pitched sounds lasting longer during inspiration—at the lung bases. Bronchovesicular breath sounds—medium-pitched sounds that are equal in duration on inspiration and expiration—can be heard between the scapulae. Decreased or absent breath sounds may result from bronchial obstruction, muscle weakness, obesity, or pleural disease. If you hear an adventitious breath sound, note its location and whether it occurs during inspiration or expiration. Then, continue auscultating the posterior chest. After listening, instruct the patient to cough and breathe deeply. Let him rest, and listen again to the area where you heard the adventitious sound. Note any changes. Sometimes, rales

Assessing breath sounds

Normal breath sounds

Bronchial (tubular) breath sounds

Anterior

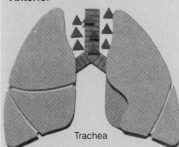

Trachea

Location
Over trachea

Ratio

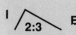
I / 2:3 \ E

Description
Loud, high pitched, and hollow, harsh, or coarse

Bronchovesicular breath sounds

Anterior

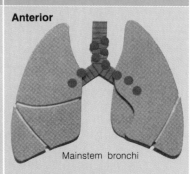

Mainstem bronchi

Posterior

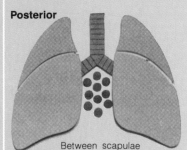

Between scapulae

Location
Anteriorly, near the mainstem bronchi in the first and second intercostal spaces; posteriorly, between the scapulae

Ratio

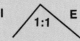
I / 1:1 \ E

Description
Soft, breezy, and pitched about two notes lower than bronchial sounds

Vesicular breath sounds

Anterior

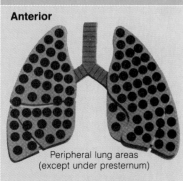

Peripheral lung areas (except under presternum)

Posterior

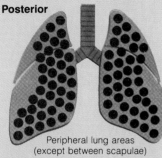

Peripheral lung areas (except between scapulae)

Location
In most of the lungs' peripheral parts (cannot be heard over the presternum or the scapulae)

Ratio

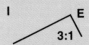
I / 3:1 \ E

Description
Soft, swishy, breezy, and about two notes lower than bronchovesicular sounds

Abnormal breath sounds

Rales	Rhonchi	Wheezes	Pleural friction rub
Location Anywhere. Heard in lung bases first with pulmonary edema, usually during inspiratory phase	**Location** In larger airways, usually during expiratory phase	**Location** Anywhere. May occur during inspiration or expiration	**Location** Anterolateral lung field, on both inspiration and expiration (with the patient in an upright position)
Cause Air passing through moisture, especially in the small airways and alveoli	**Cause** Fluid or secretions in the large airways or narrowing of large airways	**Cause** Narrowed airways	**Cause** Inflamed parietal and visceral pleural linings rubbing together
Description Light crackling, popping, nonmusical; can be further classified by pitch: high, medium, or low	**Description** Coarse rattling, usually louder and lower pitched than rales; can be described as sonorous, bubbling, moaning, musical, sibilant, and rumbly	**Description** Creaking, groaning; always high-pitched, musical squeaks	**Description** Superficial squeaking or grating

Identifying percussion sounds

To help identify the sounds you may hear when you percuss the patient's chest, keep these characteristics in mind:

Flatness
Pitch: high
Intensity: soft
Quality: extreme dullness

Dullness
Pitch: medium
Intensity: medium
Quality: thudlike

Resonance
Pitch: low
Intensity: moderate to loud
Quality: hollow

Hyperresonance
Pitch: lower than resonance
Intensity: very loud
Quality: booming

Tympany
Pitch: high
Intensity: loud
Quality: musical, drumlike

Recognizing respiratory patterns

To determine the rate, rhythm, and depth of your patient's respirations, observe him at rest. Make sure he's unaware that you're counting his respirations. Why? A person conscious of his respirations may alter his natural pattern.

Always count respirations for at least 1 minute. If you count for only a fraction of a minute and then multiply, your count may be off by as much as 4 respirations per minute. Your patient's respiratory rhythm should be even, except for an occasional deep breath. Use this chart as a guide for noting differences in respiratory rates, rhythms, and depths.

Eupnea

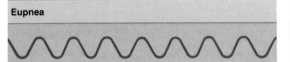

Normal respiration rate and rhythm. For adults and teenagers, 12 to 20 breaths/minute; ages 2 to 12, 20 to 30 breaths/minute; newborns, 30 to 50 breaths/minute. Also, occasional deep breaths at a rate of 2 or 3 breaths/minute.

Tachypnea

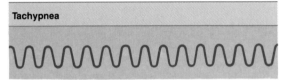

Increased respirations, as seen in fever. Respirations increase about 4 breaths/minute for every Fahrenheit degree above normal.

Bradypnea

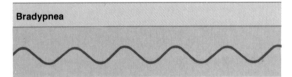

Slower but regular respirations. Can occur when the brain's respiratory control center is influenced by opiate narcotics, tumor, alcohol, metabolic disorder, or respiratory decompensation. Normal during sleep.

Apnea

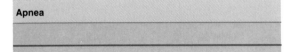

Absence of breathing; may be periodic.

Hyperpnea

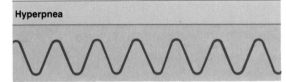

Deeper respirations; rate normal.

Cheyne-Stokes

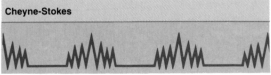

Respirations gradually become faster and deeper than normal, then slower, over a 30- to 170-second period. Alternating periods of apnea for 20 to 60 seconds.

Biot's

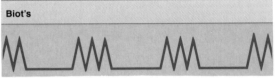

Faster and deeper respirations than normal, with abrupt pauses in between. Each breath has same depth. May occur with spinal meningitis or other CNS conditions.

Kussmaul's

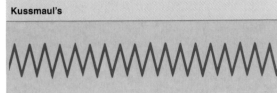

Faster and deeper respirations without pauses; in adults, over 20 breaths/minute. Breathing usually sounds labored, with deep breaths that resemble sighs. Can occur from renal failure or metabolic acidosis.

Apneustic

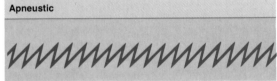

Prolonged gasping inspiration, followed by extremely short, inefficient expiration. Can result from lesions in the brain's respiratory center.

Sighing

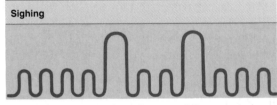

Deep, audible respirations that sound like repeated sighing.

Air trapping

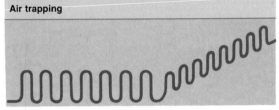

Inspiration is normal, at first, followed by forced expiration. Respirations become shallow. Occurs in obstructive pulmonary disease.

Identifying chest deformities

As you inspect the anterior chest, you may notice deviations in size or shape. The illustrations demonstrate four such deformities. Note the physical characteristics, signs, and conditions associated with each deformity.

Pectus carinatum (pigeon chest)

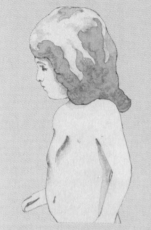

Physical characteristics
• Sinking or funnel-shaped depression of lower sternum
• Diminished anteroposterior chest diameter

Signs and associated conditions
• Postural disorders, such as forward displacement of neck and shoulders
• Upper thoracic kyphosis
• Protuberant abdomen
• Functional heart murmur

Barrel chest

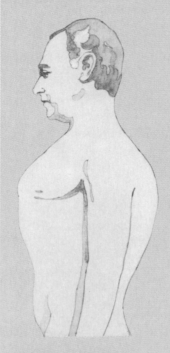

Physical characteristics
• Projection of sternum beyond abdomen's frontal plane. Evident in two variations: projection greatest at xiphoid process; projection greatest at or near center of sternum

Signs and associated conditions
• Functional cardiovascular or respiratory disorders

Pectus excavatum (funnel chest)

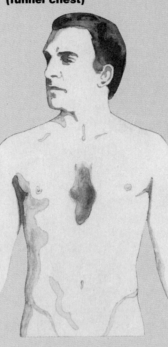

Physical characteristics
• Enlarged anteroposterior and transverse chest dimensions; chest appears barrel-shaped
• Prominent accessory muscles

Signs and associated conditions
• Chronic respiratory disorders
• Increasing shortness of breath
• Chronic cough
• Wheezing

Bifid sternum

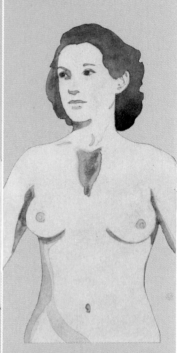

Physical characteristics
• Complete or incomplete sternal separation

Signs and associated conditions
• Missing or supernumerary ribs
• Ectopia cordis (development of heart outside thoracic cavity)

and rhonchi can be cleared by coughing; wheezes and friction rubs can't.

Assess for resonance
If you detect any respiratory abnormality during palpation, percussion, or auscultation, assess the patient's voice sounds for vocal resonance. The significance of vocal resonance is based on the principle that sound carries best through a solid, less well through fluid, and poorly through air. Normally, you should hear vocal resonance as muffled, unclear sounds, loudest medially and less intense at the lung periphery. Voice sounds that become louder and more distinct at the lung periphery signal bronchophony, an abnormal finding except over the trachea and posteriorly over the upper right lobe. To elicit broncho-

phony, ask your patient to say "99" or "one, two, three," while you auscultate the thorax systematically. Bronchophony usually accompanies enhanced fremitus, abnormal bronchial breath sounds, and dullness on percussion.

Check for whispered pectoriloquy, which is an exaggerated form of bronchophony. Ask the patient to whisper a simple phrase like "one, two, three." Normally, whispered words sound faint and indistinct. Hearing the words clearly through the stethoscope is an abnormal finding. Because whispered pectoriloquy precedes bronchophony, it aids early diagnosis of pneumonia.

Egophony is another form of abnormal vocal resonance. Ask the patient to say "ee, ee." Transmission of the sound through the stethoscope as "ay, ay," is an abnormal finding,

Sequences for percussion and auscultation

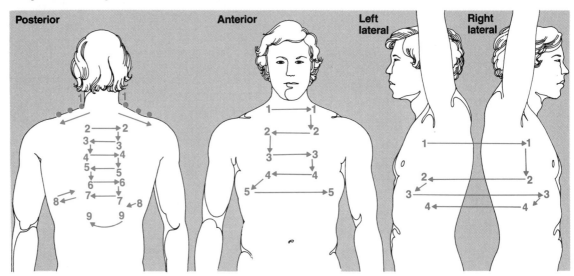

Follow the sequences illustrated here to percuss and auscultate the patient's lungs. Remember to compare sound variations from one side to the other as you proceed, and to avoid bony areas. Document any abnormal sounds and describe them carefully, including their location.

possibly indicating compressed lung tissue, as in pleural effusion. You may hear increased vocal resonance, whispered pectoriloquy, and egophony in any patient with consolidated lungs.

Inspect the anterior chest
To inspect the patient's anterior chest, place him in semi-Fowler's position. Begin by inspecting the anterior chest for draining, open wounds, bruises, abrasions, scars, cuts, punctures, rib deformities, fractures, lesions, and masses. Then, inspect the rate, rhythm, and depth of respirations. Men, infants, and children are normally diaphragmatic (abdominal) breathers, as are athletes, singers, and people who practice yoga. Women are usually intercostal (chest) breathers. The patient's face should look relaxed when he breathes. Abnormal findings include nasal flaring, pursed lip breathing, use of neck or abdominal muscles on expiration, and intercostal or sternal retractions. Inspect for local lag and impaired chest wall movement. Observe for thoracic deformities, such as pectus carinatum (pigeon chest) and bifid sternum. Check for barrel chest by noting the ratio between the anteroposterior diameter of the chest and its lateral diameter; the normal ratio ranges from 1:2 to 5:7.

Palpate the anterior chest
Begin palpating the patient's anterior chest, using your fingers and palms. Feel for areas of tenderness, muscle mass, and skin turgor and elasticity. Note any crepitus during palpation, especially around wound sites, subclavian catheters, and chest tubes. Palpate the sternum and costal cartilages for tenderness and deformities. Then, using your metacarpophalangeal joints and finger pads, palpate the intercostal spaces and ribs for abnormal retractions, bulging, and tenderness. Remember to proceed to the lateral aspects of the thorax.

Next, palpate the thoracic landmarks used to identify underlying structures. To assess for symmetrical respiratory expansion, place your thumbs along each costal margin, pointing toward the xiphoid process, with your hands along the lateral rib cage. Ask the patient to inhale deeply, and observe for symmetrical thoracic expansion.

Now, palpate for vocal or tactile fremitus, remembering to examine the lateral surfaces and to compare symmetrical areas of the lungs. (If your patient is a woman, you may have to displace her breasts to examine her anterior chest.) Fremitus will usually be decreased or absent over the precordium.

Percuss the anterior chest
Percussing the patient's anterior chest allows you to determine the location and density of the heart, lungs, liver, and diaphragm. A forceful percussion stroke penetrates through 1¼" (3 cm) of thoracic wall and about 1¼" of lung tissue. Use a forceful stroke to detect changes in the density of lung tissue (sonorous percussion). Unfortunately, this won't

detect all abnormalities, particularly if they're less than ¾" (2 cm) in diameter, deep-seated, and covered by aerated lung tissue. Use a lighter stroke to outline the borders of adjacent organs (definitive percussion). Begin by percussing the lung apices (supraclavicular areas), comparing right and left sides. Then, percuss downward in 1¼" to 2" (3- to 5-cm) intervals. You should hear resonant tones until you reach the third or fourth intercostal space (ICS), to the left of the sternum, where you'll hear a dull sound produced by the heart. This sound should continue as you percuss downward toward the fifth ICS and laterally toward the midclavicular line. At the sixth ICS, at the left midclavicular line, you'll hear resonance again. As you percuss downward toward the rib cage, you'll hear tympany over the stomach. On the right side, you should hear resonance, indicating normal lung tissue. Near the fifth to seventh ICS you'll hear dullness, marking the superior border of the liver.

To percuss the lateral chest, instruct the patient to raise his arms over his head. Percuss laterally, comparing the right and left sides as you proceed. These areas should also be resonant.

Auscultate the anterior chest
In the same way you auscultated the patient's posterior chest, auscultate the anterior and lateral chest, comparing sounds on both sides before moving to the next area. Use the open bell of the stethoscope for the intercostal spaces, supraclavicular fossa, or other narrow areas. Hold the chestpiece tightly against the skin so the skin forms a diaphragm. Make sure the entire rim of the chestpiece touches the skin to avoid introducing extraneous noise and to eliminate sounds of respiratory excursion, like the movement of intercostal muscles, which may mimic a friction rub.

Begin auscultating the anterior chest at the trachea, where you should hear bronchial (or tubular) breath sounds. Next, listen for bronchovesicular breath sounds where the mainstem bronchi branch from the trachea (near the second ICS, ¾" to 1¼" or 2 to 3 cm to either side of the sternum). Bronchial and bronchovesicular sounds are abnormal when heard over peripheral lung areas.

Now, using the standard chest landmarks, listen over the patient's peripheral lung fields for vesicular sounds. Auscultate the lateral chest walls, comparing right and left sides as you proceed. On the left side, heart sounds

diminish breath sounds; on the right side, the liver diminishes them. If you hear adventitious breath sounds, describe them and note their location and timing. After listening to several respirations in the area of adventitious sound, instruct the patient to cough and breathe deeply. Then, using the technique described for the posterior chest, auscultate the area producing the abnormal sound and, if necessary, auscultate for bronchophony, whispered pectoriloquy, and egophony.

NURSING DIAGNOSES
After completing the physical examination, you can use the collected assessment data to develop nursing diagnoses. A nursing diagnosis defines an actual or potential health problem that a nurse can treat. To develop these diagnoses, first familiarize yourself with the list of nursing diagnoses accepted by the National Group for the Classification of Nursing Diagnoses. Use these diagnoses as a model to develop new diagnoses for problems not included in the list.

Three steps to success
Developing a nursing diagnosis is actually a simple, three-step process:
1. Observe the patient for signs and symptoms that may point to a health problem. Keep in mind that the problems you identify must be ones that a nurse can treat. Label possible problems "high risk" or "potential."
2. Identify the probable cause of the problem. Keep the etiology clear and concise so it's useful at the bedside. Also phrase it to suggest interventions or a plan of care.
3. Write your diagnostic statement, using the formula "problem related to etiology." For instance, a sample nursing diagnosis might be "Hazards of immobility related to prolonged bed rest."

Following these three steps will help you develop concise nursing diagnoses and a care plan that addresses the patient's changing needs.

A final note
Assessment is the critical first step in the nursing process. When skillfully done, it provides a firm data base on which to plan and implement care. Continuing respiratory assessment helps you to evaluate and modify your care plan as needed. Most important, it ensures prompt detection of subtle changes that may herald serious respiratory dysfunction.

Points to remember

• Correct respiratory assessment ensures prompt detection of respiratory changes that might otherwise result in acid-base disturbances, tissue hypoxia, and even sudden death.
• The most common chief complaints in respiratory disorders are cough—with or without sputum production or hemoptysis—dyspnea, and chest pain.
• A good description of the chief complaint and its history is a key assessment step.
• Respiratory assessment is the basis for all nursing diagnoses that address respiratory problems.

3 UPDATING DIAGNOSTIC CONCEPTS

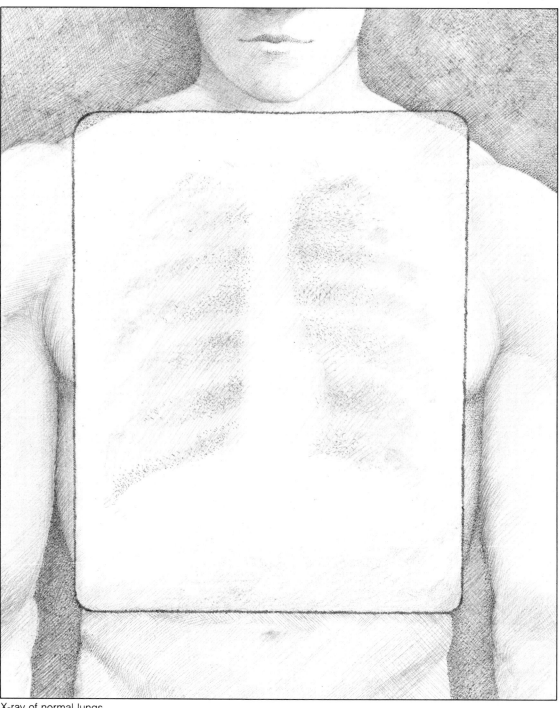

X-ray of normal lungs

f your practice often includes patients with respiratory disorders, you know that diagnostic evaluation of such disorders has become extremely complex, and your own involvement in diagnosis has become more direct. You're now performing or assisting with more tests than ever before, often at the patient's bedside. And you're expected to use the results of this perhaps baffling array of tests to form nursing diagnoses, create nursing care plans, and structure patient teaching.

Probably the most significant change in your care of respiratory patients stems from the fact that you can now receive arterial blood gas (ABG) analysis results in minutes. This speed has dramatically increased the test's importance as an assessment tool and your role in monitoring therapy. Now, you can put test results to immediate use, altering treatment regimens to reflect even minute-to-minute changes in your patient's condition. Similarly important in nursing assessment of patient progress are the pulmonary function tests made possible at bedside by the portable spirometry units.

Diagnostic respiratory tests evaluate pulmonary function, gas exchange, and the origin of respiratory disorder. The tests are interrelated; accurate diagnosis usually requires correlating the results of several tests with clinical assessment and the patient's complete health, occupational, social (smoking), and environmental history.

Whether or not you actually perform a given test, you must understand it well enough to prepare your patient. Adequate preparation and your counsel and encouragement during testing are doubly important for procedures that evaluate respiratory function, since anxiety may influence respirations and skew the test results. Thus, your efforts to promote relaxation help guarantee a successful test that provides a sound basis for continuing patient evaluation. Before you can provide effective teaching and reassurance, you must know which tests are included in respiratory evaluation, when and how they are used, what they measure, and what the test results mean.

BLOOD TESTS
Of all the laboratory analyses performed to diagnose respiratory disorder and assess degree of dysfunction, two blood tests are the most common—ABG analysis and the complete blood count (CBC). The CBC has long been an important diagnostic tool, but the ABG analysis has only recently achieved this status. Because new sophistication in analysis equipment allows almost immediate test results that keep pace with your patient's constantly changing condition, ABG analysis is used not only for initial diagnosis, but also for continuous monitoring of ventilatory status.

Arterial blood gas analysis
Since ineffective pulmonary exchange of carbon dioxide and oxygen is the central factor in all respiratory disorders, ABG analysis, which tests the quality of this exchange, is among the first diagnostic studies performed on your patient. It's also important for monitoring treatment, for supplying information for calculating response to therapy, and for deciding changes in treatment, especially regarding weaning from mechanical ventilation.

Laboratory analysis of blood gases evaluates alveolar ventilation by measuring the partial pressures of oxygen (PO_2) and carbon dioxide (PCO_2) and by measuring blood pH; PO_2 indicates the amount of oxygen the lungs deliver to the blood, and PCO_2 reflects the lungs' ability to eliminate carbon dioxide. The pH, a measurement of the hydrogen-ion concentration, shows the blood's acid-base balance. This is important, because impaired gas exchange and metabolic dysfunction can lead rapidly to acidosis or alkalosis; interpretation of ABG results distinguishes respiratory from metabolic imbalance and verifies compensatory mechanisms. ABG samples can also be analyzed for oxygen content and saturation, and for bicarbonate values.

ABG analysis is commonly ordered for patients with chronic obstructive pulmonary disease, pulmonary edema, acute respiratory distress syndrome, myocardial infarction, or pneumonia. It's also performed during shock and after cardiothoracic surgery, resuscitation from cardiac arrest, changes in respiratory therapy or status, or prolonged anesthesia.

Although ABG analysis is invaluable for gauging overall respiratory and metabolic status, it isn't diagnostically specific and doesn't necessarily detect pulmonary disease or differentiate it from cardiac disorder. ABG analysis is most useful when correlated with other factors, such as ventilation and perfusion, cardiac output, and tissue oxygenation, and with the results of other diagnostic screening tests, such as spirometry and chest X-ray.

Complete blood count
The CBC screens for gas-transport capability

and helps evaluate the amount of oxygen available for internal (cellular) respiration. Actually a series of separate blood tests, the CBC quantifies the blood's formed components and includes determinations of hemoglobin concentration, hematocrit, red and white cell counts, differential white cell count, and stained red cell examination.

The CBC is useful for patients with various pulmonary disorders, as well as for those with suspected anemia or heart disease. Besides indicating the need for additional studies, the CBC supplies valuable information. For example, comparing the hemoglobin concentration with the red cell count detects anemias and reveals the blood's oxygen-carrying capacity. Comparing the hemoglobin and hematocrit helps diagnose abnormal states of hydration (both values rise in dehydration). And comparing the differential white cell count with the total white cell count helps detect inflammation, infection, and allergic reaction; differentiates acute and chronic infections; and determines the stage and severity of infection.

White cells. Although infection usually increases the total white cell count (leukocytosis), the type of infection determines the degree of increase and the type of white cell affected. Thus, knowing the behavior of specific white cells can indicate the nature and origin of the infection. In acute infections, the number of white blood cells (WBCs), or leukocytes, usually rises sharply. Specifically involved are the polymorphonuclear leukocytes—the neutrophils and eosinophils. Neutrophils, which normally make up 50% to 70% of the total WBCs, increase in bacterial infections. Eosinophils, which normally make up less than 1% of the total WBCs, increase in allergic disorders, such as allergic asthma.

Understanding arterial blood gas measurements

PO_2

Oxygen tension. Partial pressure exerted by the small amount of oxygen dissolved in arterial blood.

Normal values
80 to 100 mm Hg

Abnormal values
Value less than 50 mm Hg indicates hypoxia. PO_2 between 50 and 80 mm Hg may or may not indicate hypoxia, depending on age of patient and oxygen concentration he's receiving. A newborn has a PO_2 between 40 and 60 mm Hg. After age 60, PO_2 may fall below 80 mm Hg without hypoxia.

PCO_2

Carbon dioxide tension. Partial pressure exerted by carbon dioxide dissolved in arterial blood. Primarily influenced by lung disorders and respiratory pattern.

Normal values
35 to 45 mm Hg

Abnormal values
Value above 45 mm Hg indicates hypoventilation (hypercapnia). Value below 35 mm Hg indicates hyperventilation (hypocapnia). PCO_2 level may also indicate respiratory (lung-regulated) acid-base imbalance. If patient's pH shows an imbalance, PCO_2 above 45 mm Hg indicates respiratory acidosis; PCO_2 below 35 mm Hg indicates respiratory alkalosis.

HCO_3

Carbonic acid, formed by carbon dioxide and water. Source of acid hydrogen ions and basic bicarbonate ions. Always 3% of PCO_2.

Normal values
1.05 to 1.35 mEq/liter
1:20 ratio with bicarbonate ions

Abnormal values
The important value here is the ratio of carbonic acid to bicarbonate. More carbonic acid, as in a 1:16 ratio, indicates acidosis. More bicarbonate, as in a 1:23 ratio, indicates alkalosis. However, a ratio of 1:19 or 1:21 may indicate compensation for acidosis or alkalosis.

H_2CO_3

Amount of bicarbonate dissolved in blood. Primarily influenced by metabolic changes. Determined by calculation involving pH and PCO_2.

Normal values
22 to 26 mEq/liter

Abnormal values
Value greater than 26 mEq/liter indicates metabolic (kidney-regulated) alkalosis. Value less than 22 mEq/liter indicates metabolic acidosis.

pH

Expression of hydrogen ion concentration. Clinical measure of blood acidity.

Normal values
7.35 to 7.45

Abnormal values
Value greater than 7.45 indicates alkalosis. Value less than 7.35 indicates acidosis. If the patient has either imbalance, check PCO_2 and HCO_3 measurements to see if it's respiratory or metabolic. Then, to see if his system has begun to compensate, look at the chart on page 41. Also check for compensation if pH is borderline (for example, 7.37).

SaO_2

Oxygen saturation (percentage of hemoglobin carrying oxygen). Hemoglobin carries most of the oxygen in the blood.

Normal values
95% to 100%

Abnormal values
If PO_2 is between 60 and 95 mm Hg, SaO_2 should remain above 85%. Sharply decreased values usually indicate drop in PO_2 below 50 mm Hg.

In chronic infections, however, the number of WBCs may rise only slightly or may even drop (leukopenia), as in tuberculosis and other chronic parenchymal diseases or in severe debilitation. Specifically affected are the mononuclear leukocytes—the lymphocytes and monocytes. Lymphocytes, which normally form 25% to 33% of the total WBCs, rise with certain viral and chronic bacterial infections. Monocytes, which normally form 4% to 6% of the total WBCs, usually rise in tuberculosis, chronic inflammation, and during recovery from infection.

Red cells. Since hemoglobin transports oxygen to the cells, any hemoglobin deficiency directly affects tissue oxygenation. The red blood cell (RBC) count, hematocrit, and hemoglobin concentration provide information for calculating any inadequacy. Normal values for all three indicators vary, depending on the patient's age and sex, type of sample drawn, and laboratory method used (see *Red cell values,* page 42).

TESTS FOR PATHOGENS

Blood culture
In patients with suspected bacteremia (bacterial invasion of the bloodstream) and septicemia (systemic spread of such infection), a blood culture can identify about 67% of pathogens within 24 hours and up to 90% within 72 hours. These results are achieved by inoculating a culture medium with a blood sample collected under sterile conditions and incubating it for isolation and identification of pathogens.

Although blood is normally sterile, a positive culture doesn't necessarily confirm septicemia, because many pathologic organisms

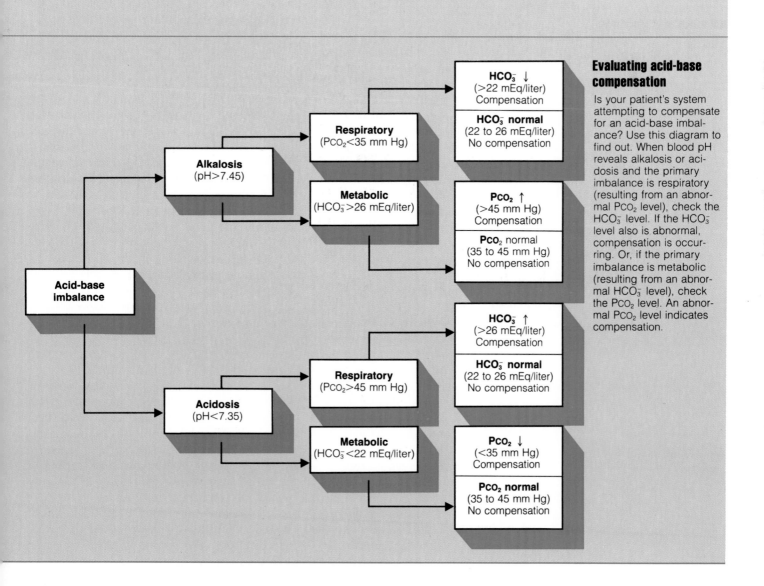

Evaluating acid-base compensation

Is your patient's system attempting to compensate for an acid-base imbalance? Use this diagram to find out. When blood pH reveals alkalosis or acidosis and the primary imbalance is respiratory (resulting from an abnormal PCO_2 level), check the HCO_3^- level. If the HCO_3^- level also is abnormal, compensation is occurring. Or, if the primary imbalance is metabolic (resulting from an abnormal HCO_3^- level), check the PCO_2 level. An abnormal PCO_2 level indicates compensation.

Acid-base imbalance

Alkalosis (pH>7.45)

Respiratory (PCO_2<35 mm Hg)

HCO_3^- ↓ (>22 mEq/liter) Compensation

HCO_3^- normal (22 to 26 mEq/liter) No compensation

Metabolic (HCO_3^->26 mEq/liter)

PCO_2 ↑ (>45 mm Hg) Compensation

PCO_2 normal (35 to 45 mm Hg) No compensation

Acidosis (pH<7.35)

Respiratory (PCO_2>45 mm Hg)

HCO_3^- ↑ (>26 mEq/liter) Compensation

HCO_3^- normal (22 to 26 mEq/liter) No compensation

Metabolic (HCO_3^-<22 mEq/liter)

PCO_2 ↓ (<35 mm Hg) Compensation

PCO_2 normal (35 to 45 mm Hg) No compensation

Red cell values

Red cell count

Men	4.5 to 6.2 million/μl of venous blood
Women	4.2 to 5.4 million/μl of venous blood

Hematocrit

Men	42% to 54%
Women	38% to 46%

Hemoglobin

Men	14 to 18 g/dl
Men after middle age	12.4 to 14.9 g/dl
Women	12 to 16 g/dl
Women after middle age	11.7 to 13.8 g/dl

may temporarily invade the bloodstream during the early stages of infection. Mild, transient bacteremia may occur during the course of many infectious diseases or may complicate other disorders. However, persistent, continuous, or recurrent bacteremia reliably confirms serious infection.

Common blood pathogens that you may see listed on laboratory reports include *Neisseria meningitidis, Streptococcus pneumoniae, Hemophilus influenzae,* Group A beta-hemolytic Streptococcus, *Staphylococcus aureus, Pseudomonas aeruginosa,* Bacteroidaceae, *Brucella,* and the Enterobacteriaceae. In addition, despite all precautions for securing a noncontaminated sample, 2% to 3% of blood samples cultured are contaminated by skin bacteria, such as *Staphylococcus epidermidis,* diphtheroids, and *Propionibacterium.* Although these bacteria are common contaminants, they may be clinically significant when isolated from multiple cultures.

Sputum culture

Bacteriologic examination of sputum can aid in diagnosis of bronchitis, tuberculosis, lung abscess, and pneumonia by isolating the offending organism. The usual method of specimen collection is expectoration, which may require ultrasonic nebulization, hydration, physiotherapy, or postural drainage to obtain an adequate specimen. Less common methods include tracheal suctioning, bronchoscopy with or without biopsy or bronchial brushing, transtracheal aspiration, and gastric aspiration. Collecting a specimen for analysis requires care; some patients expectorate a mixture of nasopharyngeal secretions and saliva, but this is not sputum and will give misleading results if cultured as a sputum specimen.

Sputum is the normal mucus secretion of the tracheobronchial tree. It helps preserve the integrity of the airways by cleansing them of inhaled particles. With its collection of trapped foreign matter, sputum is carried upward from the lungs by ciliary motion to the oropharynx, where the normal person swallows it unconsciously. Coughing and expectoration are normally unnecessary and characterize an abnormal condition; the amount of sputum produced by coughing reflects the condition's severity.

Through antibody and lysozyme activity and a slightly acid pH, sputum directly attacks invading bacteria and works to maintain airway sterility. But chronic infection can over-

whelm this respiratory defense mechanism, and changes in the sputum contribute, in turn, to the pathophysiologic process. As the white cell count and sputum volume increase in response to infection, so do sputum acidity, which checks the ciliary action, and sputum viscosity, which further inhibits normal mucus flow. Membrane permeability increases, as it does in any inflammatory condition, allowing antibiotics and certain blood components to seep into the airways and the sputum.

Pathogenic organisms commonly reported in sputum include *Streptococcus pneumoniae (pneumococcus), Mycobacterium tuberculosis, Klebsiella pneumoniae* and other Enterobacteriaceae, *Hemophilus influenzae, Staphylococcus aureus,* and *Pseudomonas aeruginosa.* In addition, the following other agents are often implicated in respiratory infections but are difficult to isolate in the average laboratory: respiratory viruses (common), *Mycoplasma pneumoniae,* and the *Legionellae* (less common).

Four different tests (see *Analyzing a sputum specimen,* page 44) may be performed on a sputum specimen to different ends. Because of the variables involved, interpretation of test results must be related to the patient's overall clinical condition. While specimens obtained through transtracheal aspiration will be "pure," expectorated sputum or bronchoscopy material is invariably contaminated with normal oropharyngeal flora, such as alpha-hemolytic streptococci, *Neisseria* species, enteric gram-negative bacilli, diphtheroids, hemophili, pneumococci, staphylococci, *Candida,* and other yeasts. Nonpathogenic in the oropharynx, such flora may be significant when found in the lung. However, isolation of some organisms, such as *M. tuberculosis,* is always significant.

Throat culture

A throat culture is most often ordered for suspected streptococcal pharyngitis. Isolating and identifying the offending organism, group A beta-hemolytic streptococcus (*Streptococcus pyogenes*), allows prompt antibiotic treatment and helps prevent sequelae, such as rheumatic heart disease and spread of infection. In the patient with excessive exudate or pseudomembranous ulcers, a culture may be important to a differential diagnosis of candidiasis (thrush), diphtheria, or Vincent's angina. A throat culture may also be used to screen for asymptomatic carriers of certain pathogens,

Interpreting fluid analysis tests

Pleural fluid analysis and the sweat test for cystic fibrosis have a common factor: nursing involvement. In the sweat test, your preparation of the patient, who's almost always a child, and your reassurance during the procedure can prevent psychological scars and contribute to the test's successful outcome. In pleural fluid analysis, your post-test monitoring of the patient is crucial to detect or prevent such complications as pneumothorax, tension pneumothorax, fluid reaccumulation, or mediastinal shift from cardiac distress or pulmonary edema.

Pleural fluid analysis. This test helps determine the cause and nature of pleural effusion and to relieve pulmonary compression and the respiratory distress that results when fluid builds up in the pleural space, such as occurs with cancer, tuberculosis, and blood and lymphatic disorders.

A sample of pleural fluid is taken by thoracentesis and examined for color, consistency, glucose and protein content, cellular composition, and the enzymes lactic dehydrogenase (LDH) and amylase. It's also examined for malignant cells and cultured for pathogens.

Normally, the pleural space maintains negative pressure and contains less than 20 ml of serous fluid. Pleural effusion results from the abnormal formation or reabsorption of pleural fluid. Certain characteristics classify pleural fluid as either a transudate (a low-protein fluid that has leaked from normal vessels, as in cirrhosis, congestive heart failure, and nephrotic syndrome) or an exudate (a protein-rich fluid that has leaked from blood vessels with increased permeability, as in neoplastic and infectious diseases, asbestosis, pulmonary infarction, and lymphatic drainage disorders).

The most common pathogens that appear in cultures of pleural fluid include *Mycobacterium*

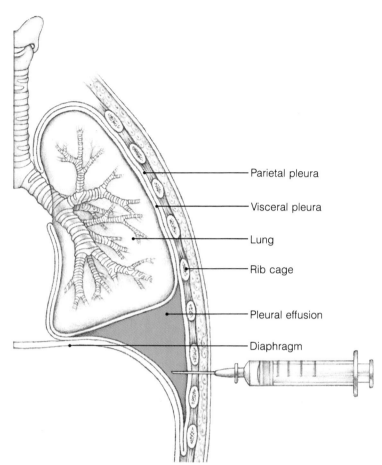

Parietal pleura

Visceral pleura

Lung

Rib cage

Pleural effusion

Diaphragm

Thoracentesis, needle puncture through the chest wall and the parietal pleura into the pleural space, produces a sample of pleural fluid for laboratory analysis.

tuberculosis, Staphylococcus aureus, Streptococcus pneumoniae and other streptococci, *Hemophilus influenzae, Legionellae,* and in the case of a ruptured pulmonary abscess, anaerobes, such as *Bacteroides*. Excess neutrophils suggest septic inflammation; excess lymphocytes suggest tuberculosis, or fungal or viral effusions. Serosanguineous fluid; elevated LDH in a nonpurulent, nonhemolyzed, nonbloody effusion; or pleural fluid glucose levels 30 to 40 mg/dl lower than blood glucose levels may indicate malignancy. Increased amylase levels occur with pleural effusions associated with pancreatitis.

Sweat test. This test measures electrolyte concentrations (primarily sodium and chloride) in sweat. It's used in children to confirm cystic fibrosis, and in

the occasional older patient suspected of the disease because of recurrent respiratory infection or malabsorption syndrome.

Quantitative analysis is performed on sweat produced locally by pilocarpine iontophoresis. Normal sodium values in sweat range from 10 to 30 mEq/liter, abnormal from 50 to 130 mEq/liter. Normal chloride values range from 10 to 35 mEq/liter, abnormal values from 50 to 110 mEq/liter. Sodium and chloride concentrations of 50 to 60 mEq/liter strongly suggest cystic fibrosis. Concentrations greater than 60 mEq/liter, with typical clinical features, confirm it. While a few other conditions, such as untreated adrenal insufficiency, also raise sweat electrolyte levels, only cystic fibrosis raises these levels above 80 mEq/liter.

Analyzing a sputum specimen

Four types of tests may be performed on a sputum specimen to identify the infecting organism or abnormal cells.

Gram's stain differentiates gram-positive bacteria, which retain the crystal or gentian violet stain after decolorization, from gram-negative bacteria, which lose the violet stain but counterstain red with safranine. The test permits rapid visualization of bacteria from a smear and indicates if the specimen is representative (many white blood cells, few epithelial cells) or if oral contamination has occurred (few WBCs, many epithelial cells). Gram's staining often provides early presumptive diagnosis of lower respiratory infection, such as bacterial pneumonia.

Acid-fast stain helps rapidly identify organisms of the genus *Mycobacterium,* since they retain carbolfuchsin stain after treatment with an acid-alcohol solution. This test provides early presumptive diagnosis of tuberculosis.

Culture and sensitivity testing allows growth and isolation of microbes for positive identification and determination of their vulnerability to specific antibiotics. The test helps diagnose lower respiratory infection or confirm earlier presumptive diagnosis from a stained smear.

Cytologic (exfoliative) testing is performed to identify tumors and other abnormal cells to help diagnose and type malignant pulmonary lesions and identify granulomas, inflammation, and other benign conditions.

---

especially *Neisseria meningitidis* and pathogenic staphylococci.

Normal throat flora include nonhemolytic and alpha-hemolytic streptococci, *Neisseria* species, staphylococci, diphtheroids, some hemophili, pneumococci, yeasts, and enteric gram-negative rods. In addition to group A beta-hemolytic streptococci *(S. pyogenes),* which can cause scarlet fever or pharyngitis, possible throat pathogens may include *Candida albicans* (thrush), *Corynebacterium diphtheriae* (diphtheria), and *Bordetella pertussis* (whooping cough). The laboratory report should identify and quantify the pathogens cultured or note their absence. Culture results should be correlated with clinical status and recent antibiotic therapy.

RADIOLOGIC AND SONOGRAPHIC TESTS

Laboratory tests on blood, sputum, and throat-swab specimens confirm infection and identify the causative organism but can't reveal the dimensions of the disease. Radiographic tests, from chest X-ray through the more complicated and invasive tests, localize the disorder, supply information for staging it, and determine its toll on your patient.

Although all the radiographic tests are performed by a technician or by the doctor, you may be asked to assist with certain ones, such as bedside chest X-rays. What's more, your ability to recognize the abnormalities these tests reveal and to understand their implications will help you monitor changes in your patient's condition and plan more effective nursing care.

Chest radiography

Chest X-ray, or radiography, is used to screen for anatomic abnormalities and to monitor progress through treatment. It may be performed with a stationary machine or at bedside with a portable machine. X-rays taken with a stationary machine generally produce a clearer image than those taken with a portable machine because the patient can more easily assume the proper position (upright posture, full inspiration) and the machine can easily be placed 6' (1.82 m) away from him. This distance is needed to show images with most sharpness and least magnification.

X-rays may be taken from various angles, depending on diagnostic intent. The most common views are frontal, with the patient upright and the X-ray beam positioned posteriorly or anteriorly, and lateral, with the patient upright and the X-ray beam positioned at his side. The posteroanterior (PA) view, with the X-ray beam directed at the patient's back, is the most common frontal view. It's preferred over the anteroposterior (AP) view because the heart is anteriorly situated in the thorax and magnified less than in an AP view. The frontal views usually show greater lung area than other views because they allow lower diaphragmatic position. The left lateral (LL) view, with the X-ray beam directed at the patient's left side, is preferred over the right lateral (RL) view because the heart is left of midline and magnified less in an LL view than in an RL view. Lateral views are used primarily to visualize lesions not apparent on a PA view.

Chest X-ray can detect pulmonary disorders, such as pneumonia, atelectasis, pneumothorax, pulmonary bullae, and tumors; and mediastinal abnormalities, such as tumors and cardiac disease. It's also ordered to determine the location and size of a lesion, to help assess pulmonary status, and to check for correct placement of an endotracheal tube. Its newest use is to help distinguish pulmonary edema from lung inflammation and infection by using gravity and serial X-rays to detect movement of lung fluid. In this procedure, called a gravitational-shift test, one chest X-ray is taken after the patient has remained supine or semi-erect for 2 hours. Then the patient is turned on one side for 2 to 3 more hours and returned to his original position for a second X-ray. The two X-rays are compared for evidence of fluid shift. If the patient has pulmonary edema, gravity causes the infiltrate to shift toward the lower (dependent) lung while the upper lung clears or remains stable. By contrast, in the patient with inflammation, the X-ray shows no fluid shift. (See *Locating landmarks in the chest X-ray* and *Clinical implications of chest X-ray films* on pages 46 and 47.)

Although chest X-ray was once routinely performed as a cancer screening test, the associated risk of exposure to radiation has caused many authorities to question its usefulness. The American Cancer Society now recommends sputum analysis over X-ray.

You should be aware of the limitations of chest X-rays. An X-ray may appear normal in patients with bronchial asthma or chronic bronchitis, even in its severe form, and in patients with emphysema until they reach an advanced stage. Chest X-rays appear normal when respiratory insufficiency stems from extrapulmonary abnormalities, such as brain and spinal cord damage, unless pulmonary infection is present; from neuromuscular disorders (poliomyelitis, myasthenia gravis); and from respiratory depression resulting from sedative overdose. In addition, chest X-rays usually fail to detect primary lung cancer until the tumor has grown to 1 cm in diameter, a process that may take 10 years, and may even overlook large tumors if they're growing in "blind" areas of lung tissue hidden by the heart, great vessels, diaphragm, or other solid organ. Because accurate diagnosis depends on correlating X-ray findings with other radiologic and pulmonary tests, such tests as tomography and ultrasonography may compensate for X-ray's shortcomings.

Fluoroscopy

Fluoroscopy is a dynamic chest X-ray using an image intensifier rather than a photographic plate. A stream of X-rays directed through the patient causes the screen to emit light and allows continuous viewing of thoracic structures during breathing. As the patient breathes, the image displayed on the screen changes, revealing shape and density of the lungs, heart, diaphragm, and other cardiopulmonary structures and their motion throughout inspiration and expiration. Special equipment that intensifies the images and projects them onto a viewing screen, and the possibility of making spot X-rays or a videotape recording for later study, have made fluoroscopy more useful in recent years.

Chest fluoroscopy is performed to assess lung expansion and contraction during quiet breathing, deep breathing, and coughing; to assess movement and paralysis of the diaphragm; and to detect bronchiolar obstructions and pulmonary disease. In addition, fluoroscopy defines location and movement of mediastinal lesions during breathing and swallowing more effectively than X-ray and is used in such procedures as transbronchial lung biopsy, transthoracic needle aspiration (biopsy), and thoracentesis.

Normal diaphragmatic movement is synchronous and symmetric, with an excursion ranging from ¾" to 1⅝" (2 to 4 cm). Diminished diaphragmatic movement may indicate pulmonary disease. Increased lung translucency may indicate loss of elasticity or bronchiolar obstruction. In elderly persons, the lowest part of the trachea may be displaced to the right by an elongated aorta. Diminished or paradoxical movement of the diaphragm may indicate diaphragmatic paralysis; however, fluoroscopy may not detect such paralysis in patients who compensate by aiding expiration with forceful contraction of their abdominal muscles.

Ultrasonography

Because it's more sensitive than X-ray to differences in soft-tissue densities and is considered a safe procedure even during pregnancy, ultrasound may be used to detect pulmonary abnormalities. In A-mode presentation, the technique used for thoracic diagnosis, energy pulsing from a transducer beams cross-sectionally through the patient. Each time the sound beam strikes the border of a mass with different density, the reflected sound is detected by a transducer, which converts

X-rays and tissue density

In a chest X-ray, a high-voltage current passing through a Coolidge tube produces short wavelength "X" rays. These rays either pass through the chest and react on a photographic plate as light does on film or are partially or fully absorbed by body structures of varying densities before reaching the plate.

Normal densities
Those internal structures filled with gas, like the lungs and airways, are the least dense body parts. They allow nearly all X-rays to pass through them and burn into the photographic plate, creating the darkest areas on the film. Tissue with the density of water (heart, muscle, blood vessel) absorbs some of the X-rays and prevents them from reaching the film, creating deep gray areas on the film. Fat tissue absorbs even more rays, leaving paler gray areas on the film. Bony structures have a density equal to metal and absorb nearly all the X-rays, leaving white or underexposed areas on the film.

Abnormal densities
Abnormalities appear as changes in normal densities. Since normal pulmonary tissue is radiolucent, foreign bodies, infiltrates, fluids, tumors, and other abnormalities show as white spots in a normally dark area. And a disorder like pulmonary edema changes lung tissue from gas-density to fluid-density, making the lungs merge on film with adjacent water-density structures—heart, blood vessel, and muscle tissue. A chest X-ray is most useful in detecting changes when compared with the patient's previous films.

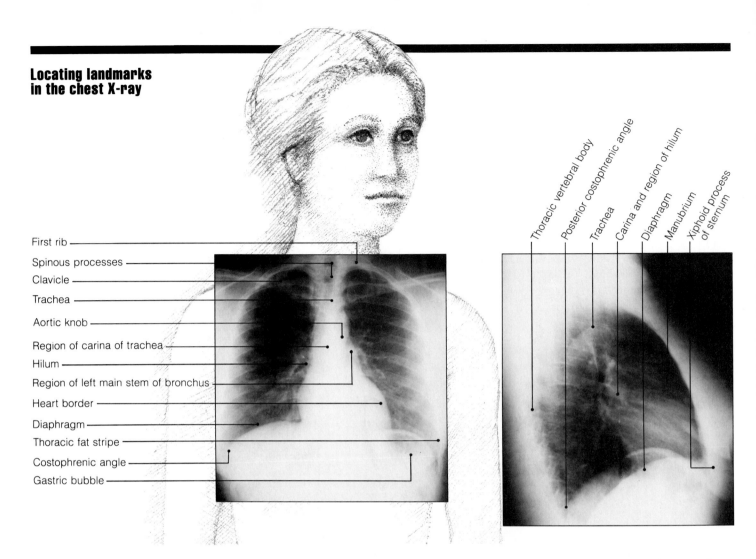

First rib
Spinous processes
Clavicle
Trachea
Aortic knob
Region of carina of trachea
Hilum
Region of left main stem of bronchus
Heart border
Diaphragm
Thoracic fat stripe
Costophrenic angle
Gastric bubble

Thoracic vertebral body
Posterior costophrenic angle
Trachea
Carina and region of hilum
Diaphragm
Manubrium
Xiphoid process of sternum

sound to electrical impulses that are displayed on an oscilloscope. The return echo is timed to reveal the precise location of any abnormal mass.

Lung tissue reflects sound waves, so they don't penetrate deeply; therefore, this test is insensitive to deep-lying structures. However, repeating this test from several angles may ultimately reveal a hidden tumor. This procedure can detect pleural effusion and establish its boundaries when chest X-ray or thoracentesis fail, and it can locate an appropriate site for pleural aspiration. In addition, it identifies mediastinal and near-chest-wall lesions as either fluid or solid.

Tomography

With greater clarity than ultrasonography, but with the associated hazard of radiation, tomography uncovers lesions hidden from view by other body structures. Also called laminagraphy, planigraphy, stratigraphy, and bodysection roentgenography, this procedure consists of a series of cross-sectional X-rays focused at different depths, producing exposures in which a selected body plane appears

sharply defined while the areas above and below it are blurred.

Tomograms can demonstrate pulmonary densities (for detecting cavitation, calcification, and presence of fat), tumors (especially those obstructing the bronchial lumen), or lesions (especially those located deep within the mediastinum, such as lymph nodes).

A normal chest tomogram shows structures equivalent to those in a normal chest X-ray film. Central calcification in a nodule suggests a benign lesion; an irregularly bordered tumor suggests malignancy. Evaluation of the hilum can help differentiate blood vessels from nodes; identify bronchial dilation, stenosis, and endobronchial lesions; and detect tumor extension into the hilar lung area. Tomography can also identify extension of a mediastinal lesion to the ribs or spine.

Pulmonary angiography

This invasive test involves radiographic examination of the pulmonary circulation after injection of a radiopaque iodine contrast agent through a catheter inserted into the pulmonary artery or one of its branches. It allows

Clinical implications of chest X-ray films

Normal anatomic location and appearance	Possible abnormality	Implications
Trachea Visible midline in the anterior mediastinal cavity; translucent, tubelike appearance	• Deviation from midline • Narrowing, with hourglass shape and deviation to one side	• Tension pneumothorax, atelectasis, pleural effusion, consolidation, mediastinal nodes • Substernal thyroid
Heart Visible in the anterior left mediastinal cavity; solid appearance due to blood contents; edges may be clear in contrast with surrounding air density of the lung	• Shift • Hypertrophy of right heart • Cardiac borders obscured by stringy densities ("shaggy heart")	• Atelectasis • Cor pulmonale, congestive heart failure • Cystic fibrosis
Aortic knob Visible as water density; formed by the arch of the aorta	• Metal densities (possible calcifications within aorta) • Tortuous shape	• Atherosclerosis • Atherosclerosis
Mediastinum (mediastinal shadow) Visible as the space between the lungs; shadowy appearance that widens at the hilum of the lungs	• Deviation to the nondiseased side; deviation toward the diseased side by traction • Gross widening	• Pleural effusion or tumor, fibrosis or collapsed lung • Neoplasms of esophagus, bronchi, lungs, thyroid, lymph nodes; mediastinitis; cor pulmonale
Ribs Visible as thoracic cavity encasement	• Break or misalignment • Widening of intercostal spaces	• Fractured sternum or ribs • Emphysema
Spine Visible midline in the posterior chest; straight bony structure	• Spinal curvature • Break or misalignment	• Scoliosis, kyphosis • Fractures
Clavicles Visible in upper thorax; intact and equidistant in properly centered X-ray films	• Break or misalignment	• Fractures
Hila (lung roots) Visible as small, white, bilateral densities above heart where pulmonary vessels, bronchi, and lymph nodes join the lungs	• Shift to one side • Accentuated shadows	• Atelectasis • Emphysema, pulmonary abscess, tumor, enlarged lymph nodes
Mainstem bronchus Visible to about 1" (2.5 cm) from hila; translucent, tubelike appearance	• Spherical or oval density	• Bronchogenic cyst
Bronchi Usually not visible	• Visible	• Bronchial pneumonia
Lung fields Usually not visible throughout, except for fine white areas from the hilum	• Visible • Irregular, patchy densities	• Atelectasis • Resolving pneumonia, silicosis, fibrosis, metastatic neoplasm
Hemidiaphragm Rounded, visible; right side ⅜" to ¾" (1 to 2 cm) higher than left	• Elevation of diaphragm (difference in elevation can be measured on inspiration and expiration to detect movement) • Flattening of diaphragm • Unilateral elevation of either side • Unilateral elevation of left side only	• Active tuberculosis, pneumonia, pleurisy, acute bronchitis, bilateral phrenic nerve involvement, atelectasis • Asthma, emphysema • Possible pneumothorax or unilateral pulmonary infection, unilateral phrenic nerve paresis • Perforated ulcer, gas distention of stomach or splenic flexure of colon, free air in abdomen

measurement of pressures at various sites during catheter insertion—right atrium, right ventricle, pulmonary artery—along with cardiac output and pulmonary vascular resistance. Because this test involves more risk than other imaging techniques, newer scanning tests have largely supplanted or replaced it for diagnosing lung tumors, blebs, and other lung tissue changes. Its use is largely restricted to identifying defects in pulmonary vascular perfusion—such as aneurysms, vessel displacement, and diminished blood flow. But even in these conditions, pulmonary angiography may be superseded by the less hazardous ventilation/perfusion scan.

In certain instances, however, pulmonary angiography may be more conclusive and therefore worth the risk. It is now used most commonly to confirm symptomatic pulmonary embolism when lung scans show no abnormalities, especially in the patient for whom anticoagulant therapy is contraindicated. It also helps evaluate pulmonary circulation preoperatively in the patient with congenital heart disease. Normally, the contrast medium flows symmetrically and uninterrupted through the pulmonary circulatory system. Any interruption of blood flow may result from a pathological condition, such as embolism, vascular filling defect, or stenosis. Complications of pulmonary angiography include arterial occlusion, myocardial perforation or rupture, ventricular dysrhythmias from myocardial irritation, and an allergic reaction to the contrast medium or the local anesthetic.

NUCLEAR STUDIES
Radionuclide imaging, the injection or inhalation of radiopaque contrast medium and the external tracing of its dispersal through the system to detect abnormal distribution, provides more information with greater sensitivity and less risk than older respiratory tests. Its impact on diagnostic testing has come through steady improvements in equipment and the use of computers, which have made the techniques more accurate.

Computerized tomography
Thoracic computerized tomography (CT) provides cross-sectional views of the chest by passing a narrow X-ray beam through the body at different angles. This technique differs from routine tomography in that the transmitted X-ray data are computer-processed to determine how small volumes of body tissue attenuate the X-ray beam. The data are con-verted to images of high resolution and improved sensitivity. CT scanning may be done with or without an I.V.-injected radiopaque contrast agent, which is used primarily to highlight blood vessels and to allow greater visual discrimination.

This test is especially useful in detecting small differences in tissue density. When used with a radiopaque contrast agent, thoracic CT is one of the most accurate and informative diagnostic tests. Because it's far less invasive, it may replace mediastinoscopy in diagnosis of mediastinal masses and Hodgkin's disease. Thoracic CT shows the exact dimensions and internal composition of a mass and may localize its site for biopsy or identify new growths, but it doesn't eliminate the need for a biopsy. Its clinical application in the evaluation of pulmonary pathology is still evolving.

Thoracic CT is used to locate suspected neoplasms (such as Hodgkin's disease), especially those with mediastinal involvement; to determine if solitary pulmonary nodules contain calcium (indicating an inflammatory rather than neoplastic lesion); and to distinguish tumors adjacent to the aorta from aortic aneurysms. It can also detect the invasion of a neck mass in the thorax and help evaluate primary malignancy that may metastasize to the lungs, especially in patients with primary bone tumors, soft-tissue sarcomas, and melanomas.

Black and white areas on a thoracic CT scan refer, respectively, to air and bone densities. Shades of gray correspond to water, fat, and soft-tissue densities. Among the abnormal findings that may show up are tumors, nodules, cysts, aortic aneurysms, enlarged lymph nodes, pleural effusions, and accumulations of blood, fluid, or fat.

Lung scintigraphy: Two complementary tests
Two types of scan, a ventilation scan and a lung perfusion scan (lung scan, lung scintiscan), make up lung scintigraphy. After inhalation or I.V. injection of a radiopaque agent, each produces a diffuse image of the agent's distribution throughout the lung, revealing any abnormal patterns of ventilation or perfusion. Performance of both tests yields complementary results that better detect and differentiate suspected disorders, most frequently pulmonary emboli but also tumors, emphysema, fibroses, and bronchiectasis. These results are expressed in terms of prob-

ability because the image produced is indicative rather than anatomically specific. However, the tests may provide enough evidence for diagnosis, obviating the need for more invasive tests, such as angiography. Because these scans permit easy calculation of relative ventilation and perfusion values, they've replaced bronchospirometry in pretreatment evaluation and prediction of lung function.

Ventilation scanning delineates areas of the lung ventilated during respiration after inhalation of air mixed with radioactive gas (xenon 133; krypton 85 for the patient on mechanical ventilation). It consists of serially recording gas distribution during three phases: buildup of radioactive gas (wash-in phase), maximum concentration after the patient rebreathes from a bag (equilibrium phase), and removal of the gas from the lungs (wash-out phase). Performed with a perfusion scan, the ventilation scan helps distinguish between parenchymal disease, such as emphysema, sarcoidosis, bronchogenic carcinoma, and tuberculosis, and conditions stemming from vascular abnormalities, such as pulmonary emboli.

Normal findings for the ventilation scan include an equal distribution of gas in both lungs and normal wash-in and wash-out phases. Unequal gas distribution indicates poor ventilation or airway obstruction in areas with low radioactivity. Comparison of ventilation and perfusion scans yields these findings: in vascular obstructions, such as pulmonary embolism, perfusion to the embolized area decreases, while normal ventilation continues; in parenchymal disease, such as pneumonia, ventilation is abnormal in areas of consolidation.

Lung perfusion scanning (also called lung scan and lung scintiscan) produces a visual image of pulmonary blood flow after I.V. injection of a radiopaque contrast agent—human serum albumin microspheres (particles) or macroaggregated albumin, both of which are bonded to technetium. This scan is most useful in confirming pulmonary vascular obstruction, such as pulmonary emboli. It may also be used for preoperative evaluation of pulmonary function in a patient with marginal lung reserves.

A normal lung perfusion scan shows a uniform pattern of radioactive uptake, indicating normal blood perfusion throughout the lung. By contrast, cold spots—areas of low radioactive uptake—indicate poor perfusion, such as from an embolism; however, a ventilation

Comparing normal and abnormal lung scans

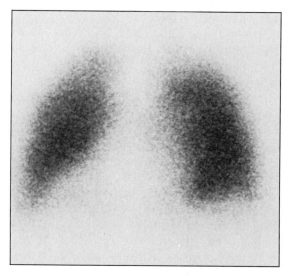

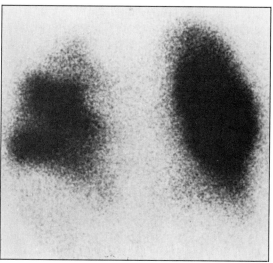

The normal posteroanterior (PA) lung scan view (top) shows smooth outlines and uniform, complete visualizations of both lung fields. The abnormal PA view (bottom) shows uneven densities, particularly in the right lung field, indicating impaired blood flow resulting from a pulmonary embolus.

scan is necessary to help confirm this diagnosis. When embolism is suspected, such conditions as chronic obstructive pulmonary disease (COPD), vasculitis, pulmonary edema, tumor, sickle cell disease, and parasitic disease may confuse the results, because they also can cause abnormal perfusion. In addition, decreased regional blood flow that occurs without vessel obstruction may indicate pneumonia.

Gallium scanning

This test, a total body scan, is usually performed 24 to 48 hours after the I.V. injection of radioactive gallium (^{67}Ga) citrate. Although the liver, spleen, bones, and large bowel normally take up gallium, so do certain neoplasms and inflammatory lesions. However, many neoplasms and a few inflammatory lesions may fail to demonstrate abnormal gallium activity. Because gallium has an affinity for both benign and malignant neoplasms and inflammatory lesions, exact diagnosis requires additional confirming tests, such as ultrasonography and CT.

Gallium scanning is usually helpful when the site of the disease (usually malignancy) hasn't been clearly defined and when the patient's condition won't be jeopardized by the time required for the procedure. The test is performed to detect primary or metastatic neoplasms and inflammatory lesions, to identify recurrent tumors after chemotherapy or radiation therapy, to evaluate suspected bronchogenic carcinoma when sputum culture proves positive for malignancy but other tests are normal, or when hydrothorax is present and bronchoscopy is contraindicated.

PULMONARY FUNCTION TESTS

These tests, a series of measurements and calculations, provide two types of information about pulmonary function. One series of tests, called ventilatory function tests, evaluates lung mechanics by measuring the volume of air the patient moves in and out during respiration and then estimating various lung capacities. They also help to distinguish between obstructive and restrictive ventilation defects. Another series of tests measures gas distribution throughout the lungs, diffusion across the respiratory membrane, and the efficiency of vascular perfusion of the alveoli. A useful test in this series is the diffusion capacity of carbon monoxide (DL_{CO}).

Pulmonary function tests measure the degree of respiratory impairment and provide a valuable baseline to evaluate treatment and monitor changes in the patient's condition. Specifically, they help determine the cause of dyspnea and, when performed while the patient exercises, determine the tolerance for exertion before dyspnea develops. The tests help determine whether a functional abnormality is obstructive or restrictive; estimate the degree of dysfunction; evaluate surgical risk; assess the effectiveness of specific therapies, such as bronchodilators or steroids; and determine the need for continued mechanical ventilation. They also help evaluate both the effect of work environment on pulmonary function and any related disability for legal or insurance purposes. Pulmonary function tests use three testing methods: spirometry, gas dilution and plethysmography, and diffusing capacity.

Distinguishing restrictive from obstructive lung disease

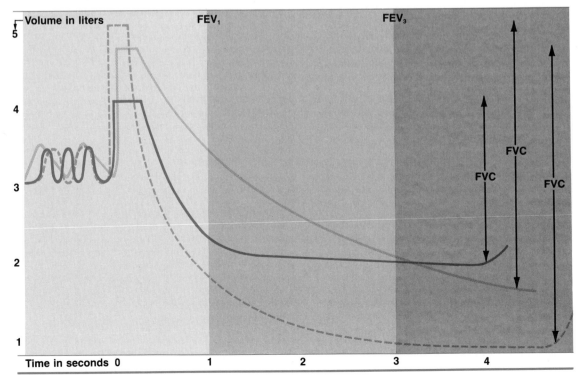

A spirogram helps determine if a lung disease is restrictive or obstructive. As these graphs of forced vital capacity (FVC) maneuvers show, FVC and forced expiratory volume (FEV) decrease in restrictive disease. But FEV decreases more in obstructive disease because airway resistance is greater and exhalation takes longer.

Key:

Normal spirogram

- - - - - - - - - - - - -

Restrictive lung disease

Obstructive lung disease
. . . .

Interpreting pulmonary function tests

Measurement of pulmonary function	Method of calculation	Implications
Tidal volume V_T—amount of air inhaled or exhaled during normal breathing	Determine the spirographic measurement for 10 breaths, and then divide by 10.	Decreased V_T may indicate restrictive disease and requires further testing, such as full pulmonary function study or chest radiography.
Minute volume—total amount of air breathed per minute	Multiply V_T by the respiration rate.	Normal minute volume can occur in emphysema; decreased minute volume may indicate other diseases, such as pulmonary edema.
Inspiratory reserve volume (IRV)—amount of air inspired above normal inspiration	Subtract V_T from inspiratory capacity (IC).	Abnormal IRV alone doesn't indicate respiratory dysfunction; IRV decreases during normal exercise.
Expiratory reserve volume (ERV)—amount of air that can be exhaled after normal expiration	Direct spirographic measurement.	ERV varies, even in healthy persons.
Residual volume (RV)—amount of air remaining in the lungs after forced expiration	Subtract ERV from functional residual capacity (FRC).	RV greater than 35% of total lung capacity (TLC) after maximal expiratory effort may indicate obstructive disease, such as emphysema or asthma.
Vital capacity (VC)—total volume of air that can be exhaled after maximum inspiration	Direct spirographic measurement; or add V_T, IRV, and ERV.	Normal or increased VC with decreased flow rates may indicate reduction in functional pulmonary tissue. Decreased VC with normal or increased flow rates may indicate decreased respiratory effort, decreased thoracic expansion, or limited movement of diaphragm.
Inspiratory capacity (IC)—amount of air that can be inhaled after normal expiration	Direct spirographic measurement; or add IRV and V_T.	Decreased IC indicates restrictive disease.
Functional residual capacity (FRC)—amount of air remaining in lungs after normal expiration	Helium dilution technique measurement; or add ERV and RV.	Increased FRC indicates overdistention of lungs, which may result from obstructive pulmonary disease.
Total lung capacity (TLC)—total volume of the lungs when maximally inflated	Add V_T, IRV, ERV, and RV; or FRC and IC; or VC and RV.	Low TLC indicates restrictive disease; high TLC indicates overdistended lungs associated with obstructive disease.
Forced vital capacity (FVC)—dynamic measurement of the amount of air exhaled after maximum inspiration	Direct spirographic measurement at 1-, 2-, and 3-second intervals.	Decreased FVC indicates flow resistance in respiratory system from obstructive disease, such as chronic bronchitis, emphysema, or asthma.
Forced expiratory volume (FEV)—volume of air expired in the 1st, 2nd, or 3rd second of FVC maneuver	Direct spirographic measurement; expressed as percentage of FVC.	Decreased FEV_1 and increased FEV_2 and FEV_3 may indicate obstructive disease; decreased or normal FEV_1 may indicate restrictive disease.
Maximal midexpiratory flow (MMEF)—average rate of flow during middle half of FVC; also called forced expiratory flow (FEF)	Calculated from the flow rate and the time needed for expiration of middle 50% of FVC.	Low MMEF indicates obstructive pulmonary disease.
Maximal voluntary ventilation (MVV)—greatest volume of air breathed per unit of time; also called maximum breathing capacity (MBC)	Direct spirographic measurement.	Decreased MVV may indicate obstructive disease; normal or decreased MVV may indicate restrictive disease, such as myasthenia gravis.
Diffusing capacity for carbon monoxide (DLco)—milliliters of carbon monoxide diffused per minute across the alveolar-capillary membrane	Calculated from analysis of amount of carbon monoxide exhaled compared with amount inhaled.	Decreased DLco in the presence of thickened alveolar-capillary membrane indicates interstitial pulmonary disease, such as pulmonary fibrosis.

Spirometry

This most common test is usually the first one attempted. The patient breathes through a mouthpiece attached to a spirometer, which has a recording device. Usually, three breathing measurements are made—forced vital capacity (FVC), maximal voluntary ventilation (MVV), and forced expiratory volume (FEV); others can then be calculated from these. Spirometry can detect mechanical airway obstruction and may also suggest its cause. For instance, decreased volume may imply a restrictive disorder; decreased measurements of FVC, MVV, and FEV may imply an obstructive disorder. Further evaluation with volume studies and spirometry, after administration of bronchodilators, give a clearer picture of the nature and degree of impairment.

Gas dilution and plethysmography

If spirometry indicates abnormal obstruction, gas dilution tests may be performed to differentiate restrictive from obstructive disease. As the patient breathes a measured amount of a relatively insoluble gas, such as helium, along with oxygen in a closed system, the test analyzes the gas's dilution in the breathing mixture. Gas dilution permits a more precise calculation of pulmonary measurements, such as residual volume (RV) and total lung capacity (TLC). If diagnosis requires more exact information, the patient may undergo testing in a body plethysmograph, an airtight glass enclosure for measuring gas volumes, airway resistance, and alveolar pressure. Plethysmography serves as an alternative or addition to the simpler gas dilution tests.

Diffusing capacity

If earlier studies showed abnormal ventilation, diffusing capacity for carbon monoxide will help determine if the problem impairs gas exchange across the alveolar membrane. This easy-to-perform test can identify and evaluate a diffusion defect by measuring the rate at which a highly soluble gas, such as carbon monoxide, transfers across the alveolar-capillary membrane. In this test, the patient first exhales and then deeply inhales a small, measured concentration of carbon monoxide. He holds his breath for about 10 seconds, allowing the gas to diffuse, and then exhales into a rubber bag. Comparison of inhaled and exhaled gas concentrations provides the rate of gas transfer.

Predicted normal values for pulmonary function tests, based on the patient's age, height, and sex, are compared with the observed measurement and expressed as a percentage. Results are considered abnormal if they're less than 80% of the predicted value. The following measurements can be performed at bedside with a portable spirometer: tidal volume, expiratory reserve volume, inspiratory capacity, and forced expiratory volume. Results of pulmonary function tests must be correlated with results of ABG analysis; a complete patient history, including job environment and smoking habits; and a physical examination.

SPECIAL SURGICAL TESTS

Special surgical tests, such as laryngoscopy, bronchoscopy, and biopsy, inherently demand greater nursing involvement than other pulmonary tests. For example, you're likely to be responsible for preparing your patient physically as well as emotionally and for monitoring his condition afterward to prevent postoperative complications.

Direct laryngoscopy

Direct laryngoscopy allows visualization of the larynx through the use of a fiber-optic endoscope or laryngoscope passed through the mouth or the nose and the pharynx. It usually follows the more common indirect laryngoscopy when that procedure fails to provide an adequate view of the larynx. (In indirect laryngoscopy, the larynx is observed at rest and during phonation, using a laryngeal mirror, a head mirror, and a light source.) Direct laryngoscopy is performed to detect lesions, strictures, or foreign bodies in the larynx; to aid diagnosis of laryngeal cancer; and to remove benign lesions or foreign bodies. It may show such benign lesions, strictures, or foreign bodies, and, with a biopsy, may distinguish laryngeal edema from radiation reaction or tumor.

Bronchoscopy

Bronchoscopy is the direct visualization of the trachea and tracheobronchial tree through a standard metal bronchoscope or the new fiber-optic bronchoscope. It has both diagnostic and therapeutic uses. Its diagnostic purposes include visually examining and identifying possible tumor, obstruction, secretion, or foreign body in the tracheobronchial tree, as demonstrated by radiography; helping to diagnose bronchogenic carcinoma, tuberculosis, interstitial pulmonary disease, or fungal or parasitic pulmonary infection, by obtaining a specimen for microbiologic and cytologic examination; helping to locate a bleeding site in the tracheobronchial tree; determining the cause of improperly functioning intubation; and detecting tracheobronchial damage after prolonged intubation. Therapeutic purposes of bronchoscopy include removal of a foreign body, localized tumor, or mucous plug; prevention or treatment of atelectasis; improvement of bronchial drainage; drainage of abscesses; and instillation of chemotherapeutic agents.

Abnormalities of the bronchial wall include inflammation, swelling, protruding cartilage, ulceration, tumors, enlargement of the mucous gland orifices or submucosal lymph nodes, or atrophy. Abnormalities of endotracheal origin include stenosis, compression, ectasia (dilation of a tubular vessel), anomalous (irregular) bronchial branching, and abnormal bifurcation owing to diverticulum. Abnormal substances in the bronchial lumen may include blood, secretions, calculi, and foreign bodies. Combined results of tissue and cell studies may indicate interstitial pulmonary disease, bronchogenic carcinoma, or tuberculosis. Bronchogenic carcinomas include epidermoid or squamous cell carcinoma, undifferentiated oat cell carcinoma, adenocarcinoma, and bronchiolar carcinoma. In every case, correlation of bronchoscopic findings with radiographic, cytologic, and clinical findings is essential.

Biopsy

Both lung and pleural biopsies involve the excision of suspect tissue for histologic examination. The biopsy technique used may be either closed (needle or endoscopic), under local anesthesia; or open (surgical), under general anesthesia.

Lung biopsy is performed to confirm diagnosis of diffuse parenchymal pulmonary disease and pulmonary lesions. Generally, lung biopsy is recommended after chest X-ray and bronchoscopy have failed to identify the cause of diffuse parenchymal pulmonary disease or of a pulmonary lesion.

The closed biopsy technique includes both needle and transbronchial biopsies; the open technique includes both limited and standard thoracotomies.

Needle biopsy is appropriate when the lesion is readily accessible, when it originates in or is confined to the lung parenchyma, or when it is affixed to the chest wall; this biopsy provides a much smaller specimen than transbronchial biopsy or the open technique.

Transbronchial biopsy, the removal of multiple tissue specimens through a fiber-optic bronchoscope, is appropriate for diffuse infiltrative pulmonary disease or when severe debilitation contraindicates open biopsy.

Open lung biopsy is appropriate for the study of a well-circumscribed lesion that may require resection.

Histologic examination of a pulmonary tissue specimen can reveal squamous-cell or oat cell carcinoma and adenocarcinoma. Such examination supplements the results of microbiologic cultures, deep-cough sputum specimens, chest X-rays, bronchoscopy, and the patient's physical history in confirming lung neoplasms or parenchymal pulmonary disease.

Pleural biopsy is performed to differentiate between tuberculosis and malignant disease, particularly in the elderly; and to diagnose viral, fungal, or parasitic disease, and collagen vascular disease of the pleura. Needle biopsy usually follows thoracentesis (aspiration of pleural fluid), which is performed when the cause of the effusion is unknown, but it may be performed separately from the aspiration. Open pleural biopsy (a small thoracotomy), performed in the absence of pleural effusion, permits direct visualization of the pleura and the underlying lung.

The normal pleura consists primarily of mesothelial cells that are flattened in a uniform layer. Layers of areolar connective tissue—containing blood vessels, nerves, and lymphatics—lie below the mesothelial cells. Histologic examination of the tissue specimen can reveal malignant disease; tuberculosis; or viral, fungal, parasitic, or collagen vascular disease. Primary neoplasms of the pleura, which may be either localized or diffuse, are generally fibrous. Localized lesions are seldom malignant.

TEST RESULTS INTERRELATED

Clearly, these diagnostic tests for respiratory disorders are closely interrelated. Usually, a single test is inconclusive; accurate diagnosis depends on the results of two or more concurrent tests or a series of successively more specific tests. Test results must always be correlated with clinical findings and the patient's medical, social, and work history.

The skillful use of pulmonary function tests enables you to monitor your patient's response to therapy and to set realistic, reachable goals for him.

Points to remember

• Diagnostic respiratory tests evaluate pulmonary function, gas exchange, and the origin of respiratory disorder.
• Patient preparation is crucial, since anxiety can alter respirations and skew test results.
• For accurate diagnosis, respiratory test results must be correlated with each other, with clinical findings, and with the patient's medical, social, and work history.

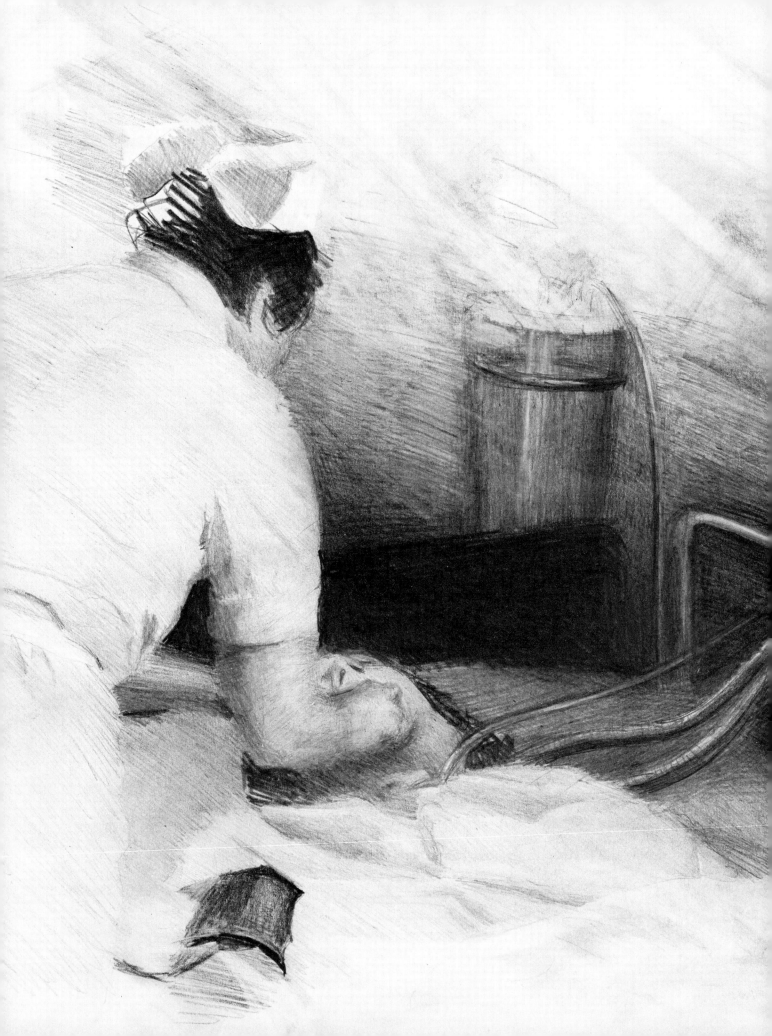

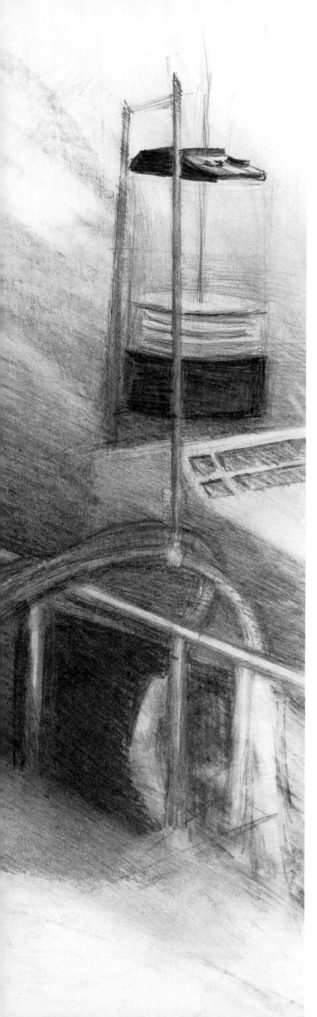

DISORDERS OF VENTILATION

4 COMBATTING ACUTE RESPIRATORY FAILURE

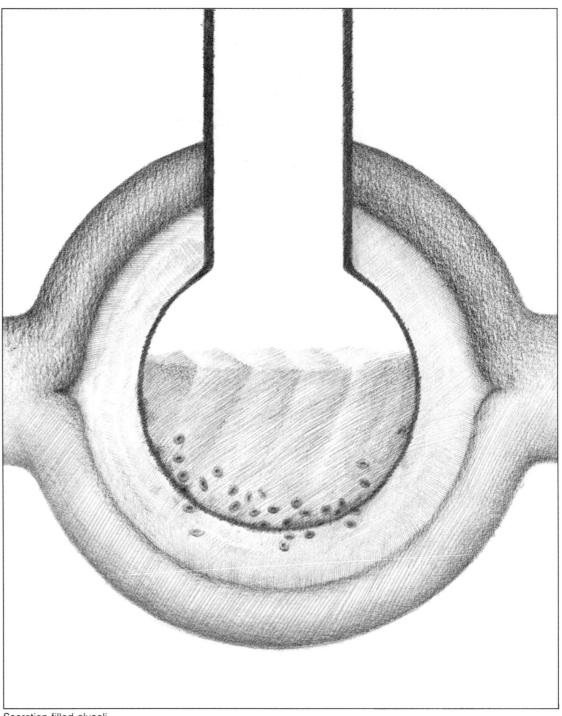

Secretion-filled alveoli

Maintaining adequate respiration is one of those ABCs of nursing that's probably second nature to you. For without the gas exchange that adequate respirations provide, all body systems quickly fail. That's why acute respiratory failure (ARF) demands early recognition and prompt treatment to improve the patient's chances of survival. Handling this life-threatening emergency effectively requires knowledge of the pathophysiology of ARF and familiarity with current treatment.

PATHOPHYSIOLOGY

Before discussing the pathophysiology of acute respiratory failure, it's important to agree on a definition and to distinguish the two basic types of this disorder. With its myriad causes and variable clinical presentation, acute respiratory failure defies easy definition. Obviously, acute respiratory failure implies that the lungs no longer meet the body's metabolic needs. Defining characteristics usually include acute dyspnea, a PaO_2 less than 50 mm Hg, a $PaCO_2$ greater than 50 mm Hg, and acidosis.

The two basic types of this disorder are hypercapnic respiratory failure and hypoxemic respiratory failure. In hypercapnic respiratory failure, hypoxemia and hypercapnia occur together. This type of respiratory failure primarily includes patients with chronic pulmonary disease or alveolar hypoventilation due to central nervous system disorders. In hypoxemic respiratory failure, hypoxemia occurs with eucapnia or hypocapnia. This type of respiratory failure primarily includes patients with acute lung injury, such as the adult respiratory distress syndrome (ARDS). But this classification isn't rigid; a patient may demonstrate both types of respiratory failure during the course of the disease. For ease of discussion, we'll consider respiratory failure in chronic pulmonary disease and in ARDS.

In patients with chronic pulmonary disease, acute respiratory failure is a leading cause of death, most commonly triggered by acute lung infection. Other causes include heart failure, myocardial infarction, pulmonary emboli, neuromuscular disorders, use of respiratory depressants, and abdominal or thoracic surgery or trauma (see *Pathogenesis of ARF in chronic pulmonary disease,* page 58). In patients without underlying pulmonary disease, diffuse lung injury from a systemic or pulmonary injury may trigger ARDS, a form of non-cardiogenic pulmonary edema that precipitates

acute respiratory failure (see *Pathophysiology of ARDS,* page 60, and *Cellular changes in ARDS,* page 61). Causes of diffuse lung injury include shock, sepsis, microemboli, inhalation of smoke or chemicals, blood transfusions, drug overdose, metabolic disease, oxygen toxicity, and aspiration of gastric contents, fresh or salt water, or hydrocarbons (see *Pathogenesis of ARDS,* page 59).

Causes of impaired gas exchange

Four pathophysiologic mechanisms—alveolar hypoventilation, ventilation/perfusion mismatch, intrapulmonary shunting, and impaired diffusion across the respiratory membrane—can impair gas exchange in acute respiratory failure. One or more of these mechanisms may operate simultaneously.

Alveolar hypoventilation. As you know, alveolar ventilation involves the exchange of oxygen and carbon dioxide across the respiratory membrane. Measurement of $PaCO_2$ helps evaluate the adequacy of alveolar ventilation. Elevated $PaCO_2$ signals inadequate alveolar ventilation, or alveolar hypoventilation.

Alveolar hypoventilation results from decreased minute ventilation or an increased dead-space ventilation. Understanding the relationship among alveolar ventilation, minute ventilation, and dead-space ventilation makes this chain of events clear. Alveolar ventilation (VA) is the difference between minute ventilation (VE) and dead-space ventilation (VD), represented by the equation $VA = VE - VD$. Factors that decrease minute ventilation or increase dead-space ventilation cause a proportionate decrease in alveolar ventilation.

Decreased minute ventilation. Because the respiratory center regulates minute ventilation, any factor that hinders transmission of the impulse—by an injury to the brain or spinal cord or by the paralysis or weakening of the respiratory muscles—can decrease minute ventilation.

Increased dead-space ventilation. Because dead-space ventilation is the sum of alveolar dead space and physiologic dead space, any factor that increases either of these volumes can increase dead-space ventilation. Ventilation/perfusion mismatch increases alveolar dead space and is the most common cause of increased dead-space ventilation.

Ventilation/perfusion mismatch. Effective gas exchange hinges on adequate perfusion and ventilation of alveoli. Mismatching occurs when some alveoli receive too little perfusion in relation to ventilation or too little ventila-

Pathogenesis of ARF in chronic pulmonary disease

Predisposing factors or injury	Pathogenesis
Acute lung infection	Acute infection increases pulmonary secretions, causing atelectasis and increased work of breathing, which, in turn, causes ventilation/perfusion mismatch.
Heart failure or myocardial infarction	In heart failure and myocardial infarction, increased left ventricular end-diastolic volume causes blood to back up in the lungs, resulting in interstitial edema and decreased compliance. Increased work of breathing follows, triggering this cycle: increased work causes increased carbon dioxide production, which stimulates increased minute ventilation. Eventually, the lungs can't work hard enough to remove excess carbon dioxide, resulting in alveolar hypoventilation.
Pulmonary emboli	Pulmonary emboli may obstruct or impair blood flow to an area of alveoli, causing ventilation/perfusion mismatch.
Neuromuscular disorders	In neuromuscular disorders, weakening or paralysis of the muscles that control ventilation results in alveolar hypoventilation.
Respiratory depressants	Administration of respiratory depressants, such as sedatives, narcotics, and tranquilizers, causes alveolar hypoventilation. Injudicious administration of oxygen may also cause respiratory depression by dampening the patient's hypoxic drive to breathe.
Abdominal or thoracic injury or surgery	Shallow breathing due to incisional pain or administration of narcotics for pain relief causes respiratory depression and alveolar hypoventilation. Accumulation of secretions due to immobility and shallow breathing causes ventilation/perfusion mismatch. Ventilation/perfusion mismatching may also occur after pneumonectomy due to hyperperfusion of the remaining lung.

tion in relation to perfusion. This impairs gas exchange by wasting available ventilation or perfusion.

Intrapulmonary shunting. A major cause of impaired gas exchange in ARDS, intrapulmonary shunting is the passage of blood from the right heart to nonventilated alveoli, causing unoxygenated blood to return to the left heart.

Impaired diffusion. The respiratory membrane—composed of the alveolar membrane, the pulmonary capillary wall, and the interstitial space between them—is normally a thin structure, freely permeable to carbon dioxide and oxygen. When diffusion across this membrane is impaired, the pulmonary capillary blood fails to equilibrate with the alveolar gas tension. But this rarely happens, since the capillary blood normally equilibrates with the alveolar gas tension quickly—within one third of the time it spends in the capillaries. Consequently, much leeway exists for changes in diffusibility before any notable impact on arterial oxygenation.

Effects of impaired gas exchange

Impaired gas exchange ultimately produces hypoxemia with or without hypercapnia and associated acidosis. The severity of impaired gas exchange varies greatly. Generally, respiratory insufficiency refers to the presence of mild to moderate hypoxemia and hypercapnia;

respiratory failure, to severe hypoxemia and hypercapnia at rest.

Signs and symptoms of impaired gas exchange vary with the onset and duration of hypoxemia, hypercapnia, and acidosis as well as with the patient's compensatory response.

Central nervous system. Of all body organs, the brain is most sensitive to oxygen deprivation. As a result, initial signs of hypoxemia—restlessness, irritability, impaired judgment—reflect cerebral hypoxia. Hypoxemia and hypercapnia trigger dilatation of cerebral vessels, a compensatory response that increases cerebral blood flow and improves oxygenation. This dilatation raises intracranial pressure and, when severe, causes cerebral edema. Acidosis depresses nerve cell function and enhances decreased level of consciousness.

Cardiovascular system. The stress of impaired gas exchange stimulates the sympathetic nervous system, which increases heart rate and contractility, a compensatory response that raises cardiac output and improves oxygenation. Increased sympathetic activity also causes vasoconstriction of peripheral blood vessels, thereby increasing blood flow to the brain and heart and raising systolic blood pressure. Arterial dilatation also occurs within the heart to improve tissue perfusion. This dilatation decreases diastolic pressure, which, in combination with increased systolic pressure, causes a wide pulse pressure. If hypoxemia goes uncorrected, dysrhythmia, chest pain, and other signs of cardiac deterioration develop.

Hypercapnia causes similar cardiovascular changes and may also cause flushing due to cutaneous vasodilatation.

Acidosis affects the heart in much the same way it affects the brain. It depresses cardiac function, decreasing contractility and automaticity. Acidosis also causes arterial dilatation, leading to decreased blood pressure.

Respiratory system. Along with the heart and the brain, the lungs respond to correct hypoxemia, hypercapnia, and acidosis. Stimulation of central and peripheral chemoreceptors increases the rate and depth of respirations, a compensatory response that increases gas exchange and improves oxygenation. Initially, this response may also cause hypocapnia, as seen in early stages of ARDS. Signs of increased work of breathing—use of accessory muscles, intercostal retractions, nasal flaring—are characteristic.

Alveolar hypoxia causes vasoconstriction of pulmonary arteries and arterioles—a major hemodynamic change in acute respiratory failure. The resulting pulmonary hypertension increases ventricular work load and may lead to right heart failure. Right heart failure secondary to lung disease is known as cor pulmonale.

Renal system. Increased sympathetic activity causes renal vasoconstriction, limiting blood flow to the kidneys, and decreasing urine formation. Renal vasoconstriction may predispose the patient to acute tubular necrosis, a complication often seen in ARDS.

Gastrointestinal system. Increased sympathetic activity causes vasoconstriction in the gastrointestinal tract, which decreases peristalsis. Prolonged vasoconstriction may cause gastric or intestinal ulceration, bowel infarction, or nutritional deficiency due to digestive disturbance.

Skin. Telltale integumentary signs of impaired gas exchange vary with the onset and

The many names of ARDS

If the signs and symptoms of ARDS sound familiar but the term "ARDS" doesn't, don't be surprised. Although ARDS is the commonly used term, its synonyms include:
• shock lung syndrome
• stiff lung syndrome
• adult hyaline membrane disease
• white lung
• wet lung
• Da Nang lung
• respiratory lung
• post pump lung
• acute pulmonary insufficiency
• acute ventilatory insufficiency
• posttraumatic pulmonary insufficiency
• noncardiogenic pulmonary edema
• hemorrhagic pulmonary edema
• post-nontraumatic pulmonary insufficiency.

Pathogenesis of ARDS

Predisposing factors or injury	Pathogenesis
Aspiration of gastric contents	The acidity of gastric contents causes direct damage to the respiratory membrane, increasing its permeability.
Aspiration of fresh or salt water	Fresh and salt water damage the alveolar epithelium by the process of osmosis. Fresh water is hypotonic and salt water is hypertonic in relation to intracellular fluid. Although both fluids increase permeability of the respiratory membrane, fresh water typically causes greater loss of surfactant.
Aspiration of hydrocarbons	Hydrocarbons spread easily within the lungs, inactivating surfactant over a large alveolar surface area. Loss of surfactant contributes to alveolar collapse and ventilation/perfusion mismatch.
Shock	Shock induces a period of hypoperfusion in the lungs that precipitates release of vasoactive substances—serotonin, prostaglandins, histamines, bradykinin, and catecholamine—which cause vasoconstriction, bronchoconstriction, and increased permeability of the respiratory membrane.
Sepsis	In sepsis, circulating endotoxins increase the pulmonary vascular resistance and the permeability of the respiratory membrane.
Microemboli	Microemboli (fat embolism, disseminated intravascular coagulation) may cause obstruction in the pulmonary capillary bed, which increases vascular resistance and the permeability of the respiratory membrane.
Inhalation of smoke or chemicals	Inhalation of smoke or chemicals may damage the respiratory membrane directly, increasing its permeability.
Blood transfusions	Particulate matter passing through the blood filter may aggregate in the pulmonary capillary bed, causing an obstruction that increases vascular resistance and the permeability of the respiratory membrane.
Drug overdose	Circulating drugs may damage the pulmonary capillary bed, increasing the permeability of the respiratory membrane.
Pancreatitis	The relationship between pancreatitis and acute lung injury isn't entirely clear. One hypothesis suggests that activation of the complement system releases endotoxins that increase the pulmonary vascular resistance and the permeability of the respiratory membrane. Another suggests that liberated pancreatic enzymes damage the respiratory membrane directly or cause lipolysis of triglycerides, releasing free fatty acid byproducts that cause the damage.
Oxygen toxicity	Administration of an FIO_2 greater than 50% may damage the respiratory membrane, increasing its permeability.

Pathophysiology of ARDS

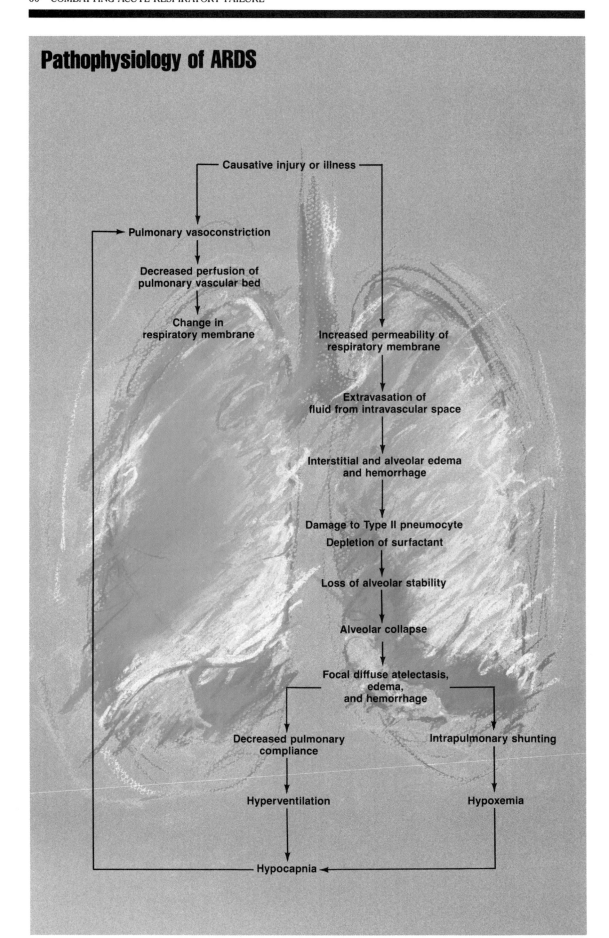

Causative injury or illness

Pulmonary vasoconstriction

Decreased perfusion of
pulmonary vascular bed

Change in
respiratory membrane

Increased permeability of
respiratory membrane

Extravasation of
fluid from intravascular space

Interstitial and alveolar edema
and hemorrhage

Damage to Type II pneumocyte

Depletion of surfactant

Loss of alveolar stability

Alveolar collapse

Focal diffuse atelectasis,
edema,
and hemorrhage

Decreased pulmonary
compliance

Intrapulmonary shunting

Hyperventilation

Hypoxemia

Hypocapnia

duration of respiratory failure. In ARDS, the skin is cool, pale, and clammy due to vasoconstriction from increased sympathetic activity. In chronic pulmonary disease progressing to respiratory failure, the skin appears dusky red due to vasodilatation from hypercapnia.

Cyanosis may also reflect impaired gas exchange, but it is usually seen only in untreated or refractory hypoxemia. Cyanosis may appear in the nail beds, the lips, the tip of the nose, the ear helices, and the underside of the tongue.

MEDICAL MANAGEMENT

Medical management of acute respiratory failure involves lifesaving measures to correct hypoxemia and stabilize the patient's condition, diagnostic tests to confirm respiratory failure and identify its cause, and supportive therapy and care to treat its cause and prevent complications.

Lifesaving support of ventilation

Because hypoxemia can depress or permanently injure the brain and other organs, lifesaving measures aim to restore adequate oxygenation as quickly as possible. Guided solely by a presumptive diagnosis, these measures often precede the results of diagnostic tests. A brief history from the patient or his family is indispensable to determine the cause of respiratory failure. Does the patient have a history of pulmonary disease? Has he recently aspirated any foreign material? Answers to such questions can separate ARDS from acute respiratory failure in chronic pulmonary disease—a crucial distinction for appropriate oxygen therapy. Meanwhile, arterial blood gas (ABG) samples can be drawn and sent to the laboratory for analysis.

For the patient with ARDS, therapy involves delivery of humidified oxygen by a tight-fitting mask, which allows use of continuous positive airway pressure (CPAP). If this approach doesn't adequately improve oxygenation, ventilatory support with intubation, volume ventilation, and positive end-expiratory pressure (PEEP) is necessary (see *Using PEEP and CPAP,* page 62). When ARDS requires mechanical ventilation, sedatives, narcotics, or neuromuscular blocking agents, such as tubocurarine or pancuronium bromide, may be ordered to minimize restlessness and facilitate ventilation.

For the patient with chronic pulmonary disease, oxygen therapy must be precisely controlled to avoid dampening the patient's

Cellular changes in ARDS

Normal alveoli

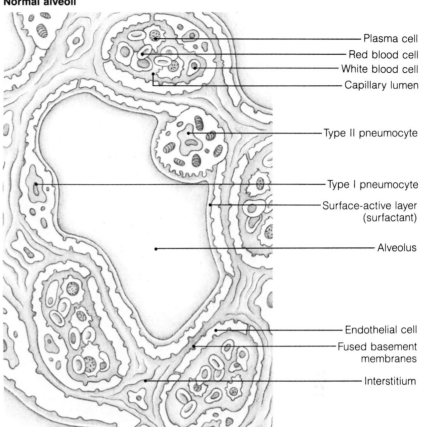

- Plasma cell
- Red blood cell
- White blood cell
- Capillary lumen
- Type II pneumocyte
- Type I pneumocyte
- Surface-active layer (surfactant)
- Alveolus
- Endothelial cell
- Fused basement membranes
- Interstitium

Alveoli in ARDS

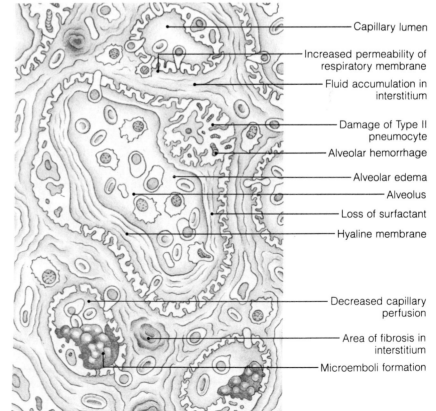

- Capillary lumen
- Increased permeability of respiratory membrane
- Fluid accumulation in interstitium
- Damage of Type II pneumocyte
- Alveolar hemorrhage
- Alveolar edema
- Alveolus
- Loss of surfactant
- Hyaline membrane
- Decreased capillary perfusion
- Area of fibrosis in interstitium
- Microemboli formation

hypoxic drive to breathe. Use of a Venturi mask allows delivery of precise, low concentrations of oxygen. By raising PaO_2 to 50 to 60 mm Hg, this method achieves 85% to 90% oxygen saturation without eliminating the patient's hypoxic drive to breathe. Although most patients respond to supplemental oxygen, some require intubation and mechanical ventilation. This decision hinges on the patient's mental and physical status, not on rigid arterial blood gas values. Generally, intubation is indicated in the patient with severe hypoxemia, acidosis, and decreased level of consciousness who fails to respond to conservative management. Other indications include

increasing patient exhaustion and, less commonly, ineffective airway clearance due to copious secretions with progressive patient deterioration.

Remember, lifesaving measures aim to bring the arterial PaO_2, $PaCO_2$, and pH to safe, but not necessarily normal, levels. In chronic pulmonary disease, rapid reversal of hypoxemia may precipitate respiratory depression; rapid reversal of hypercapnia may precipitate acute alkalosis with seizures, hypokalemia, and dysrhythmias. Consequently, ABG analysis is necessary to evaluate the effectiveness of therapy and prevent overzealous correction of altered blood gas levels.

Using PEEP and CPAP

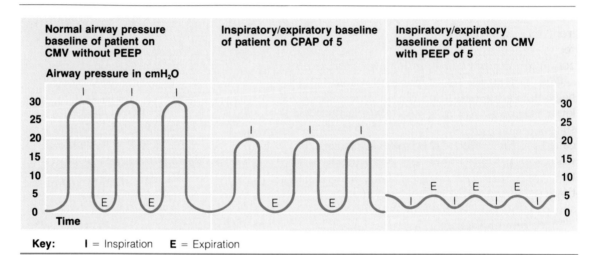

Key: **I** = Inspiration **E** = Expiration

You probably know that a fraction of inspired oxygen (FIO_2) of less than 50% is recommended to avoid oxygen toxicity. But what happens when this therapy fails to maintain an adequate PO_2 level? That's when PEEP or CPAP may be the answer for the patient with respiratory failure. Positive end-expiratory pressure (PEEP) is the application of positive pressure during expiration on a

ventilator. Continuous positive airway pressure (CPAP) is the application of positive pressure throughout the respiratory cycle during spontaneous breathing. PEEP and CPAP prevent airway pressure from returning to zero, or atmospheric pressure, as shown. This, in turn, creates an intraalveolar volume great enough to overcome the elastic forces of the lung, which helps reopen col-

lapsed alveoli and prevents small airway closure at the end of expiration. Use of PEEP or CPAP increases functional residual capacity (FRC) and substantially improves gas exchange, which decreases intrapulmonary shunting and ventilation/perfusion mismatch. As a result, PO_2 improves and FIO_2 can fall below 50% without hampering the effectiveness of therapy.

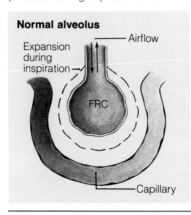
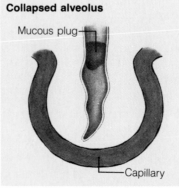
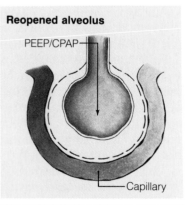

Diagnostic tests

ABG analysis and various other laboratory tests help confirm respiratory failure, determine its cause, and then monitor the effectiveness of therapy.

ABG analysis. In chronic pulmonary disease, progressive deterioration of ABGs and pH points to acute respiratory failure. In ARDS, PaO_2 falls below 50 mm Hg with a fraction of inspired oxygen (FIO_2) rate of greater than 60%. Initially, $PaCO_2$ drops to less than 35 mm Hg and the pH usually reveals respiratory alkalosis. As ARDS becomes more severe, $PaCO_2$ rises and the pH reveals respiratory acidosis. Decreased bicarbonate levels indicate metabolic acidosis due to tissue hypoxia. However, increased levels indicate metabolic alkalosis or reflect metabolic compensation for chronic respiratory acidosis.

Serum electrolytes. Hypokalemia may result from compensatory hyperventilation to correct alkalosis. Hypochloremia typically accompanies metabolic alkalosis.

Other laboratory tests. Blood lactate levels help evaluate tissue oxygenation; increased levels reflect anaerobic metabolism due to tissue hypoxia. Tests that help establish the cause of acute respiratory failure include white blood cell (WBC) count to detect infection, sputum culture and sensitivity to identify causative organisms, and toxicology screen to uncover drug ingestion.

Chest X-ray. In chronic pulmonary disease, this test shows emphysema, atelectasis, lesions, or other pulmonary pathology. In ARDS, serial chest X-rays initially show bilateral infiltrates; in later stages, a ground-glass appearance and eventually "whiteouts" of both lung fields with few visible air spaces (see *Whiteout: X-ray pattern in ARDS*). Abnormalities on the chest X-ray only appear with significant interstitial edema, long after the development of clinical signs.

Electrocardiography. Dysrhythmias are characteristic in acute respiratory failure due to underlying cardiopulmonary disease or the cardiac depressant effect of acidosis.

Pulmonary artery catheterization. This procedure helps evaluate fluid balance by determining pulmonary capillary wedge pressure (PCWP) (see *Monitoring fluid balance with PCWP,* page 64). It also allows measurement of pulmonary artery pressure and cardiac output and collection of mixed venous blood to calculate intrapulmonary shunt and to evaluate tissue oxygenation.

A-a DO₂ (alveolar-arterial oxygen tension

Whiteout: X-ray pattern in ARDS

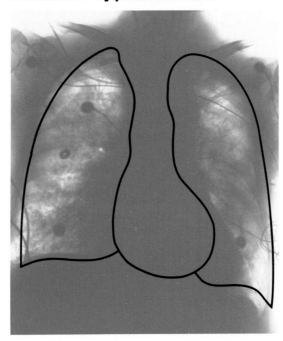

In this chest X-ray of a patient with ARDS, the lungs show the characteristic whiteout pattern associated with advanced pulmonary edema.

difference). This test estimates the extent of intrapulmonary right-to-left shunting. In ARDS, the A-a DO_2 typically exceeds 20 mm Hg and, in severe ARDS, can exceed 200 mm Hg.

Right-to-left intrapulmonary shunt (QS/QT). In ARDS, this shunt fraction increases more than 30%.

Pulmonary function tests. Four pulmonary function tests help to evaluate ARDS. *Lung compliance*, normally less than 100 ml/ cmH_2O, decreases in severe ARDS. *Vital capacity*, normally 65 to 75 ml/kg body weight, may drop to 10 ml/kg. *Functional residual capacity* also decreases below the normal range of 2 to 2.5 liters. The *dead space to tidal volume ratio* (V_D/V_T) exceeds the normal range of 25% to 40%.

Other care measures

Besides the primary goal of restoring and maintaining oxygenation, other care measures include airway management, correction of acid-base and electrolyte imbalance, drug therapy, and prevention or detection of complications.

Maintaining airway patency

Maintaining a patent airway helps ensure the effectiveness of oxygen therapy and minimize the risk of complications during recovery.

Monitoring fluid balance with PCWP

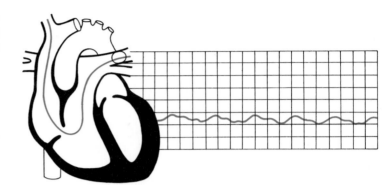

Using pulmonary capillary wedge pressure (PCWP) to evaluate fluid balance is fast becoming standard practice in the patient with ARDS—which comes as no surprise when you consider the potential dangers of fluid imbalance for this patient. For example, fluid overload may increase existing pulmonary edema, which may, in turn, increase intrapulmonary shunting and further decrease compliance. Underhydration may contribute to inadequate perfusion associated with ARDS or treatment with PEEP.

PCWP is obtained by threading a balloon-tipped, flow-directed catheter to the junction of the vena cava and right atrium. After inflation of the balloon, venous circulation carries the catheter tip through the right atrium and ventricle to a branch of the pulmonary artery, where the balloon wedges itself.

A PCWP above 12 mm Hg may indicate overhydration; below 6 mm Hg, underhydration. Monitoring this pressure guides fluid therapy and, combined with the use of vasopressors, maintains balanced perfusion.

Care measures to support the airway include adequate hydration and humidification of inspired air to keep secretions loose, coughing and deep breathing to mobilize secretions and expand collapsed airways, frequent suctioning to assist removal of tenacious or copious secretions, and chest physiotherapy to mobilize and promote drainage of secretions.

Correcting acid-base and electrolyte imbalance

Acute respiratory failure upsets the body's stores of chloride and potassium—electrolytes that play a major role in acid-base balance. The kidneys compensate for respiratory acidosis by reabsorbing bicarbonate and excreting hydrogen and chloride in the urine. The end result is hypochloremic metabolic alkalosis.

Respiratory acidosis also affects serum potassium levels. In acidosis, potassium ions migrate from the cell while hydrogen ions enter it. But compensatory alkalosis reverses this ion exchange: hydrogen ions migrate from the cell and potassium ions enter it. However, during ion exchange, the kidneys excrete some of the released intracellular potassium, causing depletion of potassium.

Administration of potassium chloride replaces these lost electrolytes and, when combined with oxygen therapy, helps restore acid-base balance.

Administering drug therapy

Drug therapy may correct the cause of acute respiratory failure or help prevent disease-related complications. In chronic pulmonary disease, drug therapy routinely includes antibiotics to destroy pathogens, bronchodilators to improve ventilation and facilitate removal of secretions, and corticosteroids to reduce airway edema and inflammation. In ARDS, careful fluid management—guided by Swan-Ganz readings, intake and output measurements, and daily weights—helps prevent fluid overload. Colloids, such as salt-poor albumin, or crystalloids, such as normal saline, may be needed to minimize the effects of hypotensive shock. When ARDS results from fat emboli or chemical injuries to the lungs, a short course of high-dose steroids may help if given early. Nonviral infections require antimicrobial drugs.

Managing complications

Unfortunately, the patient with acute respiratory failure is highly susceptible to complications—infection, pneumothorax, and pulmonary emboli are but a few. These complications can prolong the patient's recovery or, perhaps, even threaten his life. Consequently, measures to prevent complications or to detect and treat them early play a major role in nursing management of acute respiratory failure.

NURSING MANAGEMENT

Caring for the patient with acute respiratory failure is a challenge from start to finish. Typically, your patient enters the hospital in life-threatening respiratory distress and will subsequently face a long, often difficult convalescence. Effective nursing care demands keen assessment skills to keep up with the patient's many physical and psychological needs.

Sharp assessment mandatory

In acute respiratory failure, a complete history and physical examination are a must for correct diagnosis and treatment. But both of these assessment steps take considerable time—time that the breathless, dyspneic patient can ill afford to provide upon admission. That's why you'll probably have to gather this information gradually, as the patient's condition stabilizes.

Take the patient history

When taking the patient history, be sure to ask these questions: When did your present illness begin? Have you noticed a change (color, odor, amount, consistency) in your sputum recently? Has your cough worsened? Do you tire more easily than usual during physical activity? Do you have difficulty breathing? Have you felt more irritable or anxious lately? Do you feel less alert or somewhat confused?

Besides gathering this information about the present illness, review the patient's medical history. Find out if he's had previous episodes of respiratory failure. Ask about a history of conditions associated with respiratory failure, such as cor pulmonale, hypertension, renal disease, diabetes, and peptic ulcer. Determine whether members of the patient's family have a history of these conditions or any pulmonary disease. Then ask about allergies to drugs, foods, pets, dust, or pollen.

Determine if the patient smokes or has smoked. If so, ask how long and how many packs a day. Also ask the names and dosages of any over-the-counter or prescription drugs that the patient's taking.

Perform the physical exam

Because the functions of the respiratory, cardiovascular, and central nervous systems are closely integrated, these systems receive prime attention during the physical examination.

Respiratory system. Begin by determining the rate and depth of respirations. Note what position the patient assumes to breathe comfortably. Observe for signs of respiratory difficulty or increased work of breathing: use of accessory and abdominal muscles, nasal flaring, and intercostal retractions. Note the presence of thoracic abnormalities, such as barrel chest or scoliosis. Also inspect the fingers for clubbing, a sign of chronic respiratory dysfunction.

Next, use palpation to evaluate chest wall expansion. Limited or unequal expansion typically appears in chronic pulmonary disease. Palpate for vocal or tactile fremitus. Areas of enhanced fremitus point to consolidation of the lungs; areas of diminished or absent fremitus, to hyperinflation of the lungs.

Then, percuss the lungs for areas of dullness, indicating consolidation or atelectasis. Normally, the lungs produce a resonant sound on percussion. Compare percussion sounds from one side of the chest to the other as you proceed.

Finally, auscultate the lungs to evaluate bilateral aeration and breath sounds. Describe the quality and location of abnormal or adventitious breath sounds, such as rales and rhonchi, indicating atelectasis.

Central nervous system. Because of the brain's sensitivity to changes in arterial blood gases, examination of the central nervous system is especially significant in respiratory failure. Evaluate the patient's neurologic vital signs, including level of consciousness, pupil and eye movement, and motor function (muscle strength and tone, reflexes). Observe the patient for restlessness, agitation, personality changes, and other signs of hypoxia and for flapping tremor, or asterixis, a sign of hypercapnia.

Cardiovascular system. Begin by inspecting the skin and mucous membranes for pallor, cyanosis, or plethora. Look for cyanosis in the lips, the nail beds, the tip of the nose, the ear helices, and the underside of the tongue. Also inspect the neck for jugular vein pulsations to estimate central venous pressure and assess the adequacy of circulatory volume and right heart function. Palpate peripheral pulses and the extremities for edema.

Now, auscultate heart sounds. Abnormal accentuation of the pulmonic component of S_2, best heard at the pulmonic area, characterizes pulmonary hypertension. S_3, an abnormal, low-pitched sound immediately following S_2, probably results from abrupt limitation of left ventricular filling. S_4, an abnormal sound immediately before S_1, results from atrial contraction during diastolic ventricular

Common artificial airway tubes

Endotracheal tube

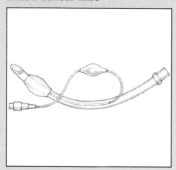

Advantages
• Quickly inserted by doctor, respiratory therapist, specially trained nurse, or anesthetist
• Inserted via nose or mouth
• Disposable

Disadvantages
• Only for short-term use (3 to 5 days)
• Oral intubation poorly tolerated by conscious patient
• May cause nasal or oral necrosis

Plastic low-pressure cuff

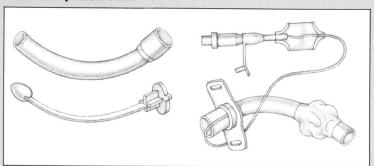

Advantages
• Cuff bonded to tube
• Distributes cuff pressure evenly; no need to deflate periodically to reduce pressure
• Disposable

Disadvantages
• More costly than other tubes

---

filling. S_3 is an early sign of heart failure, while S_4 suggests hypertension.

During auscultation, be alert for murmurs, which may indicate valvular or septal wall pathology and may precipitate heart failure, a potential cause of respiratory failure.

Abdomen. The abdominal exam can supplement your assessment of the respiratory, cardiovascular, and central nervous systems. First, inspect the abdomen for ascites, which can result from increased venous pressure. Observe for use of abdominal muscles during exhalation—a sign of increased work of breathing. Also watch for asynchronous thoracicoabdominal movement—outward motion of the rib cage with inward motion of the abdomen during inspiration—a sign of respiratory muscle fatigue.

Next, use auscultation to evaluate the frequency and character of bowel sounds. Listen in each abdominal quadrant and compare your findings. Then, use palpation to identify areas of tenderness or masses. Tenderness typically appears in the upper right abdominal quadrant due to hepatomegaly associated with right heart failure. Use percussion to estimate liver size. Normally, the liver is 2¼" to 4¾" (6 to 12 cm) at the midclavicular line.

Nursing diagnoses

As you know, nursing diagnoses define the patient's actual or potential problems that you're qualified to treat. They vary with the cause of acute respiratory failure and the chosen treatment regimen. For example, the patient with chronic pulmonary disease probably has an array of associated problems due to longstanding illness that the patient with ARDS may not face. Similarly, the patient connected to a mechanical ventilator faces a different set of problems than the patient who's receiving supplemental oxygen alone. The following nursing diagnoses with related goals and interventions address the physical, emotional, and cognitive problems you're likely to see in acute respiratory failure.

Impaired gas exchange related to alveolar hypoventilation, ventilation/perfusion mismatch, and/or intrapulmonary shunting. After formulating this nursing diagnosis, your goals are to improve respiratory function and to correct hypoxemia, hypercapnia, and respiratory acidosis. To achieve these goals, monitor vital signs and level of consciousness every 30 minutes until stable. Watch for signs of hypoxemia: tachypnea, tachycardia, elevated blood pressure, decreased level of con-

Plastic high-pressure cuff

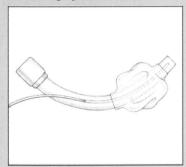

Advantages
• Cuff bonded to tube
• Disposable

Disadvantages
• More likely to cause tracheal damage or tissue necrosis than low-pressure cuff

Plastic foam cuff

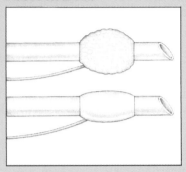

Advantages
• Cuff bonded to tube
• Maintains close to atmospheric pressure in tracheostomy tube
• Causes minimal tissue necrosis
• Doesn't require inflation and deflation
• Disposable

Disadvantages
• Those unfamiliar with device may inject air into cuff or clamp it off, which impairs function.
• Air must be aspirated from the cuff to insert this tube; if not, tracheal injury may occur.

Metal tracheal tube

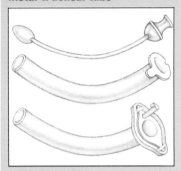

Advantages
• Reduces risk of tracheal damage
• Recommended for children because they don't require a cuff
• Permits free flow of air around tube and through larynx

Disadvantages
• In adults, lack of cuff pressure increases risk of aspiration and prevents mechanical ventilation.

sciousness, and cyanosis. If these signs develop, check arterial blood gases to evaluate severity of hypoxemia. Auscultate the lungs for adventitious sounds to help determine the cause of inadequate ventilation. Then notify the doctor.

Administer oxygen, as ordered. Frequently monitor vital signs and level of consciousness to evaluate effects of therapy. Have the patient cough and deep breathe to help expand collapsed airways and remove secretions. Describe the amount and character of secretions. If oxygen therapy, coughing, and deep breathing fail to improve the patient's condition, notify the doctor. Mechanical ventilation, often with PEEP, is typically the next treatment step to maintain adequate alveolar ventilation.

Ineffective airway clearance related to copious secretions and inadequate coughing. Your goals are to maintain airway patency and promote clearance of secretions. To achieve these goals, first assess the patient for airway obstruction. Auscultate the lungs for adventitious breath sounds that mark areas of accumulating secretions. Have the patient cough and deep breathe to mobilize and clear secretions obstructing airflow. Suction the patient, as necessary, to remove secretions and main-

tain airway patency. Ensure humidification of inspired oxygen to help thin secretions. Also, administer aerosol therapy, as ordered, to help loosen secretions. Perform chest physiotherapy 15 minutes after aerosol therapy to remove secretions. Auscultate the lungs before and after chest physiotherapy for adventitious breath sounds to pinpoint areas that need vigorous attention and to evaluate the effectiveness of physiotherapy. Monitor fluid intake and output. Monitor fluid balance to thin secretions and avoid fluid overload. Monitor pulmonary artery or central venous pressure to detect fluid overload. If the patient continues to have difficulty clearing secretions, notify the doctor. Insertion of an endotracheal or tracheostomy tube may be necessary to facilitate secretion removal.

Ineffective breathing pattern related to decreased pulmonary compliance. Your goals are to restore a normal breathing pattern that maintains adequate gas exchange and to reduce the patient's anxiety. To restore a normal breathing pattern, administer oxygen, as ordered. Monitor the rate, rhythm, and depth of respirations. Watch for use of accessory muscles during breathing and for rapid, shallow respirations. Auscultate the lungs to locate areas of inadequate airflow. Also observe for fatigue and signs of hypoxia.

Notify the doctor if the patient's breathing pattern fails to improve and signs of hypoxia and fatigue develop. Prepare for mechanical ventilation to prevent extreme fatigue and respiratory arrest.

To reduce the patient's anxiety, encourage him to express his concerns, and reassure him that a nurse is always nearby.

Inadequate nutrition related to anorexia or inability to eat. For the patient with respiratory failure, adequate nutrition is a must to maintain tissue metabolism and promote recovery. Typically, this patient requires 2,000 to 3,000 calories a day. To restore and maintain proper nutrition, administer supplemental enteral or I.V. feedings, as ordered. Accurately record intake, count calories daily, and weigh the patient daily to monitor his nutrition.

Sleep pattern disturbance related to need for continuous care. To promote sleep, plan daily rest periods for the patient, uninterrupted by nursing care or visiting hours. Dim the unit lights, avoid unnecessary noise, and provide a sedative, as ordered, to promote sleep. Check on the quantity and quality of the patient's sleep to evaluate the success of your interventions.

Knowledge deficit related to the disease, diagnostic tests, or therapy. Your goals are to teach the patient and his family about respiratory failure and its treatment, to explain necessary diagnostic tests, to prepare the patient for discharge, and to reduce anxiety. When carrying out nursing interventions to meet these goals, be sure to use words that the patient and his family can understand. Recognize that anxiety can influence their level of comprehension.

Teach the patient about respiratory failure, its symptoms, and measures to control them. Stress the importance of following the prescribed drug, dietary, and exercise regimen. Before discharge, make sure the patient understands the importance of follow-up visits and can identify reportable signs and symptoms.

Explain all diagnostic tests to the patient and prepare him, as necessary. To reduce anxiety, involve the patient and his family in planning and providing care. Also keep them current on the patient's progress.

Ineffective coping mechanisms related to effects of disease on life-style and self-image. Your goals are to provide comfort measures, to encourage expression of the patient's feelings, to outline resources available to meet his needs, and to promote independence. Achieving these goals requires a great deal of patience and understanding on your part. Keep in mind that the patient and his family may initially show anger, sadness, or depression.

Reassure the patient and encourage him to express his feelings. Listen attentively and convey an attitude of acceptance. Let him know that many patients have similar difficulty accepting such negative changes. Encourage him to draw upon his personal strength and the support of his family. And don't hesitate to refer him for psychosocial counseling.

Encourage the patient's independence to support his self-image and promote optimal function. Let him participate in treatment decisions and urge self-care whenever possible.

Potential for complications related to prolonged bed rest. Your nursing goals are to promote patient comfort, to encourage relaxation and sleep, to maintain joint mobility, to prevent skin breakdown, and to manage other complications of bed rest.

To promote patient comfort, keep bed linens clean and wrinkle-free. Position the patient comfortably, using extra pillows for support. Turn the patient at least every 2 hours.

To encourage relaxation and sleep, plan daily rest periods for the patient, uninterrupted by nursing care or visiting hours. Provide quiet during these periods and dim the unit lights.

To maintain joint mobility, perform passive range-of-motion exercises—or, if the patient's condition permits, encourage active range-of-motion exercises—at least three times daily. Observe the patient's respiratory rate and rhythm during this activity.

To prevent skin breakdown, recognize that patients with respiratory failure often have two strikes against them: poor oxygenation and poor nutrition, both of which contribute to skin breakdown. Consequently, keep the skin clean and dry. Examine skin color and integrity frequently, especially at bony prominences. Massage bony prominences and other pressure points often to stimulate circulation. Maintain proper positioning and body alignment to reduce pressure on these areas. Placing a water or foam mattress or an alternating pressure pad on the patient's bed also reduces pressure.

Be alert for other complications of prolonged bed rest: gastrointestinal bleeding, pulmonary infection, peripheral venous thrombosis, and

Weaning the patient from mechanical ventilation

Measuring vital capacity and maximal inspiratory force

Measurement of vital capacity and maximal inspiratory force (MIF) helps determine the patient's readiness for weaning and his progress once weaning is begun.

To measure the patient's vital capacity:
• Attach the Wright's respirometer and adapter to the endotracheal or tracheostomy tube with the cuff inflated. Instruct the patient to inhale deeply.
• Quickly press the respirometer's reset button to return the dial's hands to the zero mark. Then tell the patient to exhale as quickly, forcefully, and completely as possible.
• Before the patient takes his next breath, turn the control switch to the "Off" position to hold the measurement. Read the respirometer dial to determine the volume of exhaled air. The small dial measures tidal volume and vital capacity; the large dial, minute volume.

To measure MIF:
• Attach the inspiratory force meter's manifold tube to the patient's endotracheal or tracheostomy tube with the cuff inflated.
• Instruct the patient to breathe spontaneously for a few breaths.
• At the end of a normal exhalation, cover the manifold safety port with your thumb or fingertip to occlude the airway. Maintain the occlusion for 10 to 20 seconds, sufficient time for the patient to attempt inspiration.
• Instruct the patient to inhale as deeply as possible while you're blocking his airway. The unconscious patient will automatically attempt inspiration during this time.
• Note the reading on the meter dial. The red needle on the meter dial records the MIF with each inspiration. The black "memory" needle captures this reading, rising higher and locking with each greater exertion so the patient's best effort remains visible.

eaning the patient from mechanical ventilation is a complex, yet challenging, process that must address a variety of physical and emotional needs. Close monitoring during weaning prevents undue physical stress and reduces the risk of inadequate oxygenation. Careful preparation and emotional support help calm the patient and promote a smooth transition to spontaneous breathing.

A matter of timing
Proper timing contributes much to the success or failure of weaning. The patient's readiness hinges on how well he meets the following criteria:
• alert and well-oriented
• stable cardiovascular status
• adequate ventilatory function; vital capacity of at least 10 ml/kg and maximal inspiratory force of more than −25 cmH₂O
• adequate oxygenation; PO_2 of more than 70 mm Hg and PCO_2 of 35 to 45 mm Hg (Note that patients with chronic lung disease typically have a lower PO_2 and higher PCO_2.)
• FIO_2 of 40% or less
• PEEP of 5 or less.

Two approaches
Conventional weaning and intermittent mandatory ventilation (IMV) are the two basic approaches to weaning. Conventional weaning involves periodically removing the patient from the ventilator for increasing periods of time until he can breathe completely on his own. Begin weaning for 15 to 30 minutes, every 2 to 4 hours. After disconnecting the patient from the ventilator, give him supplemental oxygen through a T-piece. Evaluate his arterial blood gases within 15 minutes to ensure adequate oxygenation. Also monitor vital signs and parameters of respiratory function—vital capacity, tidal volume, inspiratory force—three or four times per hour initially, and then less frequently as the

Wright's respirometer

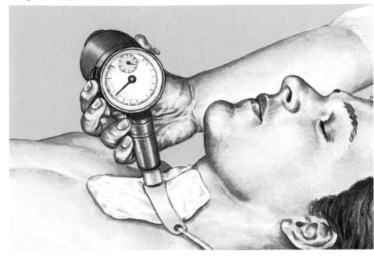

Inspiratory force meter

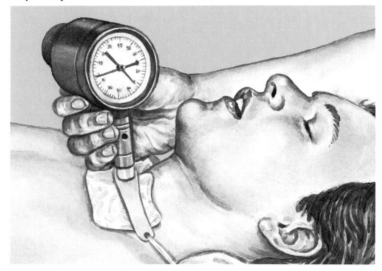

patient progresses.

IMV involves delivery of a specific number of ventilator breaths per minute, between which the patient breathes on his own. Weaning is accomplished by gradually reducing the number of ventilator breaths until the patient can breathe completely on his own. Typically, this approach is most helpful for the patient who's very dependent on the ventilator. Monitor arterial blood gases periodically to ensure adequate oxygenation as well as vital capacity, tidal volume, inspiratory force, and vital signs.

Tips for success
• Don't sedate the patient before weaning to avoid dampening his drive to breathe.
• Ensure that the patient is well rested.
• Reassure the patient that it's safe for him to breathe on his own. Encourage remaining calm.
• Warn the patient that he may experience breathlessness or dyspnea during weaning to help avoid bouts of panic that may trigger hyperventilation.
• Have the patient sitting up or leaning on a table to facilitate use of respiratory muscles.

pulmonary embolism. Gastrointestinal bleeding most commonly results from ulceration or gastritis caused by excessive acid secretion. Stress associated with prolonged illness and bed rest stimulates acid secretion.

To prevent bleeding, administer antacids and prophylactic cimetidine, as ordered. Give all drugs with meals. Recognize that supplemental nasogastric feeding helps prevent gastric bleeding while ensuring adequate nutrition. Encourage the patient to express his fears and concerns to help reduce stress. Explain all procedures carefully and involve the patient as much as possible in care decisions.

To detect gastrointestinal bleeding, monitor vital signs every 4 hours. Watch especially for a sudden rise in pulse rate. Test all stools, emesis, and nasogastric aspirate for occult blood, and watch for other signs of GI disturbance—anorexia, vomiting, abdominal distention, pain, cramps, diarrhea, or constipation. Monitor hemoglobin and hematocrit, and observe the patient for sudden dizziness or syncope. Notify the doctor if signs of GI bleeding develop.

To prevent pulmonary infection, ensure adequate removal of all secretions, which provide an excellent medium for the growth of microorganisms. Observe strict aseptic techniques when suctioning the patient. Administer prophylactic antibiotics, as ordered.

To detect pulmonary infection, watch for progressive dyspnea, fever, and a change in the amount, color, consistency, or odor of secretions. Check sputum culture and sensitivity tests, CBC for leukocytosis, and chest X-rays for evidence of pneumonia. Notify the doctor if signs of infection develop.

To prevent peripheral venous thrombosis, recognize that venostasis, vascular wall damage, and hypercoagulability of the blood contribute to thrombus formation. To prevent venostasis, apply antiembolism stockings smoothly, without wrinkles or tight areas, to avoid uneven pressure. Remove stockings for 10 to 15 minutes every 8 hours to allow filling of superficial capillaries and prevent skin breakdown. Perform or encourage range-of-motion exercises to promote circulation and turn the patient at least every 2 hours. When positioning the patient, avoid marked angulation at the groin or knee and instruct the patient not to cross his legs. Encourage ambulation as soon as tolerated.

To minimize or prevent hypercoagulability, discontinue oral contraceptives and other drugs associated with hypercoagulability, as ordered. Administer low-dose heparin for prophylaxis, if ordered. Recognize high-risk patients: those older than age 60 or those with heart failure, carcinoma, or a history of thrombophlebitis and/or embolization.

To treat peripheral venous thrombosis, administer anticoagulants and an analgesic, as ordered. Maintain bed rest during the acute period and keep the affected extremity elevated. Avoid massage or any pressure on the extremity. Place a bed cradle over the extremity and apply moist heat, if ordered. Perform or encourage range-of-motion exercises at least three times daily for the unaffected extremities and apply an antiembolism stocking, if ordered.

When planning nursing interventions to detect pulmonary emboli, recognize that signs and symptoms vary with the size, number, and location of the emboli. Observe the patient for dyspnea, perhaps with anginal or pleuritic chest pain. Also watch for tachycardia, productive cough, low-grade fever, pleural effusion and, less commonly, cyanosis, syncope, and distended neck veins. Auscultate the lungs for pleural friction rub, rales and wheezing, and accentuation of the pulmonic component of S_2. Also monitor for signs of reduced cardiac output (weak, rapid pulse, hypotension) and signs of hypoxia (restlessness, irritability).

Dependence on mechanical ventilation related to inability to maintain adequate alveolar ventilation. Your goals are to prevent ventilator malfunction, to promote synchronization of the patient's breathing with the ventilator, and to prevent or resolve complications of mechanical ventilation.

To prevent ventilator malfunction, have the respiratory therapist check ventilator function and change the tubing daily. Every 2 to 4 hours, check the ventilator settings—V_T, FIO_2 rate, sigh rate, and volume. Ensure delivery of the correct FIO_2 or PEEP level. Watch for leaks in the humidifier, tubing, endotracheal or tracheal cuff, or nebulizer connection. Check the connections and patency of all tubing, and watch for condensation or kinks in the tubing. Check alarm settings to ensure proper function. Maintain temperature of water vapor at 95° to 100° F. (52.8° to 55.6° C.). Check for proper function of pressure gauge and panel light indicators. *If the ventilator malfunctions, provide manual ventilation to ensure adequate respirations.* Have someone else inspect the ventilator to determine what's wrong while you support the patient. Consult the respiratory therapist if necessary.

To promote synchronization of the patient's breathing with the ventilator, recognize that PEEP doesn't occur in normal breathing and the patient may resist the ventilator. Explaining the purpose of mechanical ventilation and the sensations the patient is likely to experience, coupled with reassurance during therapy, is vital to successful artificial ventilation. Administer a sedative, as ordered, if the patient remains uncooperative.

During therapy, monitor the patient to ensure he's breathing in sequence with the ventilator. Watch for a low and varying V_T, unless you're using intermittent mandatory ventilation. Note factors that may contribute to restlessness, such as hypoxia, acid-base imbalance, pain, anxiety, and frustration. Notify the doctor if the patient has continued difficulty adjusting to the ventilator. Reassure the patient and change the sensitivity or flow rate on the ventilator, if indicated. Switch to intermittent mandatory ventilation, if weaning is ordered (see *Weaning the patient from mechanical ventilation,* page 69).

Be alert for complications of mechanical ventilation, such as atelectasis, oxygen toxicity, pneumothorax, mediastinal or subcutaneous emphysema, reduced cardiac output with hypotension, and fluid overload.

To prevent atelectasis, recognize that immobility and primarily constant volume ventilation contribute to its development. To prevent atelectasis, keep the sigh mode at 4 to 10/hour, as ordered. Turn the patient every 1 to 2 hours and perform vigorous chest physiotherapy every 2 to 4 hours. Monitor arterial blood gases every 3 to 6 hours until stable. Take vital signs every 2 to 4 hours. Auscultate the lungs for abnormal breath sounds every 2 to 3 hours. Check serial chest X-rays for signs of atelectasis. Watch for decreased level of consciousness and other signs of hypoxemia.

To prevent oxygen toxicity, gradually decrease FIO_2 to below 50% within the first 24 to 48 hours of mechanical ventilation. Or, institute PEEP to achieve adequate oxygenation, as ordered. Maintain PaO_2 within the patient's normal limits. Monitor arterial blood gases every 2 to 3 hours until stable. Watch for decreased level of consciousness to detect hypoxemia early.

To prevent pneumothorax, a potential complication of PEEP, keep PEEP levels as low as possible to maintain adequate oxygenation.

Use intermittent mandatory ventilation to reduce mean intrathoracic pressures, as ordered. Recognize that tension pneumothorax is a medical emergency that may trigger cardiac and respiratory failure. Be alert for the high pressure alarm on the ventilator and unilateral chest expansion.

Although a small pneumothorax may resolve with conservative treatment, a significant or tension pneumothorax requires chest tube insertion to reexpand the lung. Assist with this procedure and then monitor arterial blood gases, breath sounds, and serial chest X-rays for resolution of the pneumothorax.

To detect mediastinal emphysema, check serial chest X-rays for a widened mediastinum. Auscultate the lungs for decreased expansion and observe for signs of respiratory distress. Watch for signs of reduced cardiac output (hypotension, tachycardia) and venous congestion (distended neck veins, leg edema). Notify the doctor if these signs develop.

To detect subcutaneous emphysema, check for crepitus—a crackling sensation on palpation of the skin.

Decreased cardiac output with hypotension, another potential complication of PEEP, results from decreased venous return caused by positive intrathoracic pressure. Although decreased venous return stimulates the sympathetic nervous system, causing vasoconstriction and elevated blood pressure, this stimulus may fail to normalize blood pressure in the hypovolemic patient. *To prevent decreased cardiac output with hypotension,* institute PEEP in gradual increments while administering fluids. When you institute or increase the PEEP level, watch for hypotension, tachycardia, elevated central venous pressure, oliguria, and reduced peripheral circulation. If these signs occur, notify the doctor. Administer increased fluid and/or an inotropic agent, as ordered.

To prevent fluid overload, which may stem from fluid administration in PEEP, weigh the patient daily and monitor intake and output every 1 to 2 hours. As a rule of thumb, consider one kilogram of weight gain equal to 1,000 ml of excess fluid. Also watch for signs of pulmonary interstitial edema associated with fluid overload. Auscultate the lungs for rales and wheezing, watch for signs and symptoms of hypoxemia, and check serial chest X-rays for diffuse haziness. Notify the doctor if these signs develop.

Dependence on artificial airway. When the patient fails to maintain independent ventila-

Suctioning: Tips for safety and success

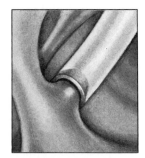

Invagination of the mucosa into the suction catheter

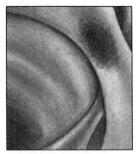

Hemorrhagic area at the site of invagination

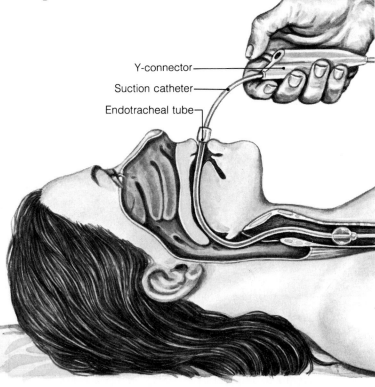

Y-connector
Suction catheter
Endotracheal tube

Maintaining airway patency is a key nursing goal in acute respiratory failure. That's why proper suctioning technique is a must. Follow these tips:
• Manually ventilate the patient's lungs with oxygen for several minutes before and after suctioning, and avoid suctioning for longer than 12 seconds to prevent oxygen depletion. Control suction by covering the open end of the Y-connector with your thumb.
• Maintain aseptic technique during suctioning. Rinse the catheter with sterile water after each use. Once a shift, deflate the cuff and suction the trachea with a sterile catheter. Don't apply suction as you insert the catheter to avoid "stealing" oxygen from the patient or snaring the mucosa and causing a hemorrhagic area, as shown.
• Suction at least every 2 hours to clear secretions and prevent mucous plugs from obstructing the tube. To evaluate the need for suctioning, listen to the air traveling through the endotracheal tube. A hissing sound in-

dicates the tube's open; a whistling sound indicates the tube's partially obstructed. Gurgling or rattling sounds also indicate some obstruction. Be alert for the high pressure alarm on the ventilator, which indicates that suctioning is needed.

• After suctioning, immediately reconnect the patient to the ventilator or oxygen delivery system. Be sure the oxygen is at the prescribed flow rate. Discard the used suction catheter, gloves, and basin. Replace equipment at the patient's bedside.

---

tion, insertion of an endotracheal or tracheostomy tube ensures unobstructed airflow in and out of the lungs (see *Common artificial airway tubes,* pages 66 to 67). Your nursing goals are to maintain a patent airway, to prevent infection and other complications, and to promote patient comfort.

To maintain airway patency, elevate the head of the bed to facilitate respirations, unless contraindicated. Auscultate the lungs for abnormal and adventitious breath sounds and for bilateral aeration to assess airway patency. Inspect the chest for respiratory rate and rhythm and for symmetrical expansion. Also monitor arterial blood gases to assess oxygenation.

To liquify thick secretions and facilitate their removal, instill normal saline solution into the endotracheal tube, as ordered, or administer vaporized air or humidified oxygen by tracheostomy collar. Turn the patient every 1

to 2 hours and perform chest physiotherapy to mobilize and help remove secretions. Suction the patient's airway as needed. If the patient has an endotracheal tube in place, also suction the oropharynx to prevent excessive accumulation of secretions above the cuff. Once every shift, deflate the cuff and suction the trachea.

The presence of an artificial airway predisposes the patient to infection and other complications. Breathing through an airway bypasses the normal filtering system of the nose and increases the risk of superimposed infection. To prevent infection, recognize that this complication usually results from poor aseptic technique during suctioning or from repeated, traumatic suctioning (see *Suctioning: Tips for safety and success*).

To detect infection, monitor vital signs every 2 to 4 hours and watch for a change in the color, amount, consistency, and odor of secretions. Obtain a sputum specimen every 3 days and send it to the laboratory for culture and sensitivity tests. Notify the doctor if signs of infection develop.

When the patient has a tracheostomy tube, infection may also occur at and around the stoma. To prevent stomal infection or peristomal skin breakdown, observe the stoma for erythema, exudate, odor, and crusts. Cleanse the stoma every 8 hours. Use a sterile, cotton-tipped applicator moistened with hydrogen peroxide to remove crusty secretions. Rinse the stoma with sterile water and apply topical antifungal or antibiotic agents, if ordered, and a dressing. Change the dressing daily or more frequently, as needed. Notify the doctor if signs of infection develop, and culture the stoma. Change the tracheostomy ties daily. Have someone else anchor the tube while you secure new ties.

For the patient with an endotracheal tube, watch for pressure sores at the corners of the mouth. Reposition the tube daily from side to side of the mouth.

Be alert for other complications associated with an artificial airway, such as tracheal erosion, tracheal esophageal fistula, and tracheal stenosis. These complications typically accompany use of high-pressure cuffs, inadequate cuff care, or concurrent use of a nasogastric tube, which places pressure on both sides of the tracheoesophageal membrane. *To prevent these complications,* use a low-pressure cuff on the endotracheal/tracheostomy tube. Keep a small air leak around the tube when it's inflated to prevent excessive pressure on the trachea. Monitor cuff pressure every 4 to 8 hours to keep it below 20 mm Hg.

Sedate or restrain the patient to prevent tube dislodgement, since frequent tube replacement causes tracheal irritation. Avoid moving the tube or twisting the tracheal collar when suctioning, changing ties, or cleansing the site. Change the tube, only as ordered, to prevent tracheal inflammation with resultant scarring and granulomatous tissue formation. Monitor tube position on the chest X-ray daily and whenever auscultation reveals unilateral aeration.

To prevent aspiration of food, encourage the patient with a tracheostomy tube to eat slowly and to refrain from talking while eating. Inflate the tube cuff before oral or nasogastric feeding. Keep the patient with an endotracheal tube N.P.O. Provide mouth care at least once every shift to promote comfort.

Impaired communication related to the presence of an artificial airway. Your goals are to help the patient find an alternative, nonverbal means of communication and to relieve his anxiety. When planning ways to help the patient communicate, consider his level of consciousness. If he's alert, place a call bell within easy reach. Provide a "magic slate" or pad and pencil for the literate patient and a communication board with illustrations for the aphasic or preverbal patient. Teach the tracheostomy patient to briefly occlude the airway to speak, as appropriate.

To relieve anxiety, reassure the patient that a nurse is always nearby. Also explain all procedures to the patient and his family.

Evaluate your care plan
You'll know that your care plan was successful when the patient:
• maintains adequate oxygenation and arterial blood gas values at his "normal" levels
• achieves effective clearance of secretions through coughing and deep breathing, chest physiotherapy, and administration of humidified oxygen
• maintains a patent airway with bilateral aeration of the lung fields and absence of adventitious breath sounds
• maintains normal body weight with adequate daily caloric intake
• communicates effectively despite the presence of an artificial airway
• achieves rest and adequate sleep
• demonstrates reduced anxiety
• demonstrates no evidence of disease or therapy-related complications
• can explain the effects of acute respiratory failure on the lungs and the accompanying treatment measures
• adheres to prescribed medical regimen and understands the importance of follow-up visits
• can list factors that precipitate symptoms and knows which symptoms require immediate medical attention.

A final word
Acute respiratory failure occurs suddenly, worsens rapidly, and kills without prompt intervention. But you can take two steps toward improving the patient's chances of survival. The first is recognizing those at risk—patients with chronic pulmonary disease or a history of systemic or pulmonary injury. The second is understanding the signs of deteriorating pulmonary function and taking measures to halt or reverse them.

Points to remember

• Defining characteristics of acute respiratory failure usually include acute dyspnea, a PaO_2 less than 50 mm Hg, a PaO_2 greater than 50 mm Hg, and acidosis.
• Recognition of high-risk patients is the key to early detection and successful treatment of respiratory failure.
• Four pathophysiologic mechanisms are responsible for impaired gas exchange: alveolar hypoventilation, ventilation/perfusion mismatch, intrapulmonary shunting, and impaired diffusion across the respiratory membrane.
• The signs and symptoms of hypoxemia, hypercapnia, and acidosis are widespread, involving all major body systems.
• Oxygen therapy must be precisely controlled in hypercapnic respiratory failure to avoid dampening the patient's hypoxic drive to breathe.

5 COMPENSATING FOR C.O.P.D.

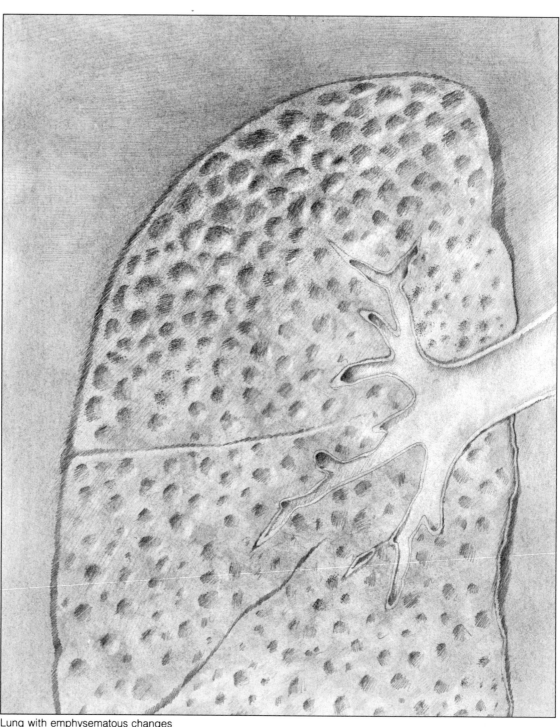

Lung with emphysematous changes

Chronic obstructive pulmonary disease (COPD) usually results from chronic bronchitis, emphysema, or asthma. In recent years, the incidence of COPD has reached epidemic proportions. It creates 3.8 billion dollars in medical costs annually and ranks fifth among the major causes of death in the United States.

Because of its chronic and debilitating nature, COPD has a profound effect on the patient. He must learn to cope with drastic changes in his life-style and body image. Consequently, the disease can lead to emotional problems, which may include severe depression. These problems extend to the patient's family, too.

Your job is to help the patient adjust to the physical and emotional changes caused by COPD and to comply with treatment, particularly home care and the inevitable life-style changes that it entails. To perform skillfully and efficiently in this critical role, you must know how to assess the quality of the patient's home care, to suggest any necessary changes, and—most important—to offer the patient the support he needs.

What is COPD?
COPD (also called chronic obstructive lung disease [COLD]) is an umbrella term for chronic airway obstruction, usually caused by chronic bronchitis, emphysema, or asthma. However, it also includes chronic airway obstruction caused by less common disorders, such as bronchiectasis and cystic fibrosis. Any of these underlying disorders may occur separately or together and may vary in severity from relatively mild, static, and reversible conditions to progressively severe, incapacitating respiratory failure. All these disorders can cause obstruction of bronchial airflow.

What causes COPD?
Predisposing factors to COPD include cigarette smoking, air pollution, occupational exposure to irritating dusts or gases, familial and hereditary factors, infection, allergies, aging, and potentially harmful drugs and chemicals.

Habitual cigarette smoking is by far the most important of these factors; COPD rarely occurs in nonsmokers. Cigarette smoking impairs ciliary action and macrophagic activity. It also causes inflammation of the airways, increased mucus production, destruction of alveolar septae, and peribronchiolar fibrosis. Air pollution, combined with the effects of

cigarette smoking, exacerbates COPD by inducing bronchospasm and mucosal edema, which increase airway resistance.

Although less common than cigarette smoking and air pollution, occupational exposure to irritating dusts or gases also aggravates COPD. Exposure to silica and other nonorganic dusts may cause lung fibrosis and focal emphysema, severely altering pulmonary function. Exposure to certain organic dusts, such as cotton fiber, may increase airway resistance, sometimes causing permanent respiratory difficulty. Pulmonary edema and bronchiolitis—and, occasionally, permanent parenchymal damage—may result from exposure to irritating gases, such as chlorine. Occupational asthma may develop, too, from exposure to irritating dusts or gases.

COPD can also result—at least partially—from familial and hereditary factors. For example, familial emphysema results from an inherited deficiency of alpha$_1$-antitrypsin, a nonspecific proteolytic enzyme inhibitor. Without this enzyme inhibitor, proteolytic enzymes derived from blood leukocytes, alveolar macrophages, and bacteria cause lysis of lung tissue. Cystic fibrosis, a congenital disorder transmitted as an autosomal recessive trait, is another hereditary factor that can contribute to development of COPD.

Aging, yet another predisposing factor for COPD, may be associated with mild panlobular emphysema, a common condition in the elderly. Many elderly patients show no outward signs of emphysema, but histopathologic examination confirms this condition. Kyphosis, a structural abnormality of the dorsal spine, may lead to emphysema.

Infection is the primary cause of bronchiectasis. It usually results from cystic fibrosis, whooping cough, influenza, tuberculosis, or cancer. Infection also contributes to the exacerbation of all forms of COPD. Viruses and *Mycoplasma pneumoniae* cause most acute episodes. *Streptococcus pneumoniae* commonly causes bacterial pneumonia; *Hemophilus influenzae* causes acute exacerbations of COPD.

The primary predisposing factor in extrinsic asthma is exposure to allergens. Since immunoglobulin E (IgE) is produced in allergic individuals in response to exposure to an allergen, they may have high serum levels of IgE antibodies. These antibodies attach to mast cells in the submucosa of bronchial epithelium. When an allergic individual is exposed to the specific sensitizing allergen, an antigen-antibody reaction occurs, releasing IgE from the mast cell and causing asthma.

Harmful drugs for some asthma patients include aspirin and various nonsteroidal anti-inflammatory drugs, such as indomethacin; potentially harmful chemicals include a yellow food dye. Exercise exacerbates asthma and, in some individuals, may actually cause the condition (exercise-induced asthma), probably from heat and moisture loss in the upper airways.

PATHOPHYSIOLOGY

In all forms of COPD, narrowing of the airways obstructs airflow to and from the lungs. Such obstruction markedly increases the work of breathing and resistance to airflow. This narrowing impairs ventilation by trapping air in the bronchioles and alveoli. The trapped air, in turn, hinders normal gas exchange and distends the alveoli. Other pathology of COPD varies with each form of the disease.

Chronic bronchitis

In this form of COPD, tissue irritation usually results from exposure to cigarette smoke or air pollution. Tissue irritation causes hypertrophy of mucus-producing cells in the bronchi, thus increasing mucus production. This, in turn, activates the cough reflex, leading to progressive destruction of smaller bronchioles, increased susceptibility to respiratory infection, airway obstruction, and inadequate gas exchange.

Because of these pathologic changes, the patient becomes increasingly dyspneic and short of breath on exertion, which forces him to restrict his physical activities. The sputum produced by his cough becomes increasingly tenacious, mucoid, and copious, particularly in the morning after secretions have accumulated during the night.

As bronchitis progresses, more alveoli become inadequately ventilated, further disrupting gas diffusion and causing first a decreased PaO_2 level and later an elevated $PaCO_2$. The patient now develops hypoxia and hypercapnia. Compensatory hyperventilation, however—common in some other forms of respiratory dysfunction—doesn't usually occur because of the insensitivity of the respiratory center in the brain stem to the sustained hypercapnia and the reactions of peripheral chemoreceptors in the aortic arch and carotid body to the evolving hypoxia.

Eventually, inadequately oxygenated hemoglobin may cause cyanosis. Also, pulmonary vasoconstriction may occur secondary to a decreased PaO_2. If this occurs, increased pulmonary vascular pressure causes resistance to the blood ejected by the right ventricle. In time, this may cause right ventricular hypertrophy and failure, with edema. Because of his cyanosis and edema, the patient with chronic bronchitis is often called a "blue bloater."

Emphysema

Emphysema may develop after a long history of chronic bronchitis, during which air becomes trapped in the alveoli because mucus is blocking the small terminal bronchioles and airway walls have collapsed. The increase in mucus production, though slight, causes the chronic nonproductive cough characteristic of emphysema. The patient usually only raises small amounts of sputum from his spasmodic and fatiguing cough. Typically, even such minimal exertion as talking initiates coughing, particularly in the morning. Severe paroxysms of coughing may cause nausea and vomiting.

Subsequently, recurrent inflammation, associated with the release of proteolytic enzymes from cells in the lungs, breaks down the alveolar walls and ducts and the respiratory bronchioles. Clusters of alveoli then merge, forming larger airspaces and reducing the total number of alveoli. The creation of these airspaces causes even more air to become trapped from collapsed airway walls. The effort required to exhale trapped air causes dyspnea on exertion. Eventually dyspnea occurs even at rest.

Meanwhile, destruction of the alveolar walls disrupts parts of the pulmonary capillary bed, located in the walls. This reduces the total alveolar capillary membrane area of the lungs available for gas exchange. The combined effects of trapped air and alveolar distention change the size and shape of the patient's chest. Eventually he develops a characteristic barrel chest—that is, a round, bulging chest with increased anteroposterior diameter. Unlike the blue bloater with chronic bronchitis, the patient with emphysema isn't usually hypoxic or cyanotic, but his expiratory effort does become markedly increased. For this reason, he's called a "pink puffer."

Asthma

Unlike bronchitis and emphysema, asthma is characterized by bronchospasms, caused by infections, hypersensitivity to irritants or psy-

Pathophysiology of bronchial asthma

Bronchial asthma is characterized by smooth muscle spasms which narrow airways. An inflammatory response further narrows airways by engorging blood vessels and swelling mucous glands and goblet cells. Eventually, epithelial denudation of the airway surface and thickening of the basement membrane result. Also, mucous secretions containing neutrophils, eosinophils, Charcot-Leyden crystals, Curschmann's spirals, clusters of epithelial cells, and bacteria or viruses plug the already narrowed airways.

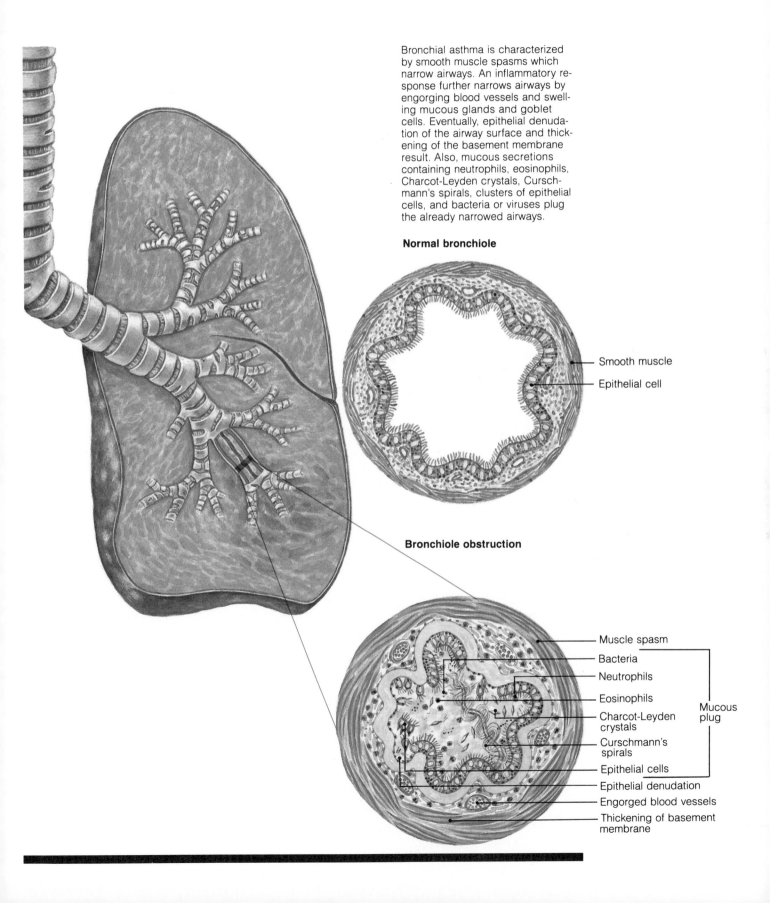

Normal bronchiole

Smooth muscle

Epithelial cell

Bronchiole obstruction

Muscle spasm

Bacteria

Neutrophils

Eosinophils

Charcot-Leyden crystals

Curschmann's spirals

Epithelial cells

Epithelial denudation

Engorged blood vessels

Thickening of basement membrane

Mucous plug

Chronic bronchitis

Because of cyanosis from insufficient arterial oxygenation and edema from right ventricular failure, the patient with chronic bronchitis is often called a "blue bloater" (shown at left).

In bronchitis, partial or complete blockage of the airways from mucous secretions causes insufficient oxygenation in the alveoli.

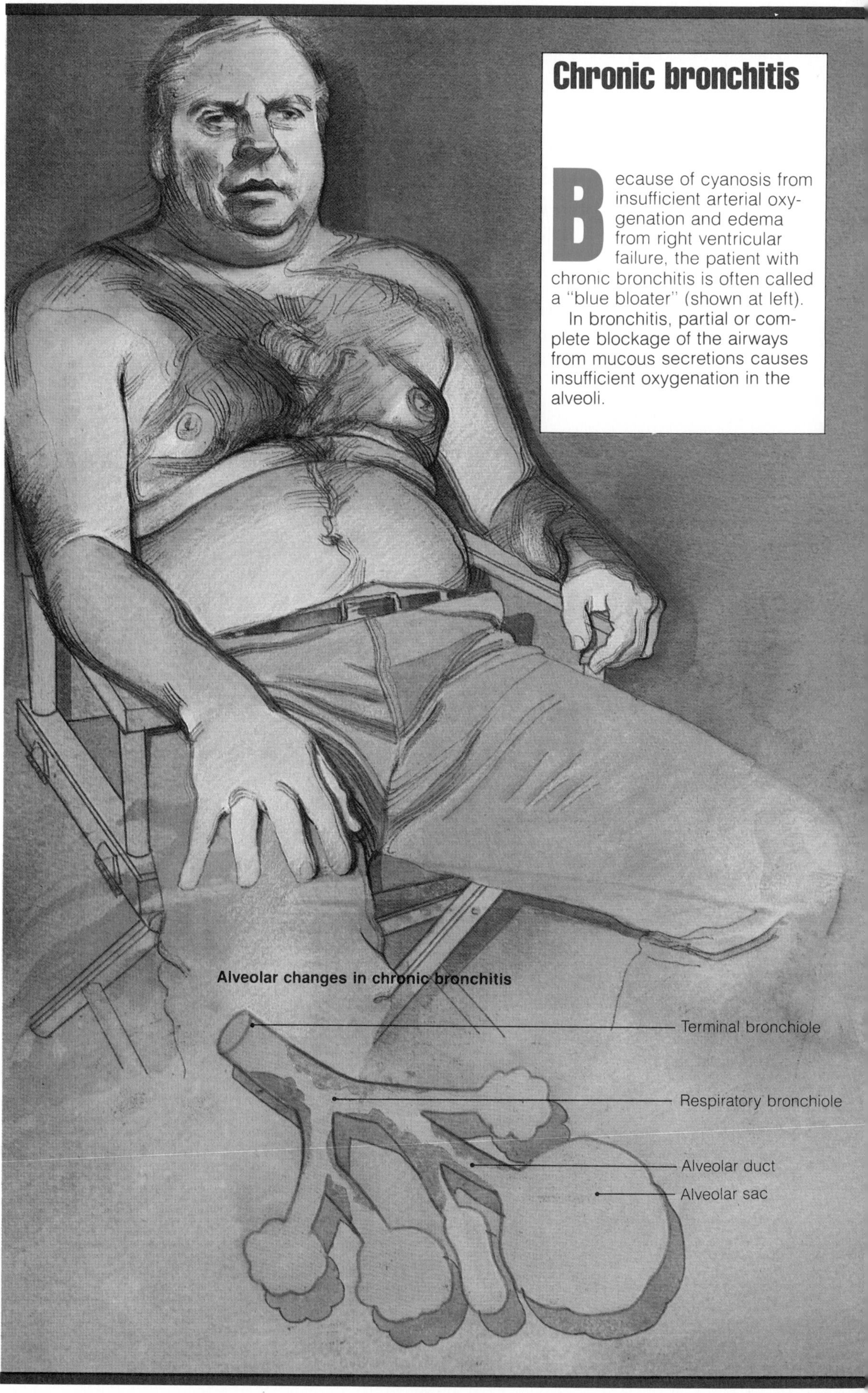

Alveolar changes in chronic bronchitis

Terminal bronchiole

Respiratory bronchiole

Alveolar duct

Alveolar sac

Three types of emphysema

A patient with severe emphysema can usually match ventilation to perfusion, avoiding cyanosis and edema. Because such a patient maintains relatively normal oxygen saturation and a pink color while his expiratory effect increases, he's sometimes called a "pink puffer" (shown at right).

Emphysema may be classified as *centrilobular* (or centriacinar), the most common type, which produces destructive changes in the respiratory bronchiole, usually in the upper portions of the lung; *panlobular* (or panacinar), which produces destructive changes and generalized dilatation of the air spaces in the secondary lobules, usually in the lower portions of the lung; or *paraseptal*, which produces destructive changes in the periphery of the lobule.

Paraseptal emphysema results from any condition that causes scarring or fibrosis in the lungs. Characterized by alveolar wall destruction and alveolar distention adjacent to fibrotic pulmonary lesions, it produces focal air cysts called blebs (lesions <1″ in diameter), bullae (lesions >1″ in diameter), or pneumatoceles.

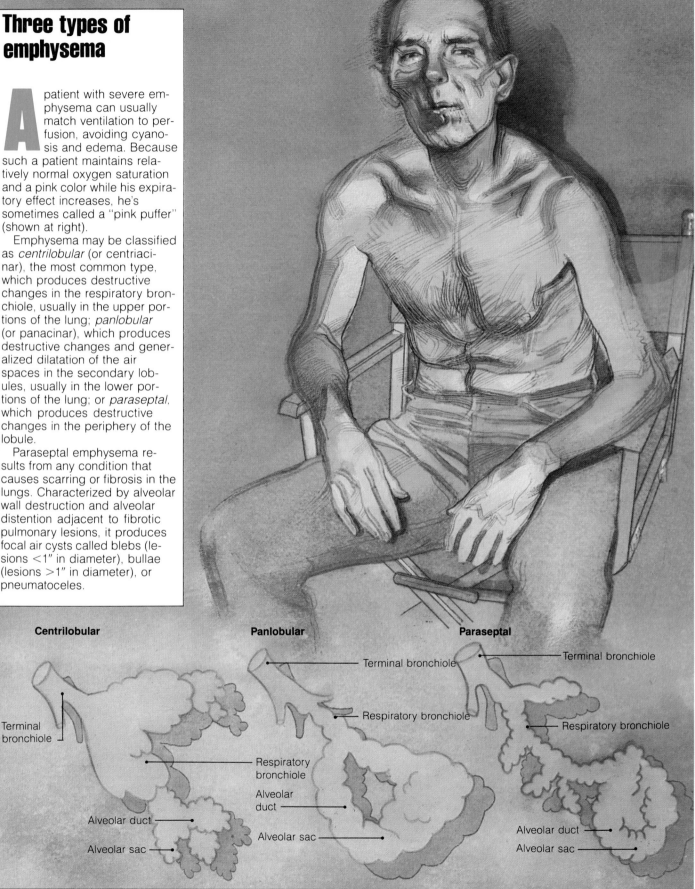

Centrilobular

Terminal bronchiole

Alveolar duct

Alveolar sac

Panlobular

Terminal bronchiole

Respiratory bronchiole

Respiratory bronchiole

Alveolar duct

Alveolar sac

Paraseptal

Terminal bronchiole

Respiratory bronchiole

Alveolar duct

Alveolar sac

Breathing techniques for the COPD patient

To alleviate the COPD patient's breathing difficulty, teach him the techniques of abdominal and pursed-lip breathing. Instruct him to use these techniques during all his activities. Eventually they should become second nature.

Abdominal breathing
• To relax his abdomen, have the patient lie on his back with his knees bent.
• Instruct him to press his hands lightly on his abdomen or place a 2″ (5-cm) phone book on it to create some resistance.
• Now instruct him to breathe abdominally, so that his hands or the book will rise during inspiration and fall during expiration. His chest should remain almost stationary.

Pursed-lip breathing
• Instruct the patient to inhale through his nose to prevent him from gulping air. He should take a normal breath. Taking too large a breath means he'll have to exhale much more.
• Now, instruct him to exhale slowly through pursed lips—tak-ing at least twice the time he took to inhale. He should make a soft, whistling sound when he exhales, which will help him maintain the correct ratio between inhaling and exhaling. Explain to him that exhaling through pursed lips will help him get rid of the stale air trapped in his lungs, whereas rapid, forceful exhalation will only trap more air by causing bronchial collapse.
• Advise him that when using stairs, he should inhale between steps and exhale while climbing. Also advise him to inhale before exertion, such as lifting any object or opening a door, and to exhale while performing the activity.

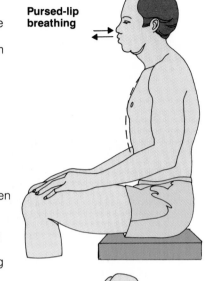

Pursed-lip breathing

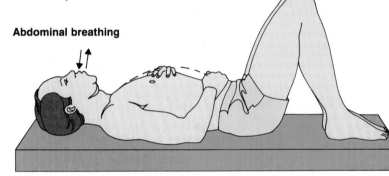

Abdominal breathing

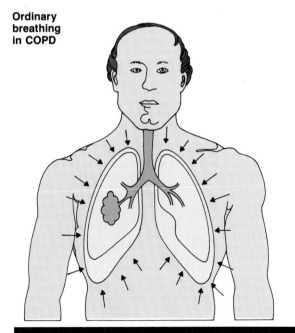

Ordinary breathing in COPD

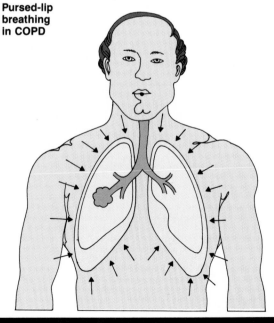

Pursed-lip breathing in COPD

chological stress, exercise, or drug use. The bronchospasms are accompanied by edema, inflammatory cell infiltrates (with many eosinophils), and hypersecretion of mucus. In chronic asthma, the amount of smooth muscle increases, inflammatory cells infiltrate the bronchial wall, the basement membrane thickens, and mucus obstructs many small airways.

As in emphysema, airway obstruction in asthma is worst during expiration. This is manifested by a prolonged expiration time (more than 4 seconds) and wheezing. (However, if the bronchospasm is severe enough to drastically reduce airflow, wheezing may be almost absent.) A productive cough, caused by hypersecretion of mucus, usually accompanies the wheezing. When the eosinophil content rises, sputum may appear purulent. It may also contain Curschmann's spirals (coiled mucinous fibrils) and Charcot-Leyden crystals (breakdown products from eosinophils). If airway obstruction is severe and the patient's fluid intake is low, mucous plugs may harden, rendering the patient's cough ineffective and causing mucoid impaction.

Overinflation of the distal airways increases as an asthmatic attack worsens. Overinflation is caused by premature airway closure, mucosal edema, mucous plugging, and increased exhalation time (from increased airflow resistance). It decreases forced expiratory volume in 1 second (FEV_1) while increasing residual volume and functional residual capacity. This is indicated by decreased diaphragmatic excursion and lateral chest expansion, widened intercostal spaces, hyperresonance, and increased work of breathing. Increased total lung capacity (TLC) is responsible for these findings. Other signs of an asthma attack include flared nostrils, the use of accessory muscles to breathe, sternocleidomastoid retraction, tachypnea, and, in a thin-chested patient, intercostal retractions during inspiration. As airway obstruction becomes more severe, anxiety increases the body's metabolic demands, inducing fatigue and respiratory failure, with mental confusion, systolic hypertension, and if extreme CO_2 elevations are present, asterixis (flapping tremor).

Most of the pathologic effects are reversible. However, chronic and sustained bronchospasms can cause smooth muscle hypertrophy and permanent narrowing of the respiratory tract, causing signs and symptoms like those that occur in emphysema and chronic bronchitis.

Cystic fibrosis
In cystic fibrosis, abnormally thick mucous secretions obstruct ducts in the pancreas, liver, and lungs, leading to trapped air, mucous stasis, and lung infection. When the patient with cystic fibrosis inhales, his airways dilate normally and air flows into the lungs and alveoli for gas exchange. During expiration, however, his airways usually collapse, trapping air and eventually causing barrel chest.

Mucus trapped in the collapsed airways increases obstruction, causing mucous stasis and predisposing the patient to infection. In turn, infection can lead to more mucus production and bronchial wall damage, exacerbating airway obstruction. Continual repetition of this cycle eventually destroys lung tissue. These pulmonary changes may produce tachypnea, chronic cough with mucus production, barrel chest, clubbing of the fingernails and toenails, shortness of breath on exertion, weight loss or failure to gain weight, cyanosis, and eventually fatal pulmonary disease.

Bronchiectasis
In bronchiectasis, chronically enlarged or dilated bronchi follow inflammatory weakening of the bronchial walls. Severely inflamed bronchial walls may produce large quantities of foul-smelling mucopurulent secretions, predisposing the patient to frequent respiratory infections and ultimately obstructing ventilation. The severity of such obstruction depends mainly on the amount of pulmonary tissue involved. Advanced bronchiectasis may cause pneumonia, cor pulmonale, or right ventricular failure.

MEDICAL MANAGEMENT
A detailed history and physical examination (see *Summary of assessment findings,* pages 88 to 89) are essential to a firm diagnosis of COPD. The results of the history and physical examination may then be confirmed by diagnostic tests. But, since onset of COPD is often insidious, early diagnosis is rare.

Diagnostic tests
Chest X-rays. While useful in diagnosing moderate or advanced bronchitis and emphysema, chest X-rays are usually not helpful in confirming bronchiectasis, asthma, or cystic fibrosis. However, bronchography, in which a radiopaque contrast medium is instilled into the tracheobronchial tree, offers a morphologic

Major complications of COPD

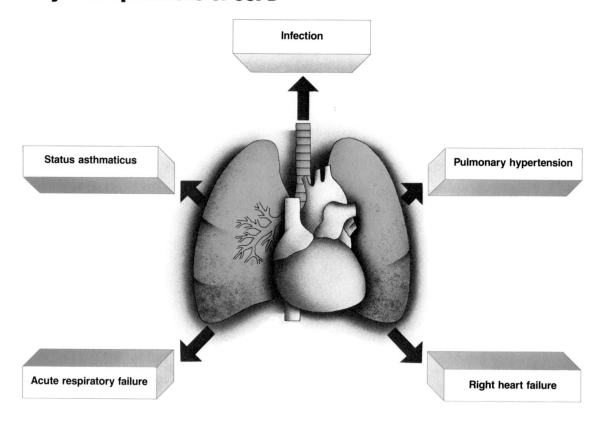

Infection

Status asthmaticus

Pulmonary hypertension

Acute respiratory failure

Right heart failure

Patients with COPD are predisposed to the major complications below. Complications often initiate a progressive cycle of deterioration, sometimes necessitating permanent changes in the patient's lifestyle.

Infection
For example, COPD increases the patient's susceptibility to infection; infection, in turn, further damages lung tissue, thus setting the stage for reinfection, respiratory irritation, and possibly an allergic reaction. The underlying pathophysiology that perpetuates this cycle includes:
• increased mucus formation
• bronchial collapse during expiration, trapping air, mucus, and germs
• ineffective coughing caused by impaired forceful expiration
• narrowed bronchial lumen
• destruction of cilia due to the loss of the body's normal mechanism for cleaning the tracheobronchial tree
• mouth breathing, which dries secretions, making them tena-

cious and difficult to expel
• retained mucus, which fosters the growth of bacteria.

Pulmonary hypertension
Pulmonary hypertension, which results from reduced space in the pulmonary vascular bed, may eventually lead to cor pulmonale. Polycythemia, which occurs in response to hypoxia, contributes to pulmonary hypertension by increased blood viscosity. That, in turn, increases the work of the heart and causes venous distention.

Right heart failure
Right heart failure (characterized by peripheral edema and venous distention) may occur in advanced COPD.

Acute respiratory failure
COPD caused by emphysema—particularly advanced emphysema—may result in severe respiratory impairment. Deficient cerebral oxygenation and elevated $PaCO_2$ levels may then produce alterations in level of consciousness, possibly leading to coma. Progression of respira-

tory impairment may be fatal.

Status asthmaticus
Status asthmaticus is a prolonged asthmatic attack that doesn't respond to usual therapy. The patient who develops this complication is usually apprehensive, pale, breathless, and exhausted from fighting for air. Other signs of this condition include tachycardia, dehydration, or wheezing (or sometimes a silent chest from mucous plugs constricting or blocking the airways). Often, the patient uses the accessory muscles of respirations so that his expirations will be active and prolonged.

Despite hypoxemia, the $PaCO_2$ level of this patient is usually normal because he compensates by hyperventilating and partially because carbon dioxide diffuses readily through the bloodstream. However, his $PaCO_2$ level may increase if he's exhausted and approaching respiratory failure. Carbon dioxide retention and accumulation of lactic acid may cause his pH to fall.

diagnosis of bronchiectasis and also shows the extent of involvement.

In moderate to advanced bronchitis, chest X-rays may show a narrow cardiac silhouette with a vertical axis and right ventricular hypertrophy secondary to pulmonary hypertension. Also, thickened bronchial walls (indicated by parallel lines) and increased bronchovascular markings may be apparent.

In emphysema, chest X-rays reflect hyperinflation of the lungs by showing an increased retrosternal airspace and a flat or scalloped diaphragm. Less specific indications of hyperinflation are a low-lying diaphragm, hyperlucent lung fields, increased intercostal spaces, and an increased anteroposterior diameter. In emphysema specifically, chest X-rays also show irregular patches of lucency and vascular changes, such as prominent hila with diminished peripheral vessels and a "pruned" vascular tree (caused by the loss of visible distal divisions).

Electrocardiography. In moderate to advanced COPD, the patient's EKG is often abnormal, showing atrial or ventricular dysrhythmias in the presence of secondary pulmonary hypertension, hypoxia, or respiratory acidosis. About one half of hospitalized COPD patients show dysrhythmias, most commonly atrial tachycardia or multifocal atrial tachycardia. Other EKG abnormalities—tall, peaked P waves; a shift to the right of the P-wave axis; and evidence of right ventricular hypertrophy—reflect secondary pulmonary hypertension. In the absence of conduction defects, right ventricular hypertrophy is shown by any combination of an S_1-Q_3 pattern, an S_1-S_2-S_3 pattern, an R/S ratio in V_6 less than 1:1, or right axis deviation greater than 110°.

Blood tests. In mixed COPD or chronic bronchitis, a *complete blood count* may show increased hemoglobin and hematocrit levels, reflecting secondary polycythemia from hypoxemia, stress, or diuretic therapy. With superimposed bacterial infection, leukocytes may be elevated; in acute allergic asthma, eosinophils may be present.

Since *arterial blood gas (ABG) analysis* reflects the extent of airway obstruction, the results will vary according to the patient's clinical status and the duration of illness. In chronic bronchitis, emphysema secondary to chronic bronchitis, bronchiectasis, cystic fibrosis, and severe asthma attacks, because of ventilation-perfusion mismatching, the patient's PaO_2 is decreased and his $PaCO_2$ is elevated. In emphysema that is not secondary to chronic bronchitis and in mild to moderate asthma attacks, the results of ABG analysis may be normal because of compensatory hyperventilation.

Sputum analysis. When a superimposed bacterial infection is present, culture and sensitivity tests on sputum may identify the infecting organism. This test may also help determine the most effective antibiotic to use in treating the infection.

Pulmonary function tests. The results of these tests vary according to the underlying disease. In the early stages of chronic bronchitis, routine pulmonary function tests are usually normal. Eventually, however, forced expiratory flow rates decrease, as does peak expiratory flow. Maximal voluntary ventilation also decreases.

In moderate to advanced emphysema, total lung capacity (TLC) and residual volume (RV) increase as a result of air trapped in distended alveoli. Because the patient takes longer to exhale, FEV_1 and the forced vital capacity (FVC) decrease.

Peak flow and FEV_1 are valuable in diagnosing and assessing asthma because they can be easily reproduced and provide reliable indications of airway obstruction. During an acute asthma attack, the FEV_1 decreases, but FVC remains normal. The ratio of FEV_1 to FVC thus decreases. Expiratory flow rates at low lung volumes decrease markedly.

After an acute asthma attack, spirometric values (FEV_1 and forced expiratory flow between 25% and 75% of vital capacity) remain abnormal. Abnormally high residual volume may persist up to 3 weeks after an attack.

Additional tests for cystic fibrosis. Elevated electrolyte concentrations (specifically sodium and chloride) in the perspiration of a patient with pulmonary disease or pancreatic insufficiency confirm cystic fibrosis. Microscopic examination of duodenal contents for pancreatic enzymes and stools for trypsin can confirm pancreatic insufficiency; trypsin is absent in over 80% of children with cystic fibrosis.

Treatment

Treatment of COPD is designed to help the patient maintain optimal breathing function and activity level. The key to successful treatment is avoiding bronchopulmonary irritants, especially during exacerbations of respiratory symptoms. Above all, the patient should avoid smoking, which contributes to bronchospasm, mucus production, decreased ciliary motion, and elevated carboxyhemoglobin levels. Other goals of COPD therapy include relieving airway obstruction with drug therapy, providing adequate arterial oxygenation, reducing coughing and sputum production, treating infections, preventing complications, managing acute respiratory insufficiency and, for asthma, preventing acute attacks.

Avoiding bronchopulmonary irritants. Avoiding bronchopulmonary irritants, particularly cigarette smoking, is essential in preventing complications and exacerbations of COPD. The patient who quits smoking cigarettes will often reduce his coughing and sputum production. Other bronchopulmonary irritants include occupational exposure to dusts and fumes, extreme heat or cold, environmental air pollution, and house dust. The asthmatic patient especially should try to keep his house, particularly his bedroom, as dust-free as possible. The patient who suffers from occupational exposure to dusts and fumes may have to consider changing jobs. If COPD is related to environmental air pollution, the patient should avoid exercise outdoors and, when possible, should stay indoors.

Avoiding such precipitating factors as stress or allergens, as well as bronchopulmonary irritants, is particularly important for the patient with asthma. When stress is the precipitating factor, relaxation techniques or tranquilizers may help prevent asthma attacks. When specific allergens are known to precipitate asthmatic attacks, desensitization may help some patients, but most asthma patients probably would not benefit from this form of therapy.

Besides avoiding bronchopulmonary irritants, all COPD patients need to minimize the risk of contracting respiratory infection. This is important because respiratory infection can lead to acute respiratory insufficiency. The COPD patient should avoid crowds during the cold-and-influenza season and should receive an annual immunization for influenza.

Drug therapy. Drug therapy for COPD consists primarily of oral bronchodilators, adrenergic agonists, and steroids. Oral bronchodilators—specifically theophylline or other xanthines—are typically used to manage airway obstruction. Adrenergic agonists—especially selective $beta_2$ agents (such as terbutaline and albuterol)—serve as bronchodilators and facilitate mucus transport. Their use is frequently limited, however, because of side effects (such as tremors) that may occur

at therapeutic dosages. As an alternative, $beta_2$-adrenergic agonists (metaproterenol sulfate, for example) are often administered by hand-bulb nebulizers, propeller-driven nebulizers, or intermittent positive-pressure breathing (IPPB). However, IPPB isn't always the most effective method for delivering medication to the airways.

IPPB therapy with saline, detergents, or mucolytics does little good. It may even be harmful since these agents may induce rather than relieve bronchospasms. The use of oral expectorants is also questionable. Anticholinergics, such as atropine, used to be contraindicated in the treatment of COPD because of their adverse effect on sputum viscosity. But recent research suggests inhalant anticholinergics may be helpful for some asthmatic patients with COPD.

Other widely used drugs—such as cough suppressants, sedatives, and hypnotic agents—not only promise little benefit, but can actually cause respiratory depression in patients with severe chronic bronchitis, particularly those with hypercapnia. Cough suppressants may lead to retention of pulmonary secretions, with resultant worsening of hypoxia and hypercapnia. This in turn can cause central nervous system depression.

Corticosteroids can sometimes be helpful in the treatment of COPD. When used with bronchodilators, parenteral corticosteroids have been shown to improve FEV_1 in hospitalized patients with chronic bronchitis. Also, oral corticosteroids used with bronchodilators may improve FEV_1 in some stable outpatients. However, the long-term use of corticosteroids in chronically ill patients can cause many side effects. Often, these side effects can be minimized with alternate-day therapy, which doesn't reduce the therapeutic effect.

Steroids can also be administered in aerosol form, the drug of choice being beclomethasone. Such topical administration delivers the anti-inflammatory agent directly to the bronchial wall. When used in therapeutic doses, this form of steroid administration has no systemic side effects but may cause thrush.

When COPD is complicated by infection, antibiotic therapy is necessary. Though ampicillin and tetracycline are the most commonly administered antibiotics, culture and sensitivity testing may be done to ensure effective drug therapy.

An acute asthma attack also requires specialized drug therapy. Traditionally, acute asthma attacks have always been treated ini-

Domestic bronchopulmonary irritants

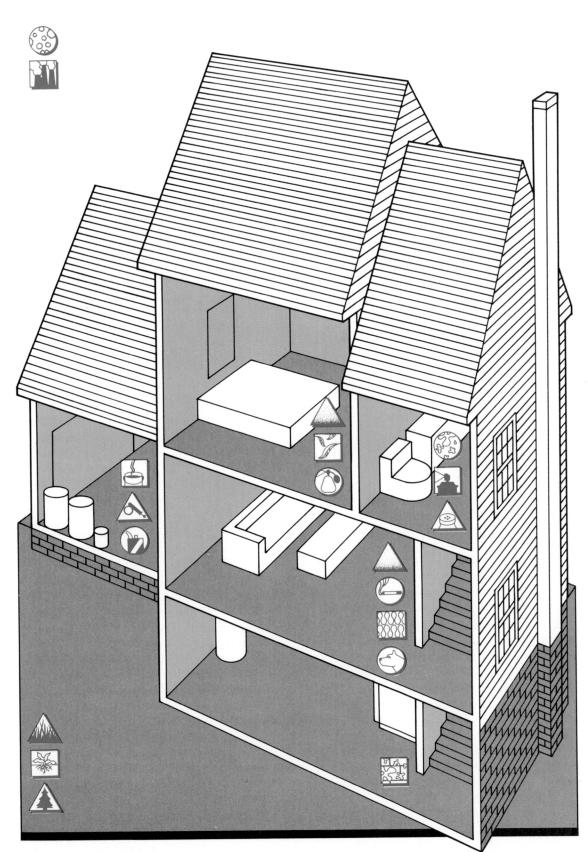

Key:

Bedroom

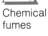 Dust

 Feathers

 Perfume

Bathroom

 Molds

 Powder

 Aerosol sprays

Living room

 Furniture stuffing

 Animal hair

 Tobacco smoke

 Dust

Garage

 Paint fumes

 Chemical fumes

 Gasoline fumes

Basement

 Mold

Outside

 Pollens

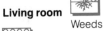 Weeds

 Trees

 Grasses

 Industrial pollutants

 Dust

tially with serial injections of adrenergic agents (such as epinephrine or terbutaline), administered subcutaneously. If broncho-spasms persist, parenteral methylxanthines (such as aminophylline) may have to be administered. Treatment may have to include oxygen administration, hydration, and aerosolized bronchodilators, particularly if the patient also has hypertension, coronary artery disease, or dysrhythmia. Two other possible treatments—both controversial—are IPPB and tranquilizers. If the above treatments fail to relieve bronchospasms, parenteral steroid therapy and hospitalization may be required.

Chest physiotherapy. This form of treatment, which includes postural drainage and chest percussion, may help to loosen and raise thick, viscous secretions in the COPD patient, clearing the airways and improving ventilation. In a patient with cystic fibrosis or bronchiectasis, this is the primary form of treatment, repeated several times a day. Chest physiotherapy is also important in patients with decreased cough and severe debilitation. Before postural drainage, preparatory treatments—such as the use of mist tents, bronchodilators, or decongestant aerosols—can mobilize secretions to facilitate their removal.

Oxygen therapy. This may be necessary in moderate to severe COPD when arterial oxyhemoglobin is significantly reduced. Oxygen may be used to provide total ventilatory support, or to counteract breathlessness or hypoxemia only during exercise. Oxygen is usually administered continuously by nasal cannula at 1 to 2 liters/minute. (A higher rate can be harmful to the patient with emphysema, because he depends on a rising $PaCO_2$ level to trigger breathing.) Continuous administration is expensive, however, and patient compliance often sporadic. As an alternative, oxygen may be administered for 12 to 16 hours daily. This reduced regimen may help prevent cor pulmonale, pulmonary hypertension, secondary polycythemia, nocturnal hypoxemia, and dysrhythmia.

NURSING MANAGEMENT
Begin your assessment of the COPD patient with a carefully detailed history. Remember that while most COPD patients complain of coughing and dyspnea, many patients with mild forms of the disease are asymptomatic or have symptoms they think aren't significant, so they fail to mention them. That's why it's a good idea to ask the patient's family the same questions you ask him.

To start with, ask the patient and his family:
• Does he smoke? If so, obtain a smoking history in pack years.
• Does he cough? Does the cough produce sputum? What does the sputum look like? When did the cough begin? What time of day does it occur? Does it worsen at any particular time?

A chronic productive cough usually develops insidiously, beginning most often in middle age. Coughing is often worse in the morning because secretions accumulate during the night. The patient's sputum is usually clear, but it may become mucopurulent or purulent if an infection develops. In bronchiectasis, sputum is usually copious and three-layered—pus on the bottom, saliva in the center, and mucus on the top. In pulmonary emphysema, the patient's cough may be nonproductive. It usually precedes development of exertional dyspnea and may exist for years without significant respiratory impairment.

Next, ask the patient and his family:
• Does he ever experience breathlessness?
• Does breathlessness worsen at any time of day or with any particular activity? Does it limit his activities?
• Does he have difficulty breathing when lying down?

Dyspnea is common in COPD patients, but many patients may attribute it to aging or obesity. Dyspnea often worsens during acute bronchitis attacks, as well as in the morning, in high humidity or altitudes, and after large meals.

You may have trouble differentiating dyspnea caused by COPD from dyspnea caused by heart disease, especially in an elderly patient. A patient with severe COPD, hiatal hernia, or gastric reflux with chronic aspiration may have paroxysmal nocturnal dyspnea.
• Does the patient's work expose him to respiratory irritants? Did the patient experience such exposure in the past?

Explore the patient's susceptibility to allergies. Ask him and his family:
• Are his symptoms constant or episodic?
• Does he have a history of nasal allergies? Does his family have a history of allergies?
• Was he exposed recently to a specific allergen, a nonspecific respiratory irritant, or unusual emotional stress? If the patient suffered an acute asthmatic episode, did he take aspirin or indomethacin before his attack?

Ask the patient and his family about other diseases, past or present, which could be

Improving nebulizer technique

To benefit from nebulizer treatments, your patient must administer an adequate concentration of the medication to his bronchial receptors. Because his rate and depth of inhalation and the positioning of the nebulizer affect the concentration administered, you'll want to make sure he uses the right technique to maximize the benefits of these treatments.

Begin by teaching the patient to hold the nebulizer about 2″ away from his open mouth. He should then tilt his head back slightly. This will help ensure that the medication penetrates deep into his airways.

Now instruct the patient to exhale normally, then to inhale deeply and slowly for about 5 seconds while holding down the top of the metal canister. The concentration of the medication that'll reach his lungs after a deep, slow inhalation is much greater than the concentration he'd receive after a quick inhalation lasting only 1 or 2 seconds (see illustration). A deep, slow inhalation allows more medication to reach the small airways; it also helps the lungs to retain the medication.

To prevent the patient from exhaling medication that would otherwise reach his lungs, tell him to hold his breath for 3 to 5 seconds after inhaling. If a second inhalation is needed, he should allow 5 to 10 minutes for the first dose to take effect before repeating the procedure.

After the treatment, he should clean the nebulizer thoroughly. Tell him to first remove the metal canister by pulling it up firmly. Then he should rinse the plastic container under warm running water and dry it thoroughly.

Note: If the patient takes both a bronchodilator (such as metaproterenol) and a corticosteroid (such as beclomethasone), he should always take the bronchodilator first. This will dilate the airways so the corticosteroid can be inhaled more deeply into the lungs.

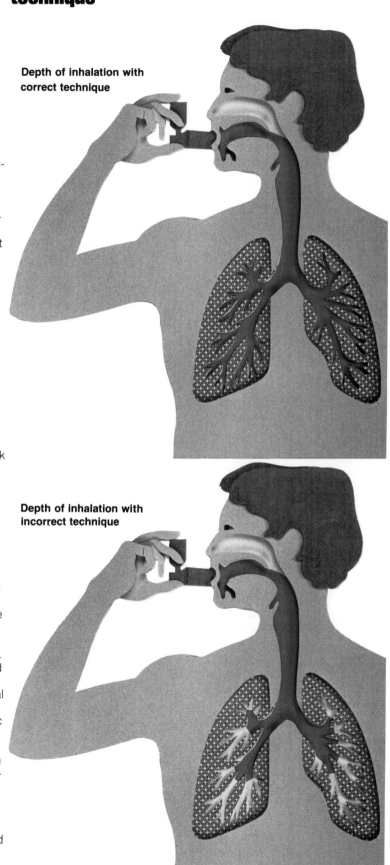

Depth of inhalation with correct technique

Depth of inhalation with incorrect technique

Summary of assessment findings

Assessment method	Chronic bronchitis	Emphysema
History	• Long-term cigarette smoking • Long-term exposure to air pollutants • Productive cough (with clear sputum) that worsens in morning • Gradual onset of shortness of breath	• Long-term cigarette smoking • Long-term exposure to air pollutants • Nonproductive cough • Progressive shortness of breath leading to dyspnea on exertion • Recent weight loss
Inspection	• Cyanosis and edema ("blue bloater") • Digital clubbing (in later stages) • Tachypnea • Use of accessory muscles to breathe • Occasional intercostal retractions • In advanced stages, patient sits leaning forward, hands on thighs • Decreased diaphragmatic excursion	• Prolonged, labored expirations, without cyanosis or edema ("pink puffer") • Use of accessory muscles to breathe • Digital clubbing (in later stages) • Decreased chest expansion • In advanced stages, patient sits leaning forward, hands on thighs
Auscultation	• Normal breath sounds • Fine to coarse rales; clear after coughing, wheezing, and/or rhonchi • Prolonged expiration	• Decreased breath sounds • Fine rales at bases and occasional wheezing, rhonchi • Prolonged expiration
Percussion	• Dull or flat sounds over areas of mucous plugging • Resonant sounds	• Hyperresonance
Palpation	• Normal voice sounds and fremitus • Decreased diaphragmatic excursion	• Decreased vocal and breath sounds and tactile fremitus • Decreased diaphragmatic excursion

confused with COPD. Also, ask if anyone else in the family has COPD.
• Has the patient ever had chronic interstitial pneumonitis or fibrosis, recurrent pulmonary thromboembolism, polycythemia vera, myxedema, or obesity-hyperventilation syndrome?
• Has he ever had any disease or condition (such as laryngeal disease) or undergone any procedure (such as tracheostomy or prolonged endotracheal intubation) that could cause extrathoracic airway obstruction?

Ask the patient about nonrespiratory symptoms. For example:
• Does he experience aerophagia (swallowing of air), gastric distention, or early satiety? Does he have a peptic ulcer (20% to 25% of COPD patients do)?
• Does he experience decreased mental ability, memory, or judgment? Has he been irritable lately? Does he have headaches, insomnia, drowsiness, confusion, or tremors? All these symptoms develop quickly with acute changes in pH or ABGs.

Explore the patient's chief complaint:
• Does he suffer from unusual fatigue, anterior chest pain, and palpitations on exertion (all signs of cor pulmonale)?
• Does he suffer from ankle edema, increased epigastric fullness, and upper abdominal aching (possible signs of right ventricular failure)?

Conduct the physical examination
After taking the patient's history, begin the physical examination by noting the patient's overall appearance. The COPD patient usually

Asthma	Bronchiectasis	Cystic fibrosis
• Allergic predispositon • Attack precipitated by exposure to allergen, emotional stress, or ingestion of aspirin or indomethacin • Dyspnea during attack	• Frequent respiratory infections • History of cystic fibrosis or cancer • Frequent, productive cough with copious, foul-smelling sputum • Hemoptysis	• Family history of cystic fibrosis • Productive cough (with copious sputum) • Shortness of breath on exertion • Weight loss or failure to gain weight
During attack: • Dyspnea • Tachypnea • Patient sits leaning forward, hands on thighs • Intercostal retractions during inspiration; intercostal bulging during expiration • Use of accessory muscles (especially abdomen and neck) to breathe • Flaring nostrils • Cyanosis *Chronic:* • Digital clubbing	• Cyanosis • Dyspnea • Digital clubbing	• Barrel chest • Cyanosis • Digital clubbing
During attack: • Wheezing and rhonchi; "silent chest" in severe attack • Unequal breath sounds over chest • Tachycardia • Paradoxical pulse	• Fine rales and coarse rhonchi	• Fine rales and coarse rhonchi
• Hyperresonance	• Dull or flat sounds over areas of mucous plugging	• Hyperresonance • Dull or flat sounds over areas of mucous plugging
• Decreased vocal and tactile fremitus • Decreased diaphragmatic excursion	• Increased vocal and tactile fremitus over middle and lower lobes • Decreased diaphragmatic excursion	• Decreased vocal and tactile fremitus • Decreased diaphragmatic excursion

sits in a characteristic posture—leaning forward with his hands on his thighs to help elevate his rib cage and facilitate expiration. On inspection, look for:

• *barrel chest*, which is common in COPD patients because of air trapped in the lungs. With barrel chest, the anteroposterior diameter of the chest increases. The angle between the ribs and the sternum and vertebrae also increases from 45° to 90°.

• *increased respiratory rate*, which occurs as the COPD patient tries to compensate for airway resistance. As lung compliance and the amount of trapped air increase, expirations become prolonged and labored and often require use of accessory muscles. Also, increased inspiratory resistance to airflow with decreased lung compliance may cause intercostal retractions during inspiration.

• *cyanosis and edema*, which result from arterial hypoxemia due to a severe ventilation-perfusion mismatch. In advanced COPD, these symptoms (which characterize the blue bloater) appear with clubbed fingers. Cyanosis and edema are common in severe bronchitis that is accompanied by arterial hypoxemia, in secondary erythrocytosis, and in cor pulmonale with right ventricular failure. The blue bloater's edema may progress to anasarca; usually, he'll have neck vein distention and hepatojugular reflex, too. The patient with severe emphysema (the pink puffer) can usually match ventilation to perfusion so he doesn't develop cyanosis and edema.

On auscultation, listen for:

• *decreased breath sounds*, which result from

Relieving gastrointestinal problems of cystic fibrosis

If your patient's problem is *decreased absorption of fats and proteins:*
• Instruct the patient's family to give him a diet that is high in carbohydrates, high in proteins, and low in fats.
• Teach the parents to mix supplemental pancreatic enzymes with carbohydrates, not with proteins, since the enzymes would immediately break down proteins. To facilitate absorption of fats and proteins, instruct the parents to give the enzymes at the beginning of a meal. To avoid skin breakdown, caution the parents not to let the enzymes remain on the child's lips or skin.

If your patient's problem is *decreased absorption of fat-soluble vitamins and iron:*
• Instruct the parents to give their child twice the usual dosage of fat-soluble vitamins. To facilitate absorption of these vitamins, they should give one dose of vitamins at breakfast and one at dinner. And since the supplemental pancreatic enzymes the patient will be taking decrease iron absorption, advise the parents to give iron supplements daily.

If your patient's problem is *frequent, foul-smelling stools:*
• Instruct the parents to increase the child's normal dosage of supplemental pancreatic enzymes if a greasy meal can't be avoided.

If your patient's problem is *diarrhea:*
• Rule out other causes of diarrhea unrelated to cystic fibrosis.
• Instruct the parents to decrease the child's usual dosage of supplemental pancreatic enzymes. If the child is being maintained on the same diet, advise the parents not to change the dosage more than once every 24 hours.

Note: Verify these recommendations with the patient's doctor before instructing the family.

decreased airflow, particularly in the lung bases. Decreased airflow may be caused by mucus accumulation or bronchospasm. If the airway is severely obstructed, you won't hear any breath sounds at all ("silent chest"). This finding may result from a severe asthma attack, for example.
• *fine and coarse rales*, which are common in COPD patients. Fine rales result from reinflation of collapsed alveoli. Coarse rales, which result from fluid accumulating in the airways, sometimes clear after the patient coughs. That'll help move accumulated fluid into the larger airways, where it can be expelled.
• *rhonchi and wheezing*, which occur with partial obstruction. Rhonchi may be diffuse or localized over the affected area.
• *changed heart position*—specifically, a vertical position behind the sternum. Air-filled lungs, interposed between the chest and heart wall, may make auscultation difficult. You'll hear the apical impulse and other heart sounds best in the subxiphoid area.
• *tachycardia*, which is a compensatory response to poor tissue oxygenation.
• *loud pulmonary closure sound*, which results from pulmonary hypertension.
• *right-sided gallop*, which may result from right ventricular failure.

On palpation and percussion, you'll find:
• *decreased vocal and tactile fremitus*, which results from lung hyperinflation.
• *decreased diaphragmatic excursion*, which results from trapped air and lung hyperinflation.
• *altered sounds*—that is, hyperresonant sounds over areas of trapped air and dull, flat sounds over areas of mucoid impaction.

Nursing diagnosis and intervention

After assessment, the data you've gathered will help you determine correct nursing diagnoses, which lead to realistic nursing goals and appropriate interventions. The following characteristic nursing diagnoses are related to appropriate nursing goals and interventions.

Impaired gas exchange related to inadequate airflow into and out of the alveoli. Your goal is *to maintain adequate tissue oxygenation.* To accomplish this, administer drugs and oxygen, as ordered. Administer supplementary oxygen at low flow rates, as ordered. Make sure the initial rate doesn't exceed 1 to 2 liters/minute nasally. Higher levels of PO_2 could depress the patient's respiratory drive and cause CO_2 narcosis. Remember that the COPD patient's respiratory impairment often results

from inability to exhale carbon dioxide, not from insufficient oxygen. The patient thus depends on a rising PCO_2 level to stimulate respiration. Monitor ABG levels during oxygen administration. The doctor may change the initial oxygen flow rate according to ABG results. Make sure the patient's PO_2 levels remain between 50 to 60 mm Hg and his oxygen saturation near 100%.

To cleanse and dilate the tracheobronchial tree, administer drugs by small-volume nebulizer or IPPB machine, as ordered. Prescribed drugs may include aerosolized bronchodilators or mucolytics, wetting agents, detergents, expectorants, antibiotics, and steroids.

To prevent exacerbations of COPD, encourage the patient to avoid bronchopulmonary irritants, particularly smoking, and to avoid exposure to infection, air pollution, high altitudes, and environments that are very hot or very cold. You'll know your interventions have been successful when the patient shows signs of adequate tissue oxygenation without complications or exacerbations.

Ineffective airway clearance related to copious mucoid secretions in the bronchi and inability to effectively expectorate mucus. Your goals are *to decrease bronchial secretions, to effectively drain mucus from the airways, and to provide adequate humidification of secretions.* To achieve these goals, administer drugs, as ordered, and perform chest physiotherapy.

Administer bronchodilators and mucolytics by small-volume nebulizer or IPPB machine to thin secretions and facilitate drainage. Antibiotics and steroids may also be ordered to reduce infection and inflammation, which will further decrease secretions.

Perform chest physiotherapy to help raise secretions into the larger airways and facilitate expectoration. Encourage the patient to cough and perform deep-breathing exercises, which will also help to mobilize secretions and clear the airways. Warn the patient, however, to avoid forceful, nonproductive coughing, which could irritate the tracheobronchial tree. If chest physiotherapy, coughing, and deep breathing fail to clear the airways, you may have to suction them. You'll know your interventions have been successful when the patient's cough is productive, breath sounds are present in all lobes, and he shows signs of adequate tissue oxygenation.

Ineffective breathing patterns related to increased lung compliance and trapped air. Your goal is *to increase the amount of air ex-*

PATIENT-TEACHING AID

Relaxation exercises

Dear _____

If you have difficulty falling asleep, try the following relaxation exercises. Breathe slowly, inhaling through your nose and exhaling *completely* through pursed lips, when you perform these exercises. You should take longer to exhale than to inhale.

Head rolls

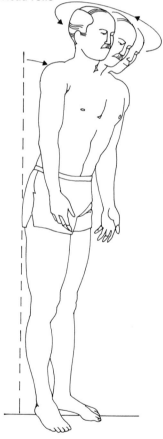

Shoulder rolls

Arm swings

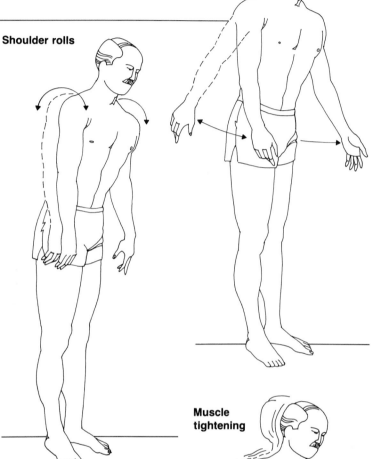

Muscle tightening

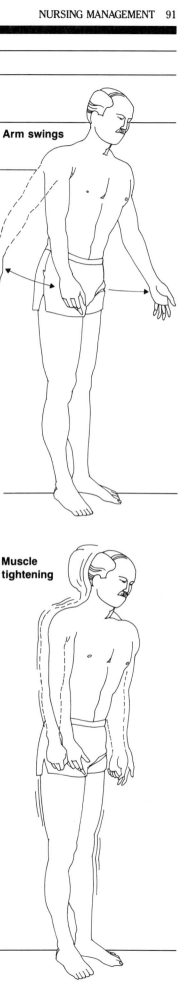

Head rolls: Slowly roll your head to the left and around to the right in a circular pattern. Inhale as you roll your head from left to right; exhale as you roll your head from right to left.

Shoulder rolls: Roll your shoulders backward and forward in time with your breathing. Inhale as you roll your shoulders backward; exhale as you roll your shoulders forward.

Arm swings: Swing your arms backward and forward in time with your breathing. Inhale as you swing your arms forward; exhale as you swing your arms backward.

Muscle tightening: Tighten all your muscles from head to toe while inhaling. Relax the muscles while exhaling.

pired from the patient's lungs. To achieve this goal, teach the patient effective breathing techniques, such as abdominal and pursed-lip breathing (see *Breathing techniques for the COPD patient,* page 80). To make these techniques beneficial, the patient must use them during daily activities. He must also perform supplementary exercises to maintain good muscle tone. Assure the patient that as he learns to control his breathing, he'll reduce the breathlessness brought on by anxiety.

Before teaching the patient abdominal and pursed-lip breathing, help him clear his respiratory tract. Suction if necessary, or stimulate productive coughing by first giving aerosol treatments to open his air passages and loosen tenacious mucus. Or you can use postural drainage to loosen secretions. Also, have the patient clear his nasal passages by blowing his nose. Some patients may benefit from a nasal decongestant.

After you've taught the patient abdominal and pursed-lip breathing, observe him carefully to ensure that he's practicing these techniques correctly. Double-check by assessing the patient for increased forced vital capacity.

Activity intolerance related to shortness of breath on exertion. Your goal is *to increase exercise tolerance and thus enhance the patient's well-being and self-esteem.* To achieve this goal, emphasize the importance of progressive exercise in achieving physical and mental wellness. Progressive exercise improves exercise tolerance by stimulating muscle tissue to make better use of the oxygen available for tissue metabolism. Remind the patient to use correct breathing techniques while exercising.

Fear of inducing respiratory failure by engaging in physical activity often compels the COPD patient to lead a more sedentary life than necessary. Discourage this notion as much as possible. Tell the patient to avoid too much bed rest. Encourage him to walk at least 15 to 20 minutes a day. (For the patient with severe COPD, suggest that he start out with 2- to 5-minute daily walks. Walking is particularly beneficial since it stimulates deep breathing and coughing.

Modify the suggested exercise program to fit the patient's life-style and environment. Make sure the exercise goals you set for the patient are realistic. You'll know your interventions have been successful if you see a noticeable improvement in the patient's exercise tolerance.

Knowledge deficit related to COPD and its treatment. Your goal is *to increase the patient's understanding of COPD.* To achieve this goal, make sure he understands the importance of avoiding bronchopulmonary irritants. Help the patient understand how and why specific irritants affect him as they do. Teach appropriate breathing techniques, and help the patient establish a progressive exercise program. Advise the patient to rest between activities to minimize fatigue. To reduce depression associated with inactivity and dependence on others, remind the patient to focus on the activities still available to him. To evaluate your interventions, assess the patient's knowledge of COPD and its treatment, as well as his use of breathing techniques and progressive exercise.

Sleep pattern disturbance related to anxiety about breathing. Your goal is *to improve the patient's sleep pattern.* To achieve this goal, encourage the patient to establish a consistent bedtime. Suggest that he keep a night table by his bed so he can have a lamp or flashlight, a box of tissues, an aerosol device, a glass of water, and perhaps a radio handy. A glass of water is particularly important if the patient requires oxygen, which can dry his mouth. In cold weather, if the patient's home has central heating, suggest a humidifier to eliminate dry air and increase patient comfort. If the patient tends to awaken during the night, suggest that he not lie there worrying about not sleeping but that he read for a while, or get out of bed and engage in some other light activity, until he feels sleepy again.

The patient may sleep more comfortably with his head elevated. Suggest that he use a wedge pillow under his regular pillow to elevate his neck or shoulders. To ensure a comfortable temperature throughout the night, the patient should use lightweight bedcovers, which can be easily pulled up or folded down.

To induce relaxation before bedtime, the patient may want to follow a standard routine of reading, listening to music, performing relaxation exercises (see *Relaxation exercises,* page 91), or drinking warm milk. (Milk contains the amino acid L-tryptophan, a precursor of serotonin, which is thought to induce sleep.) To check the effectiveness of your patient teaching, ask the patient if his sleep pattern has improved, and observe him to see if he looks well-rested.

Anxiety related to dyspnea. Acute exacerbations of COPD or advanced stages of the disease can understandably induce profound anxiety. Your goal is *to decrease anxiety.* To achieve this goal during an acute attack, reassure the patient continuously and explain the various treatments that will relieve his breathlessness.

If dyspnea and shortness of breath are chronic, however, you must realize that much of the patient's anxiety will stem from drastic impairments in life-style, such as changes in his occupational or financial status. To help decrease anxiety in these patients, try to identify the life-style changes that distress him the most so you can try to help him cope with them. Talk to him about his family to learn how these life-style changes are affecting them. The family may respond with rejection or overprotection. Evaluate the various relationships within the family, and encourage the patient and other family members to talk about their problems. If appropriate, recommend a patient support group in your hostial or in his community. To assess the effectiveness of your interventions, observe the patient to see if he seems less anxious and distressed. Also, try to determine whether the patient and his family are coping effectively.

Inadequate nutrition related to a change in appetite or problems in food metabolism. Nutritional problems—such as weight loss, muscle wasting, or anorexia—are common in patients with severe COPD, especially those with emphysema. Your goal is *to promote adequate nutrition.* To achieve this goal, instruct the patient to eat small, frequent meals with high-calorie and high-protein supplements. Eating small, frequent meals can relieve abdominal distention and shortness of breath that commonly develop after meals. For the same reason, advise the patient to avoid all gas-forming foods.

Two other problems related to nutrition are obesity and constipation. Obesity may occur in patients with chronic bronchitis because of their sedentary life-style and because of steroid therapy, which causes these patients to overeat. To minimize the dangers of this complication, teach the patient with chronic bronchitis to maintain a low-calorie diet. In the patient with COPD, constipation can have serious effects, as distention within the GI tract can elevate the diaphragm and restrict breathing. To prevent this problem, teach the patient to eat foods that are high in fiber, to ensure adequate fluid intake (which will also help to liquefy bronchial secretions), and to use stool softeners. In the patient with cystic fibrosis, deficient pancreatic enzymes are likely to cause additional GI problems (see

Relieving gastrointestinal problems of cystic fibrosis, page 90).

Find out how much fluid the patient normally drinks so you can help him set realistic goals. If he normally drinks 2 to 3 glasses of fluid daily and he needs to drink 10 to 12, help him set a schedule to slowly increase fluid intake one day at a time. Instruct him to keep track of fluid intake. Advise him to drink low-calorie, low-salt fluids (preferably water) and to avoid salty fluids (such as milk, V-8, or tomato juice). (Of course, you'd first want to make sure the patient doesn't have a condition—such as hyponatremia, renal failure, or congestive heart failure—that contraindicates fluid overload.) No matter what the patient's condition, advise him to reduce salt intake so the extra fluids will cause minimal edema.

Monitor fluid and electrolyte balance carefully. Be alert for conditions that increase fluid loss, such as fever, diaphoresis, diarrhea, diuretic therapy, or diabetic ketoacidosis. Compensate for fluid loss by increasing the patient's fluid intake; this will help liquefy secretions. If the patient has a condition that causes fluid retention, such as cor pulmonale, liver failure, or kidney failure, fluids may have to be restricted.

To check the effectiveness of your interventions, make sure the patient is maintaining an adequate weight and excreting body wastes normally. Check for peripheral edema and confirm that his nasal secretions are loose and thin.

Plan effective teaching

After you've helped the COPD patient through an acute crisis, your skillful teaching will enable him to return home and enjoy a near-normal life-style. Because COPD affects the patient's family as well as the patient, be sure to include family members in your teaching. Keep your instructions for home care simple and realistic. To make your teaching points easier to follow, relate them to the patient's activities of daily living before hospitalization. Ask him what problems he foresees in carrying out your instructions. Provide written instructions so the patient can refer to them at home.

Your COPD patient can't rid himself entirely of his breathing difficulty, but with your help he can control it. Learning how to control this problem will boost his self-confidence, promote his well-being, and significantly decrease his anxiety. You'll know then that your interventions have been successful.

Points to remember

- Habitual cigarette smoking is by far the most common cause of COPD; COPD rarely occurs in nonsmokers.
- Because onset of COPD is often insidious, early diagnosis is rare. Symptoms usually don't occur until the disease is advanced.
- Avoiding bronchopulmonary irritants, especially during exacerbations of respiratory symptoms, is the key to treatment of COPD. The goal of treatment is to help the patient maintain optimal breathing function and activity level rather than to cure the disease.

6 DEALING WITH RESTRICTIVE DISORDERS

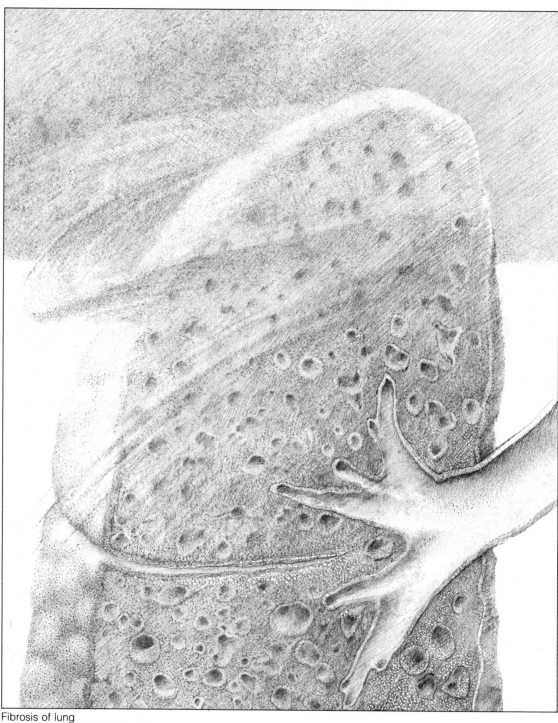

Fibrosis of lung

Restrictive lung disease is rapidly gaining attention as a significant health problem. Although this chronic condition usually lends itself to home treatment, noncompliance often poses a major obstacle to maintaining optimal respiratory function. Typically, patients are discouraged about the prospect of adhering to a lifelong treatment plan or fear making the necessary life-style changes. Your role in caring for these patients is obvious and critical. Thorough teaching of the patient and his family can provide them with a clear understanding of the disease, its potential complications, and reasons for treatment, thereby promoting compliance. To provide such teaching, you'll need to understand the pathophysiology of restrictive lung disease, its characteristic signs and symptoms, and current treatments.

What is restrictive lung disease?

Restrictive lung disease comprises a heterogeneous group of disorders that restrict lung expansion and sometimes prevent adequate pulmonary ventilation. Usually, it results from an underlying *interstitial* or *extrapulmonary* disease.

More than 100 interstitial lung diseases have been identified. Over time, these diseases gradually obliterate the lung's normal elasticity, causing it to become stiff and noncompliant. In about 70% of patients, the underlying cause of interstitial lung disease remains unknown. Rarely, toxins may cause acute interstitial disease. For example, use of marijuana tainted with the herbicide paraquat can cause lung fibrosis within 2 weeks.

Certain chemotherapeutic drugs, such as bleomycin, may cause interstitial lung fibrosis.

In extrapulmonary restrictive lung disease, the lungs are normal but their expansion is limited. For example, skeletal disorders can increase the rigidity of the thoracic cage, impairing the lungs' ability to expand fully.

In restrictive lung disease, the progress and mortality usually reflect the underlying cause.

Death may result from the primary disease or from respiratory failure caused by infection. Indeed, infection poses the greatest threat to respiratory function in patients with restrictive lung diseases. Because of limited lung expansion, these patients are unable to cough productively. Secretions then remain in the airways, causing obstruction, ventilation-perfusion mismatch, and sometimes respiratory failure.

PATHOPHYSIOLOGY

The two hallmarks of restrictive lung disease are reduction in air volume and capacity (particularly, vital capacity and total lung capacity) and noncompliant lungs.

Interstitial restrictive disease

All chronic interstitial lung diseases share certain pathologic characteristics. The major pathology is the accumulation of fluid and various inflammatory and immune effector cells within the extravascular lung tissues and spaces. During the course of inflammation, interstitial collagen becomes deranged, gathers in the interstitial spaces, and undergoes fibrosis; stiff, fibrotic scar tissue thus replaces normal elastic tissue, decreasing lung compliance. These fibrotic changes primarily affect the alveolar septa, but may also affect the bronchioles—presumably because of the variable tension exerted on them by areas of uneven elasticity.

In advanced stages of interstitial disease, constriction of fibrotic tissue may cause air sac dilation. The dilated areas alternate with constricted fibrotic areas, giving the lung a honeycomb appearance. In addition, fibrosis may narrow the pulmonary capillaries and impair blood flow to the affected areas. Also, the presence of cells, fluids, or fibrotic tissue in the interstitial spaces alters the alveolar-capillary membrane. Normally, alveolar cells and pulmonary capillaries lie so close together that their basement membranes appear fused. However, infiltration of the interstitial space may widen the basement membranes. In addition, fibrous tissue may thicken the interlobar septa and visceral pleurae.

Extrapulmonary restrictive disease

In extrapulmonary restrictive disease, lung dysfunction results from neurologic, neuromuscular, thoracic cage, or pleural disorders.

Neurologic and *neuromuscular disorders* cause loss of respiratory muscle tone or function, making the muscles unable to contract sufficiently to expand the lungs. Impaired expansion makes it difficult for the lungs to maintain sufficient alveolar ventilation. As a result, atelectasis may occur in underventilated areas, thereby stiffening the lung. Such atelectasis is an acute, reversible problem.

Skeletal disorders, such as kyphoscoliosis, may increase the rigidity of the thoracic cage, which in turn reduces chest wall compliance and restricts lung expansion.

Pleural disorders may also restrict lung expansion. In inflammatory pleural disorders,

Interstitial causes of restrictive lung disease

Fibrotic disorders
Idiopathic pulmonary fibrosis
Bronchiolitis with interstitial pneumonitis
Desquamative, giant cell, or lymphocytic interstitial pneumonitis

Granulomatous disorders
Sarcoidosis
Wegener's granulomatosis

Collagen-vascular disorders
Progressive systemic sclerosis
Rheumatoid arthritis
Sjögren's syndrome
Systemic lupus erythematosus

Lymphocytic infiltration disorders
Immunoblastic lymphadenopathy
Lymphangitic metastatic cancer
Lymphomatoid granulomatosis

Vascular disorders
Hypersensitivity angiitis
Idiopathic pulmonary hemosiderosis
Pulmonary veno-occlusive disease

Renal disorders
Goodpasture's syndrome

Inherited disorders
Familial pulmonary fibrosis
Neurofibromatosis
Tuberous sclerosis

Occupational disorders
Hypersensitivity pneumonitis (extrinsic allergic alveolitis)
Pneumoconiosis such as silicosis and asbestosis

Drug and toxins
Paraquat
Bleomycin

inspiration causes so much pain that the patient takes shallow breaths to prevent its onset. Shallow breathing may lead to underventilated alveoli. In pneumothorax, hemothorax, and pleural effusion, the pleural space fills with air or fluid, preventing lung expansion and decreasing surface area for blood gas exchange.

Altered breathing patterns
Reduced lung compliance changes normal breathing patterns. First, the respiratory muscles contract more forcefully to maintain tidal volume, thereby increasing the work of breathing. Then, the respiratory system tries to compensate through shallow, rapid breathing, thereby reducing tidal volume and the work of breathing. However, minute volume and alveolar ventilation increase sharply, resulting in greater exhalation of carbon dioxide. Supposedly, this alveolar hyperventilation results from increased transmission of afferent nerve impulses in the diseased lung, and not from hypoxemia. As a result, oxygen therapy doesn't completely reverse hyperventilation.

As restrictive lung disease progresses, compensatory mechanisms fail, lung compliance decreases, and respiratory muscle fatigue occurs. All these factors may lead to inadequate alveolar ventilation and retention of carbon dioxide.

Ventilation-perfusion mismatch
In most restrictive lung diseases, ventilation-perfusion mismatch is apparently the primary cause of hypoxemia. It results from variable lung compliance because of fibrosis, atelectasis, chest wall deformity, or neuromuscular dysfunction and causes altered movement of gas into the affected areas. It also results from impaired blood flow to ventilated alveoli because of fibrotic narrowing of the pulmonary capillaries or from compression of the lung tissue by a chest wall deformity.

Ventilation-perfusion mismatch causes the shunting of blood from underventilated to ventilated alveoli, increasing pulmonary vascular pressure. Resulting chronic pulmonary hypertension may eventually lead to right ventricular failure and cor pulmonale.

Mechanisms of hypoxemia
In restrictive lung disease, many patients do not experience hypoxemia at rest until the disease is well advanced. However, these patients may experience hypoxemia during exercise when ventilation exceeds cardiac output.

Also, pulmonary vascular resistance increases because of fibrotic narrowing of the pulmonary capillaries. Thus, with increased cardiac output, red blood cells flow too rapidly through the narrowed capillaries, allowing insufficient time for oxygenation.

Another pathologic mechanism also causes hypoxemia. Fibrosis and interstitial collagen accumulations widen the interstitial spaces, thereby increasing the distance that oxygen must diffuse from the alveolus to the capillary bed, leading to poor gas diffusion or impaired gas exchange.

MEDICAL MANAGEMENT
Detecting the underlying cause of restrictive lung disease is essential to set treatment goals. The patient's history, physical examination, and certain diagnostic tests can provide crucial information about the cause and extent of restrictive lung disease.

Radiologic tests: Helpful in detecting underlying disorder
In restrictive lung disease, the chest X-ray and fluoroscopy provide valuable baseline information.

The *chest X-ray* may appear normal in a small percentage of patients. In interstitial lung disease, this test frequently shows involvement of all lobes, with a worsening of the disease in the lower lobes. Characteristically, it shows reduced lung size and an elevated diaphragm. Reduced lung size primarily results from decreased lung compliance and may serve as a rough guide to the disease's progression or remission.

The chest X-ray may show various patterns:
• *reticular* or *interstitial pattern*—straight or curved densities distinguished from normal vascular markings by their irregular distribution in the lung
• *nodular pattern*—rounded densities of various sizes, usually with fluffy, ill-defined margins
• *reticulonodular pattern*—the most common pattern, combining reticular and nodular patterns, with individual nodules remaining small
• *honeycomb pattern*—fibrotic areas alternating with dilated air spaces; usually associated with advanced disease
• *ground-glass pattern*—homogeneous, hazy, soft appearance; usually associated with intra-alveolar filling and early disease
• *miliary pattern*—small, round, regular densities, usually caused by acini filled with fluid
• *Kerley's lines*—A lines: long, linear shadows,

centrally located in the upper lobes; B lines: short, thin, horizontal shadows at the periphery of the lung near the aortophrenic angles; C lines: a spiderweb network of fine lines that may cover the entire lung. These shadows are thought to represent thickened interlobular septa.

The chest X-ray may also help determine extrapulmonary disorders, such as hilar adenopathy, skeletal deformities, pneumothorax, hemothorax, or pleural effusion. It may also show right ventricular enlargement, indicating end-stage disease with resulting pulmonary hypertension and right ventricular failure.

Fluoroscopy of the diaphragm may prove more valuable for detecting extrapulmonary disease than for interstitial disease. Normally, fluoroscopy shows the diaphragm's descent during inspiration. In unilateral paralysis caused by tumor, trauma, or neurologic disorders, one hemidiaphragm moves paradoxically upward during inspiration. In bilateral paralysis, fluoroscopy is of limited value when the intercostal, abdominal, and accessory muscles remain intact.

Pulmonary function tests: Important to diagnosis and treatment
Pulmonary function tests help to determine the type and extent of functional abnormality and to monitor the effectiveness of treatment. However, these tests alone cannot detect the underlying cause of restrictive lung disease.

In restrictive lung disease, vital capacity and total lung capacity fall to less than 80% of the predicted value. However, flow rates usually remain normal; so the ratio of the 1-second forced expiratory volume to the forced vital capacity usually exceeds 70%, a normal finding. In interstitial lung disease, this ratio may rise because of airway dilatation.

Diffusion (DLCO) abnormalities can result from diffuse fibrosis, interstitial infiltration, or resection. In interstitial disease, DLCO may fall to less than 50%.

Measurement of maximal inspiratory and expiratory pressures helps detect neuromuscular disorders. In Guillain-Barré syndrome and amyotrophic lateral sclerosis (ALS), these pressures may fall to 30 cmH_2O—the result of diaphragm and abdominal muscle weakness. If these pressures fall below 20 cmH_2O, respiratory failure is imminent.

ABG analysis detects hypoxemia
Measurement of arterial blood gas (ABG) levels with the patient at rest, during sleep, and during exercise can detect the presence and extent of hypoxemia. Typically, PO_2 is less than 80 mm Hg, and SaO_2 is less than 95%. Hypocapnia (PCO_2 less than 35 mm Hg) appears commonly, except in severe disease accompanied by hypercapnia (PCO_2 greater than 45 mm Hg) and respiratory acidosis.

Special tests pinpoint diagnosis
Biopsies and immunologic and neurologic tests may pinpoint a diagnosis that eludes customary respiratory tests. *Biopsy* of the lymph nodes, kidney, or mucocutaneous lesions may reveal sarcoidosis, Wegener's granulomatosis, or Goodpasture's syndrome. When no other organ appears to be involved, lung biopsy may be performed.

Immunologic tests may detect increased globulins and autoantibodies in collagen diseases. Skin tests for tuberculosis, coccidioidomycosis, histoplasmosis, and other diseases caused by organic dusts may aid diagnosis.

In suspected Guillain-Barré syndrome or ALS, *neurologic tests* (such as cerebrospinal fluid analysis and electromyography) may pinpoint diagnosis. In suspected hypoventilation syndrome, *sleep studies* help determine the ventilatory response to hypoxemia and hypercapnia, thereby characterizing the defect and guiding therapy. In suspected systemic or hematogenous infection, *blood* and *bone marrow cultures* may be needed.

Treatment
In restrictive lung disease, treatment addresses the underlying cause, if identified. Depending on the patient's condition, it can also include oxygen, mechanical ventilation, and drugs. For patients with severe restrictive disease limited to the lungs, such as smoke inhalation, lung transplant may be the only option, even though lung transplant has not been perfected to the same extent as other organ transplants.

Oxygen therapy. Such therapy is indicated when PaO_2 is at or below 55 mm Hg at rest or during exercise, or if pulmonary hypertension or erythrocytosis develops. A liter flow that achieves an SaO_2 greater than 90% can prevent or relieve pulmonary hypertension. Type II respiratory failure (pH less than 7.2, PCO_2 greater than 50 to 60 mm Hg, and PO_2 less than 50 to 60 mm Hg) indicates the need for intubation and mechanical ventilation—and may pose a moral dilemma. Unless respiratory failure results from acute, reversible process, such as trauma, Guillain-Barré syndrome,

Extrapulmonary causes of restrictive lung disease

Neuromuscular and neurologic disorders
Amyotrophic lateral sclerosis
Guillain-Barré syndrome
Multiple sclerosis
Muscular dystrophy
Myasthenia gravis
Poliomyelitis

Thoracic cage disorders
Ankylosing spondylitis
Chest wall deformity
Kyphosis
Pickwickian syndrome
Scoliosis

Pleural disorders
Hemothorax
Pleural effusion
Pleurisy
Pleuritis

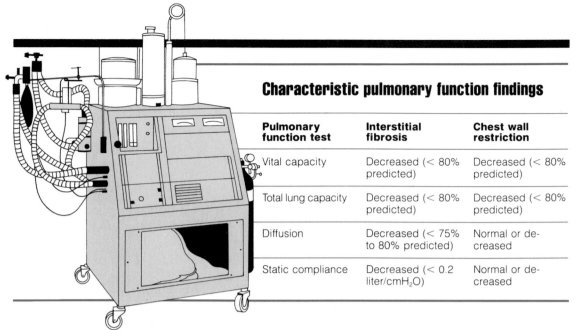

Characteristic pulmonary function findings

Pulmonary function test	Interstitial fibrosis	Chest wall restriction
Vital capacity	Decreased (< 80% predicted)	Decreased (< 80% predicted)
Total lung capacity	Decreased (< 80% predicted)	Decreased (< 80% predicted)
Diffusion	Decreased (< 75% to 80% predicted)	Normal or decreased
Static compliance	Decreased (< 0.2 liter/cmH$_2$O)	Normal or decreased

or pneumonia, the need for positive-pressure mechanical ventilation usually heralds severe, end-stage disease.

With underventilated alveoli, negative-pressure ventilators or rocking beds give nocturnal support. In central alveolar hypoventilation, phrenic pacing may be needed. (See *Respiratory assist devices,* pages 100 and 101.)

A permanent tracheostomy may relieve upper airway obstruction resulting from obstructive sleep apnea. When obesity contributes to hypoventilation, weight loss may decrease the frequency and severity of apneic episodes, snoring, and daytime somnolence. However, weight loss may be ineffective for patients with pickwickian syndrome because of their abnormal ventilatory response to hypoxemia and hypercapnia. For these patients, progesterone, a respiratory stimulant, may be useful.

Drug therapy. Immunosuppressives, the cornerstone of drug therapy for interstitial lung disease, are recommended for patients with significant or progressive respiratory symptoms. Azathioprine appears to be helpful in correcting active inflammation or when steroid therapy fails to stop progressive illness. Antimicrobial drugs provide aggressive treatment for acute infections. With concomitant airway obstruction, such bronchodilators as aminophylline may be needed. With debilitating cough, antitussives provide relief.

NURSING MANAGEMENT
Successful nursing management of restrictive lung disease requires a thorough history and accurate assessment. After collecting this subjective and objective data and correlating it with the results of diagnostic tests, you'll be ready to form nursing diagnoses, set goals, and plan and evaluate your interventions.

Patient history: Always ask about dyspnea
Begin the patient history by asking about dyspnea and the kind of activities that cause it. Dyspnea may range from mild during vigorous exercise to severe during rest, depending on the disease's severity. Its onset may be insidious, as in progressive kyphoscoliosis, or sudden, as in traumatic injury. In advanced disease, paroxysmal nocturnal dyspnea may result from ventricular failure.

Ask the patient if he experiences dyspnea in the lateral, prone, or supine positions. Dyspnea in the lateral position may indicate unilateral diaphragmatic paralysis. Dyspnea in the prone or supine positions may occur with severe kyphoscoliosis, bilateral diaphragmatic paralysis, or ALS. The absence of dyspnea, however, in such disorders as Guillain-Barré syndrome, ALS, or myasthenia gravis should not lull you into forgetting about imminent respiratory failure. In many instances, patients with progressive neuromuscular disease do not complain of dyspnea until the diaphragm, the major muscle of respiration, becomes involved. By that time, ventilatory reserve may be severely compromised.

Ask the patient what he does when he experiences dyspnea to gain valuable insight into his coping mechanisms.

Listen to the patient's cough. Is it paroxysmal and nonproductive? Is his sputum blood-streaked or mucoid? Ask about previous or current cigarette smoking. Although smoking doesn't cause restrictive lung disease, it may cause bronchitis and further complicate or aggravate the disease.

Ask the patient about chest pain. Substernal chest discomfort may indicate right ventricular failure; pleuritic chest pain may indicate pleural effusion or pleurisy.

Ask the patient if he wheezes. Wheezing doesn't usually occur in restrictive lung disorders unless left ventricular failure or obstructive lung disease is also present. Also ask about nonspecific complaints, such as drowsiness, irritability, muscular weakness, chronic fatigue, morning headache, and disturbed sleep.

Gather environmental data

The patient's workplace, neighborhood, or home can supply clues to the primary disorder. Ask about exposure to infectious agents, such as tuberculosis. Does he tend chicken or pigeon coops? Has he traveled recently? Has he inhaled organic dusts, moldy hay, sugar cane, or air from contaminated ventilation systems? Has he been exposed to mineral dusts, such as silica and asbestos, or to toxic fumes? Has he been exposed to radiation or taken bleomycin? Has he smoked marijuana?

Perform the physical exam

Once you've completed the patient history, you're ready to perform the physical exam, using techniques of inspection, palpation, percussion, and auscultation.

Inspection. First, observe the patient's respirations, which are usually rapid and shallow. The inspiration-expiration ratio, normally 1:1.5, may be closer to 1:1 in restrictive lung disease. Because expiration is normally a passive motion, the respiratory muscles have less resting time. Inspiration may suddenly cease (the "doorstop sign") as the patient reaches the elastic limits of inspiration.

Look for central cyanosis secondary to hypoxemia. At first, cyanosis may appear only during exercise; later, as the disease progresses, it occurs even at rest. Of course, hypoxemia is present without cyanosis in many cases.

Check the fingernails for clubbing, which is associated with advanced restrictive lung disease and, commonly, with early pulmonary fibrosis. In patients with rheumatoid arthritis, look for arthritic deformities. In patients with kyphoscoliosis, note the lateral bending and rotation of the spinal column, which produces spinal column convexity on one side and concavity on the other. This rotation causes anterior displacement of the posterior ribs, decreasing the volume of one hemithorax, and posterior displacement of the anterior ribs, increasing the volume of the other hemithorax; the interspaces may be flared on the

convex side. Also, observe the patient's chest for asymmetry and his overall stature for reduced spinal length. Check for an abnormal lower thoracic spine, which can cause severe respiratory problems.

If restrictive lung disease has produced bilaterally decreased thoracic excursion (in pulmonary fibrosis, obesity, or ankylosing spondylitis) or unilaterally diminished movement (in unilateral paralysis of the diaphragm or pleural effusion), use a tape measure to verify limitation of motion.

Check if the patient uses accessory neck muscles, especially during exercise. Look for paradoxical inward movement of the chest wall in flail chest and of the abdominal wall during supine inspiration in bilateral diaphragmatic paralysis.

Palpation. In known or suspected blunt chest injury, palpate the bones and joints of the thorax for tenderness and crepitation. Crepitation is a coarse, crackling sensation that suggests the presence of air in the subcutaneous tissues or bone fracture.

Palpate for tactile fremitus. Pleural effusion, fibrosis or thickening, pneumothorax, and obesity produce "insulation" between the palpating hand and the bronchopulmonary system, and fremitus may be decreased or absent. It may also be abnormal in kyphoscoliosis.

Palpate the trachea. In most restrictive lung diseases, it's located in the midline; however, in unilateral disease, such as pneumothorax, pleural effusion, or fibrosis, it may be displaced. Palpate the axillary and supraclavicular lymph nodes to detect a localized or generalized inflammation or malignancy.

Palpate for the point of maximum impulse (PMI). It may shift toward the affected side in unilateral fibrosis or atelectasis and away from the affected side in large pleural effusions or pneumothorax. The PMI is also displaced in kyphoscoliosis.

Percussion. Diaphragmatic movement may be decreased or absent in extrapulmonary disorders that produce unilateral or bilateral paralysis and in obesity when the diaphragm is elevated because of increased volume of the abdomen. Percussion may be normal; dull to flat in pleural effusion; hyperresonant to tympanic in pneumothorax; or dull to hyperresonant in kyphoscoliosis and atelectasis.

Auscultation. Breath and voice sounds may be diminished or absent in obesity, pleural thickening and effusion, or pneumothorax. Breath sounds may be bronchial if fluid com-

Oxygen delivery devices

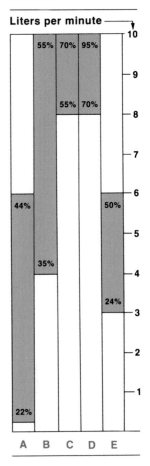

Liters per minute

	A	B	C	D	E
10		55%	70%	95%	
8			55%	70%	
6	44%				50%
4		35%			
3					24%
	22%				

Key:

A Nasal cannula

B Simple mask

C Partial rebreathing mask

D Nonrebreathing mask

E Venturi mask

Note: Fraction of inspired oxygen (FIO$_2$) values, except for the Venturi mask, are approximations. Actual FIO$_2$ values depend on the oxygen delivery device; the liter flow; and the rate, depth, and I:E ratio of breathing.

Respiratory assist devices

Most respiratory assist devices use either positive or negative pressure to improve respiration. An alternative device, a phrenic pacemaker, may be implanted surgically to correct chronic respiratory dysfunction.

Iron lung

Positive-pressure ventilators
The most common type of mechanical ventilation in use today is positive-pressure ventilation. These devices improve severe ventilation-perfusion mismatch by opening alveoli not previously involved in gas exchange. With positive-pressure ventilation, alveolar ventilation and arterial blood gas levels improve and inspired air distributes more evenly, reducing the work of breathing.

Positive-pressure ventilators are classified according to the type of preset limit—either pressure or volume—that ends the inspiratory cycle.

A *pressure-cycled* or *pressure-limited ventilator* (such as Bird Mark 7 or Bennett PR-

2) is primarily used for short-term (less than 24 hours) mechanical ventilation in patients without underlying lung disease. With this type of ventilator, tidal volume may vary from breath to breath, depending on changes in lung compliance and airway resistance. Also, a pressure-cycled ventilator allows regulation of three settings: peak airway pressure, inspiratory flow, and sensitivity. These settings allow measurement of tidal volume, depending on lung compliance and airway resistance.

A *volume-cycled* or *volume-limited ventilator* (such as Emerson 3-PV, Bourns Bear, or Bennett MA-2 + 2) is used for patients requiring ventilatory assistance for more than 24 hours and for patients with underlying lung disease who require a constant, reliable minute volume. It allows delivery of a preset tidal volume and respiratory rate.

Negative-pressure ventilators
These devices replace or aid spontaneous ventilation by applying intermittent negative (sub-

Volume-limited ventilator

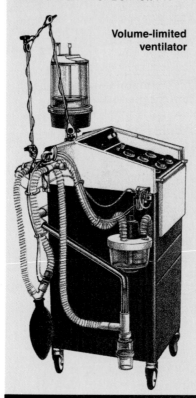

Pressure-limited ventilator

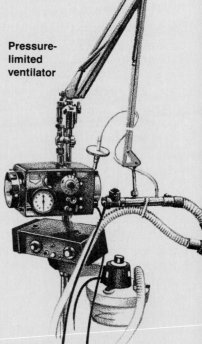

atmospheric) pressure to the trunk or the entire body, expanding the chest wall and causing atmospheric air to enter the lungs. They're used for patients with neuromuscular disease who have normal lungs but lack sufficient vital capacity to maintain adequate ventilation. These ventilators don't require artificial airway placement.

An *iron lung* or *tank ventilator* is an airtight tank that encloses the entire body, except for the head. A rubber diaphragm circles the patient's neck to seal the tank. An electric motor creates negative pressure inside the tank, making air flow into the patient's lungs. A calibrated gauge on the tank measures the amount of negative pressure. If a power failure occurs, a handle beneath the tank allows manual operation.

An iron lung is rugged, dependable, and easy to operate. However, its drawbacks include its large size, noisiness, the inaccessibility of the patient and restrictions on his activity, difficulty in sterilization, venous pooling in larger abdominal vessels, and decreased cardiac output from negative pressure on the abdomen. Also, an iron lung may be inadequate for ventilating patients with lung disease because of inability to achieve a pressure gradient.

Rocking bed

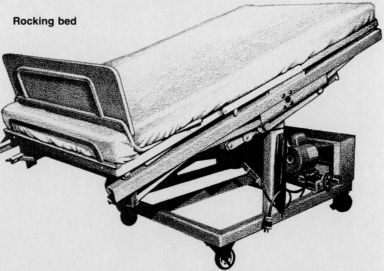

Cuirass ventilator

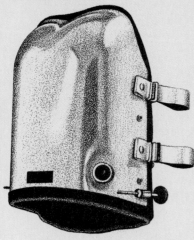

The *cuirass ventilator*, a rigid shell that covers the anterior thorax and abdomen, may be used to wean patients from tank ventilators or to allow rest periods for patients with residual respiratory muscle paralysis. A flexible hose extending from the shell to a power source creates negative pressure on the thorax, sucking the chest wall outward and causing atmospheric air to enter the lungs.

A cuirass ventilator has many advantages—it's less cumbersome and smaller than an iron lung; it doesn't place negative pressure on the abdomen; and it accommodates a flow sensor to assist ventilation. However, its disadvantages include skin irritation, noisiness, and difficulty in maintaining a tight seal and in regulating the inspiration/expiration (I:E) ratio.

A *rocking bed* offers an alternative to conventional mechanical ventilation for patients with alveolar hypoventilation. Its slow, rocking movements improve ventilation by using the weight and gravity of the abdominal contents to move the diaphragm up and down.

Phrenic pacing
A third type of respiratory assist device, the *phrenic pacemaker*, uses neither positive nor negative pressure. It induces respiration by means of a surgically implanted device, which, when electrically stimulated by an external transmitter and antenna, stimulates the phrenic nerve. This stimulation causes the diaphragm to descend and air to be pulled into the lungs. When stimulation stops, the muscles relax, the diaphragm ascends, and air is exhaled as with normal breathing.

A phrenic pacemaker is most commonly implanted in patients with central alveolar hypoventilation and spinal cord lesions or trauma. It's usually attached to the left phrenic nerve because any damage here affects pulmonary function less than damage to the right phrenic nerve, which controls ventilation of the larger right lung.

Phrenic pacemaker

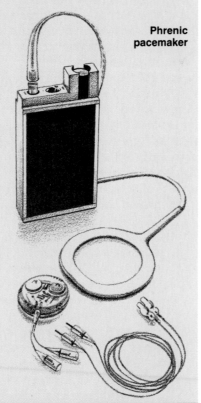

Relieving the distress of dyspnea

No matter what causes restrictive lung disease, the patient's chief complaint is always dyspnea. And, if unchecked, dyspnea can lead to ever-deepening distress. First, the patient becomes anxious, fearing that he'll lose the ability to breathe. Then, anxiety produces muscular tension, and tense muscles consume more oxygen, perpetuating the distress of dyspnea.

You can help relieve the patient's distress by reassuring him that he won't lose his ability to breathe. Also, to reduce muscle tension, teach relaxation and energy conservation techniques and proper positioning.

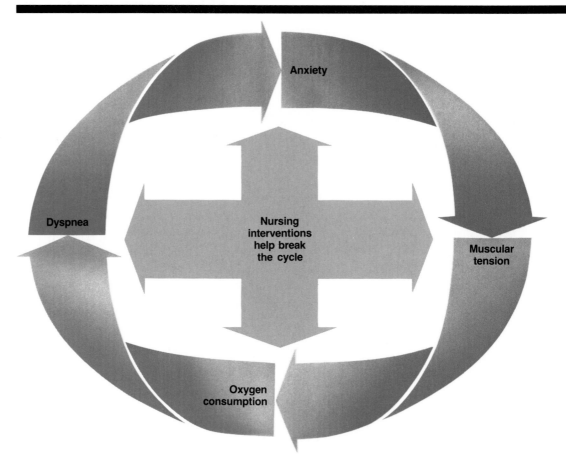

Anxiety

Muscular tension

Nursing interventions help break the cycle

Oxygen consumption

Dyspnea

presses the underlying lung tissue. Bronchophony, egophony, and whispered pectoriloquy may also be present.

Late inspiratory crackles (crepitations, rales) are characteristic in interstitial lung diseases. These are thought to result from the opening of the bronchioles during inspiration.

In pleural disorders, listen for a pleural friction rub. Auscultate for sibilant rhonchi, which occur rarely with bronchial involvement in sarcoidosis. Also, auscultate for rhonchi or rales if secretions are being retained because of ineffective coughing. Be sure to listen for heart sounds: an accentuated pulmonic S_2—accompanied by left parasternal heaves, neck vein distention, hepatomegaly, and peripheral edema—signals cor pulmonale.

Formulate nursing diagnoses

After collecting subjective data from the patient interview and objective data from the respiratory assessment, you're ready to formulate nursing diagnoses that clearly explain the patient's problem and allow you to plan appropriate goals and interventions.

Ineffective airway clearance related to retained secretions from nonproductive coughing. Your goals are to teach effective coughing techniques, to remove retained secretions, and to prevent or correct complications. To achieve these goals, demonstrate effective coughing techniques. But if noncompliant lungs make productive coughing impossible, evaluate the need for other bronchial hygiene. Encourage adequate fluid intake to thin secretions. Give aerosol therapy, chest physiotherapy, and suctioning to remove secretions.

Watch for signs of acute respiratory infection. Note the quantity and character of sputum. Arrange for routine sputum culture and sensitivity studies to detect respiratory infection. If infection does occur, give antibiotics, as ordered, to avoid respiratory failure. Encourage the patient to refrain from smoking, to avoid exposure to other respiratory irritants, and to recognize the signs and symptoms of acute infection.

Evaluate your interventions. Consider them effective if:
• the patient demonstrates effective coughing techniques, or therapy has removed retained secretions.
• his sputum is clear and thin, and culture and sensitivity studies are negative.
• auscultation reveals no coarse rales or decreased breath sounds.
• the patient's temperature is within normal limits.
• infection, if present, has been corrected by antibiotics.

Impaired gas exchange. Your goals are to ensure optimal respiratory function and to explain all procedures to the patient. To achieve these goals, monitor ABGs for PO_2 at or below 55 mm Hg, pH less than 7.35, and PCO_2 greater than 45 mm Hg. Assess and report signs of respiratory failure: altered blood pressure and heart rate, dysrhythmias, chest pain, tachypnea, cyanosis, flushing, dyspnea, restlessness, insomnia, nightmares, confusion, headache, disorientation, excitement, paranoia, lethargy, drowsiness, coma, or fine tremors. Avoid respiratory depressants if hypercapnia or acidosis is present.

Give oxygen, as ordered. Be sure to explain the reasons for oxygen therapy to the patient, because he may not get relief from it. Remember that even though oxygen improves PO_2 levels, hyperventilation may continue because afferent nerve impulses continue to be transmitted in noncompliant lungs.

If respiratory failure occurs, prepare for intubation, mechanical ventilation, or phrenic pacing. Explain these procedures to the patient to allay his anxiety.

If ordered, deliver a high concentration of oxygen by continuous positive airway pressure. This form of therapy can be given by mechanical ventilation and intubation, tight-fitting face or nasal masks, or specially designed nasal cannulas.

If appropriate, consider using biofeedback to wean a paralyzed patient from a respirator. Teach him to reduce his respiratory rate and increase tidal volume and vital capacity. Allow him to view respiratory volumes on an oscilloscope screen and mark target goals to promote weaning.

Evaluate your interventions. Consider them successful if:
• ABGs remain within normal limits.
• the patient accepts the need for ventilatory support.
• the paralyzed patient uses biofeedback to wean himself from a respirator.

Impaired gas exchange related to nocturnal hypoventilation or sleep apnea. To promote adequate ventilation during sleep, assist with sleep assessment studies, such as transcutaneous PO_2 monitoring, apnea monitoring, and impedance pneumography. If necessary, prepare the patient for tracheostomy or phrenic pacing. Also, if appropriate, instruct the patient and his family in the use of mechanical ventilation and suctioning. If obesity causes hypoventilation, promote weight loss through correct diet and weigh the patient weekly.

Evaluate your interventions. Consider them successful if:
• the patient and his family use suctioning and mechanical ventilation properly.
• the obese patient complies with the prescribed diet and loses weight.

Ineffective breathing patterns related to decreased lung and chest wall compliance. Your goal is to teach energy conservation and relaxation techniques. For example, teach the patient to assume positions that decrease the work of breathing, such as sitting on a stool when taking a shower.

Evaluate your intervention. Consider it successful if the patient learns and uses energy conservation and relaxation techniques.

Activity intolerance related to dyspnea on exertion. To gradually raise the patient's activity level and to reduce his anxiety, allow frequent rest periods during patient-care activities, and encourage the patient to gradually increase activity, using portable oxygen if needed. Allow him to express his fears about dyspnea, and help him set and accept realistic limitations on activity.

Evaluate your interventions. Consider them successful if:
• the patient gradually increases his activity level, with minimal dyspnea.
• the patient expresses his fear of dyspnea and accepts realistic activity limitations.

Sleep pattern disturbances. The disturbance may stem from fear of death, of awakening in acute distress, or of diagnostic tests or treatments. First, make sure the patient's sleep disturbance doesn't stem from blood gas abnormalities. If the patient's sleep disturbance stems from one of the causes above, relieve his anxiety, encourage him to express his fears, and fully explain all tests and treatments. Before he sleeps, reduce environmental stimuli and provide comfort measures, such as a massage, to promote relaxation.

Evaluate your intervention. Consider it successful if the patient sleeps restfully without fear or anxiety.

A final word

Restrictive lung disease presents a formidable nursing challenge. At times, it can demand all the patience and skills at your command. But with few other diseases are the results so immediately gratifying as when, simply because of your reassuring presence and calm ministrations, an air-starved, apprehensive patient finds that he can breathe easier and no longer fears breathlessness.

Points to remember

• Restrictive lung disease usually results from an underlying interstitial or extrapulmonary disorder.
• Most interstitial lung disorders result from unknown causes.
• Despite possible side effects, immunosuppressive drugs are the cornerstone of pharmacologic treatment of interstitial lung disease.
• Acute respiratory infection, with its threat of respiratory failure, poses the greatest danger to patients with noncompliant lungs.
• Effective nursing management requires keen history-taking and assessment skills as well as thorough patient teaching.

7 INTERVENING IN PLEURAL DISORDERS

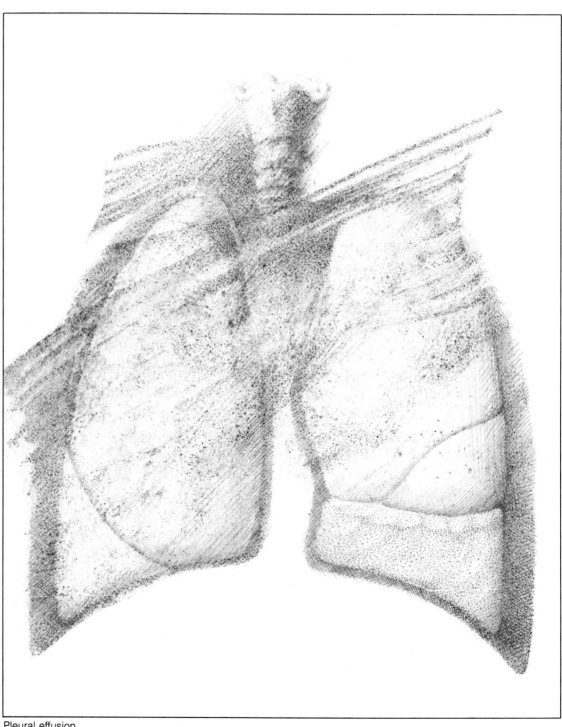

Pleural effusion

Acute and chronic pleural disorders occur so often that sooner or later you'll probably see and treat them all. These disorders may restrict chest or lung expansion because of inflammation; fibrosis; or the accumulation of air, blood, fluid, or purulent matter in the pleural cavity. But most importantly, certain pleural disorders, such as tension pneumothorax, can suddenly and unexpectedly threaten the lives of even apparently healthy people. That's why accurate assessment and prompt, skillful nursing interventions are crucial in managing pleural disorders. Equally crucial, too, is an understanding of pleural pathophysiology and current treatment measures.

What causes pleural disorders?

Pleural disorders can result from many causes, but generally fall into three categories. They can result from inflammation or can arise spontaneously, usually without apparent cause. They can also result from trauma—either iatrogenic (resulting from medical or surgical treatment) or noniatrogenic (resulting from some other cause).

Pleural disorders can be classified by their effect as inflammatory disorders, disorders that increase pleural fluid pressure, and disorders that increase intrapleural gas pressure.

Inflammatory disorders

Inflammation of the pleura (pleurisy, pleuritis) most often develops as a complication of pneumonia, tuberculosis, viral infection, collagen vascular disease, uremia, Dressler's disease, malignancy, pulmonary infarction, or chest trauma. It can also result when an irritating or infectious agent invades the pleural cavity, as in pancreatic pleurisy.

Increased pleural fluid pressure

Disorders that result in pleural effusion, the collection of fluid in the pleural cavity, cause a rise in pleural fluid pressure that compresses the lung. A pleural effusion may be a transudate, an exudate, a hemothorax, or a hydrothorax.

Transudates. A transudative effusion develops when increased pulmonary venous pressure or decreased serum protein alters normal osmotic and hydrostatic pressure balance and promotes movement of fluid across intact capillaries into the pleural cavity. This fluid transudate, an ultrafiltrate of plasma, contains low concentrations of protein (less than 3%).

Transudative pleural effusions often result from congestive heart failure, hepatic disease with ascites, hypoalbuminemia, and disorders resulting in overexpanded intravascular volume.

Exudates. An exudative effusion develops when capillary permeability increases, with or without changes in hydrostatic or colloid osmotic pressures, and protein-rich fluid exudes into the pleural cavity. Such effusions may occur with inflammation, tuberculosis, subphrenic abscess, pancreatitis, malignancy, pulmonary embolism, collagen vascular disease, myxedema, and chest trauma.

Differentiated by composition, types of exudative pleural effusions include empyema, chylothorax, pseudochylous effusion, and sterile exudates. Empyema denotes the presence of pus, and is most commonly related to pneumonitis, metastasis, or esophageal perforation or rupture. Chylothorax denotes the presence of chyle (digested triglycerides arising from the intestinal lymph vessels), resulting from trauma or disease of the thoracic duct. Pseudochylous effusion denotes the presence of excessive amounts of cholesterol, resulting from the degeneration of cells in chronic pleural effusion associated with tuberculosis and rheumatoid arthritis. Sterile exudates result from noninfectious inflammation, such as pancreatitis, malignancy, pulmonary embolism, or collagen vascular disease.

Hemothorax. Different from a hemorrhagic pleural effusion, a hemothorax involves bleeding into the pleural cavity from rupture at such sites as the heart, great vessels, lungs, or chest wall vessels. It usually follows blunt or penetrating chest trauma; about 25% of patients with such trauma have this condition. Less often, it results from thoracic surgery, pulmonary infarction, neoplasm, dissecting thoracic aneurysm, or anticoagulant therapy.

Hydrothorax. This type of pleural effusion results from iatrogenic causes. For example, a displaced central venous catheter permits serum, total parenteral nutrition, or other intravenous fluid to enter the pleural cavity.

Increased intrapleural gas pressure

Disorders that allow air to enter the normally airtight pleural cavity raise intrapleural gas pressure and compress the lung. Pneumothorax, the presence of air in the pleural cavity, can be classified according to cause as either spontaneous or traumatic. In turn, spontaneous pneumothorax may be either primary or secondary, and traumatic pneumothorax

Normal pleural fluid mechanics

Pressure	Parietal pleura	Pleural cavity	Visceral pleura
Hydrostatic pressure	30	−5	11
Colloid osmotic pressure	34	−8	34
	Systemic capillaries	Pleural fluid	Pulmonary capillaries

Pleural fluid forms and passes through the pleural cavity at a daily rate of up to several hundred milliliters, its movement controlled by certain pressure gradients. Hydrostatic pressure in the parietal pleural capillaries far exceeds the pressure in the visceral pleural capillaries. This gradient forces fluid to filter from systemic blood and lymphatics, move into the pleural cavity, and then be reabsorbed into pulmonary blood and lymphatics. Eighty to ninety percent of pleural fluid is reabsorbed this way; the remainder returns to the blood via the lymphatic system. Colloid osmotic pressure works in reverse. Its low level in pleural fluid, compared with its level in the blood, guards against colloid leakage out of the capillaries and into pleural fluid.

Any abnormal change in these two pressure patterns will change the amount and character of pleural fluid.

may be either iatrogenic or noniatrogenic. Both spontaneous and traumatic pneumothoraces may lead to tension pneumothorax.

Spontaneous pneumothorax. This disorder can occur for no apparent reason (primary) or result from an existing disease (secondary). In this condition, the chest wall remains intact (closed), but air enters the pleural cavity from the respiratory tree through an opening on the lung surface.

Primary spontaneous pneumothorax. Often striking seemingly healthy men aged 20 to 40, primary spontaneous pneumothorax occurs suddenly and for no apparent reason. However, its usual cause is an undetected bleb (small vesicle) or bulla (larger vesicle) on the visceral pleura or underlying lung surface. The bleb ruptures under stress, such as coughing, and allows air to leak from the lung into the pleural cavity. Such blebs are most likely to occur in the lung apices. They may develop from areas of existent but undetected paraseptal emphysema that border the pleura, a common condition revealed at autopsy.

Secondary spontaneous pneumothorax. Occurring equally unexpectedly, secondary spontaneous pneumothorax has an identifiable or probable cause. Usually, it results from a disorder that causes lung hyperinflation, such as asthma, chronic obstructive pulmonary disease (COPD), or emphysema, or from an anatomic deformity, such as pulmonary fibrosis. It may also result from malignancy.

Traumatic pneumothorax. This form of pneumothorax follows an external injury. It may be closed if the chest wall remains intact, or open if direct communication exists between the atmosphere and the pleural cavity because of an opening in the chest wall. Traumatic pneumothorax may result from a noniatrogenic cause, such as a stab or gunshot wound or a blow that fractures a rib and drives it inward to lacerate the lung. It may also follow iatrogenically from a medical procedure, such as thoracentesis, percutaneous lung biopsy, cardiopulmonary resuscitation, or mechanical ventilation with positive end-expiratory pressure (PEEP).

Tension pneumothorax. A life-threatening sequela of either spontaneous or traumatic pneumothorax, tension pneumothorax occurs when a large volume of air becomes trapped in the pleural cavity. As a result, air and tension build up in the chest cavity, compressing the lung and mediastinum and shifting them toward the opposite lung. This shift can collapse the other lung and the great vessels and, if unchecked, quickly cause death.

UNDERSTANDING PLEURAL PATHOPHYSIOLOGY

The pleurae consist of a thin membrane that doubles back on itself at the hilum so that one (visceral) layer encases the lungs and the other (parietal) layer lines the inner chest wall. Composed of connective tissue, these layers contain blood and lymph vessels and smooth muscle fibers; the parietal layer alone has pain fibers. The two layers are held together by negative (subatmospheric) pressure that results from the natural tendency of lung and chest wall tissue to pull in opposite directions. A thin layer of lymphatic (pleural) fluid lubricates the pleural surfaces to prevent friction during breathing. (See *Normal pleural fluid mechanics* on page 106.) Between the layers, the airtight pleural "cavity" becomes a true space only under abnormal conditions.

Mechanics of inflammation

With inflammation, the pleurae become swollen and congested, hampering pleural fluid transport. This increases friction between the pleural surfaces and causes sharp, stabbing pain that mounts with inspiration. The pain results from inflammation or irritation of sensory nerve endings in the parietal pleura and is aggravated during respiration as the pleurae shift against each other. Inflammation may stimulate the production or hinder the reabsorption of pleural fluid, leading to pleural effusion.

Mechanics of increased pleural fluid pressure

Pleural effusion, when not caused by hemothorax or hydrothorax, usually results from an abnormal change in the dynamics of pleural fluid transport that causes the rate of fluid production to exceed the rate of removal. This change may reflect increased permeability of parietal pleural capillaries, increased hydrostatic pressure, altered colloid osmotic pressure, or reduced lymphatic drainage.

Increased capillary permeability in the parietal pleura commonly results from inflammation, either through damage to pleural capillaries or the influence of histamines and other products of inflammation or malignancy. This action increases the flow of pleural fluid into the pleural cavity, taxing the reabsorptive capacity of the visceral pleura and the lymphatic system. The accumulating exudate has a high protein content because increased capillary permeability has allowed large protein molecules to leak into the pleural fluid.

Increased systemic hydrostatic pressure commonly results from such conditions as congestive heart failure or occlusion of the superior vena cava, leading to excessive fluid filtration into the pleural cavity. In the absence of pulmonary venous hypertension, visceral pleural capillaries may adequately reabsorb the excess fluid to prevent pleural effusion. However, the presence of pulmonary venous hypertension creates effusion by reducing visceral reabsorption. In this case the fluid accumulation, caused by changes in pressure rather than changes in capillary permeability, shows normal or low protein concentration.

Changes in plasma colloid osmotic pressure also disrupt pleural fluid transport. For example, hypoproteinemia can increase fluid influx. A plasma albumin level below 1.5 g/dl promotes pleural edema, which apparently leads to pleural effusion. At extremely low albumin levels, visceral pleural capillaries intensify the problem by failing to reabsorb the transudate, leaving it to be reabsorbed by the lymphatic system.

Disorders that disrupt lymphatic drainage often result in pleural effusion. Because this system acts as the sole pathway for systemic reabsorption of protein, any disorder that impairs its ability to drain pleural fluid—such as systemic venous hypertension—produces an effusion high in protein. The pleural lymphatics also help drain lymphatic vessels in the peritoneal cavity, increasing the risk of pleural effusion in diseases such as cirrhosis.

Mechanics of increased intrapleural gas pressure

In both closed and open pneumothoraces, air enters the pleural cavity until the normally negative intrapleural pressure rises to equal atmospheric pressure and lung collapse stabilizes. When ruptured tissues allow only one-way airflow into the pleural cavity, trapping incoming air in the cavity and increasing intrapleural pressure, a tension pneumothorax develops. (See *Mechanics of tension pneumothorax* on page 108.) Large and tension pneumothoraces can cause mediastinal shift and its fatal complications.

Intrapleural air compresses the lung, increases the work of breathing, and decreases ventilation, but plays no part in pulmonary

Special tests for underlying disorders

Because pleural effusion usually reflects an underlying disorder, blood, sputum, and pleural fluid tests can provide important diagnostic information. The complete blood count (CBC) may show increased numbers of white cells typical of infection, or decreased hemoglobin levels secondary to chronic disease or tumor infiltration. Cytologic study of sputum detects tumor, and a sputum culture detects infection caused by fungi, bacteria, or acid-fast bacilli. In addition, an EKG excludes recent myocardial infarction, and tuberculin testing with purified protein derivative detects previous exposure to tuberculosis.

Thoracentesis and, if appropriate, pleural biopsy provide specimens for glucose, protein, and lactic dehydrogenase (LDH) determinations; cell count and differential; cytologic studies; culture for fungi, acid-fast bacilli, and aerobic and anaerobic bacteria; Gram's stain; cholesterol and triglyceride determinations (for a chylous sample); and pleural pH (for suspected parapneumonic effusion or esophageal rupture). Simultaneous testing of serum glucose, protein, and LDH provides comparison values.

Mechanics of tension pneumothorax

In tension pneumothorax, negative intrapleural pressure during inspiration draws air into the pleural cavity, but positive pressure during expiration prevents its escape. As a result, intrapleural air volume increases, and the lung collapses more with each breath. This can shift the mediastinal contents (heart, great vessels, trachea, and esophagus) to compress the other lung, causing acute respiratory distress. By twisting or stretching the great vessels, this mediastinal shift lowers venous return, cardiac output, and blood pressure. Failure to reverse this progressive cardiac and respiratory distress can quickly cause death.

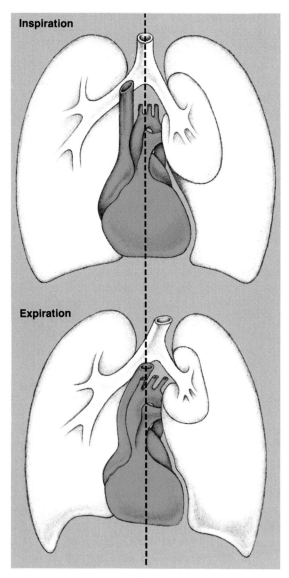

Inspiration

Expiration

pleural disorder, radiographic and blood studies provide important diagnostic information and help guide treatment.

Radiographic tests detect pneumothorax and effusion

Chest X-ray confirms the presence of air or fluid in the pleural cavity, allows diagnosis of pneumothorax, and may detect mediastinal shift. Because radiographic contrast is less marked with fluid than with air, chest X-ray usually reveals pleural effusion only after 200 to 300 ml of fluid have accumulated in the pleural cavity. This test may also demonstrate pleural calcification, an indication of asbestosis and related pleural tumor.

Despite increased lung density on the affected side, chest X-ray reveals pneumothorax as hyperlucency over the entire hemithorax—the result of an increased volume of thoracic air and reduced pulmonary vasculature. An expiratory X-ray enhances air-lung contrast, taking advantage of further lung compression and reduced intrapulmonic air volume during expiration to emphasize the lung boundary and the size of the pneumothorax. A lateral X-ray may show the lateral air-lung border if an upright view fails to detect the apical border. It may also demonstrate pneumomediastinum, rare with spontaneous pneumothorax but more common with traumatic pneumothorax, and mediastinal shift. Pleural adhesions from an earlier pleural disorder can complicate diagnosis by creating pleural air pockets. These air pockets, along with small deviations of pleural layers that disguise relatively large volumes of air, make it difficult to determine the size of a pneumothorax.

Chest X-ray shows pleural effusion as a radiopaque density in dependent areas, a meniscus, a pocket resembling an elevated diaphragm, or as a mass along fissures or the chest wall. In the lateral view, the shifted pleural fluid may allow visualization of an underlying tumor or other mass; in fact, up to 45% of pleural effusions result from malignancies. At times, though, a computerized tomography scan is necessary to confirm diagnosis. In large effusions, chest X-ray shows mediastinal shift; however, a shift to the affected rather than the opposite side suggests bronchogenic carcinoma, which causes up to 24% of pleural effusions.

gas exchange. Breathing becomes labored for several reasons. Intrapleural pressure expands the chest wall on the affected side, making its contracted muscles less able to expand the chest further on inspiration; this delays and reduces ipsilateral chest movement. Counterpressures needed to ventilate shrunken airways mount exponentially as airway diameter shrinks and resistance grows.

But arterial hypoxemia, which initially follows pneumothorax, is usually mild and self-limiting in the first few hours. Initial hypoxemia from decreased ventilation causes vasoconstriction and increased pulmonary vascular resistance. So, reduced perfusion parallels reduced ventilation, keeping ventilation/perfusion mismatch to a minimum.

MEDICAL MANAGEMENT
Although a history and physical examination are essential in identifying the cause of a

ABG levels evaluate ventilatory status
Significant lung collapse alters arterial blood gas (ABG) levels in proportion to the degree

of ventilatory dysfunction. Acidosis develops as blood pH falls below 7.35; oxygen saturation falls; hypoxemia and hypercapnia result as PO_2 falls below 80 mm Hg and PCO_2 rises above 45 mm Hg.

Treatment
Treatment of pleural disorders aims to correct the underlying cause and any complications.

Inflammation. Treatment is usually symptomatic and includes anti-inflammatory agents, analgesics, and bed rest. However, severe pain, particularly during coughing and deep breathing, may require an intercostal nerve block. Acute inflammation resulting in chronic adhesive pleuritis, marked by restrictive thickening of the pleurae and sometimes secondary to empyema, hemothorax, or tuberculosis, may require surgical decortication. Inflammation with resultant pleural effusion requires thoracentesis to aid treatment and diagnosis. Recurrent effusion after thoracentesis, common with a metastasizing tumor, may require closed chest drainage without suction. A nonpyogenic effusion may resolve spontaneously with bed rest, but a pyogenic effusion requires chest intubation to drain purulent fluid, antibiotics, and oxygen.

Lung collapse. Minimal lung collapse, from either air or fluid accumulation, may resolve spontaneously. However, a large collapse, or any collapse with complications, requires more aggressive treatment.

Pneumothorax. Treatment is conservative for spontaneous asymptomatic pneumothorax: without signs of increased pleural pressure (indicating tension pneumothorax), with limited lung collapse (usually under 20%), and without dyspnea or other signs of respiratory distress. Such treatment consists of bed rest; careful monitoring of blood pressure, pulse rates, and respirations; oxygen administration (at low flow rates for patients with hypercapnia due to COPD or emphysema, to avoid stifling the hypoxic drive to breathe); and possibly, needle aspiration of air. Spontaneous reabsorption of air usually occurs at a daily rate of 1.5% of the pneumothorax volume.

Treatment to reexpand the lung in symptomatic pneumothorax is more complex. It includes placement of a thoracostomy tube in the second or third intercostal space in the midclavicular line (since gravity causes air to rise in the chest cavity) and connecting it to an underwater seal or suction system. A small, slowly resolving pneumothorax may be treated with a one-way flutter valve, such as the

Significance of pleural fluid analysis

Test	Interpretation
Gram's stain culture and sensitivity	Positive result may mean the early stages of bacterial infection. In the later stages of bacterial infection, the fluid may look grossly purulent with a positive Gram's stain, yet cultures may be negative from antibiotic therapy.
Acid-fast stain and culture	Positive result may indicate tuberculosis.
Red blood cell count	If count is about 10,000/mm³ and the specimen's pink or light red, may indicate tissue damage. If count is above 100,000/mm³ and the specimen's grossly bloody, suggests intrapleural malignancy, pulmonary infarction, tuberculosis, or closed chest trauma. If a hemothorax is present, the hematocrit of the pleural fluid will be similar to that of capillary blood.
Leukocyte count	If count is above 1,000/mm³ or above 50% neutrophils, may indicate septic or nonseptic inflammation.
Lymphocyte count	If count is over 50%, may indicate tuberculosis, lymphoma, or other form of cancer.
Blood clots	May indicate neoplasm, tuberculosis, or infection.
Specific gravity	If measurement exceeds 1.016, may indicate neoplasm, tuberculosis, or infection; if less than 1.104, may indicate congestive heart failure.
Total protein	Level below 3 g/dl may indicate congestive heart failure or other transudates. Level above 3 g/dl suggests neoplasm, tuberculosis, or infection.
Lactic dehydrogenase (LDH)	Levels rise in cancer and other conditions associated with exudates; decrease in heart failure and other conditions associated with transudates.
Glucose	If less than serum glucose level, may suggest cancer, bacterial infection, or nonseptic inflammation.
Sediment	May represent cancerous cells, cellular debris, or cholesterol crystals.
Biopsy	May reveal a tumor.

Recognizing tension pneumothorax

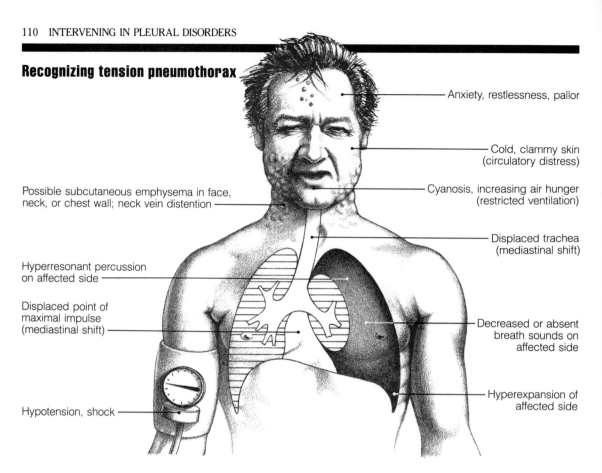

Possible subcutaneous emphysema in face, neck, or chest wall; neck vein distention

Hyperresonant percussion on affected side

Displaced point of maximal impulse (mediastinal shift)

Hypotension, shock

Anxiety, restlessness, pallor

Cold, clammy skin (circulatory distress)

Cyanosis, increasing air hunger (restricted ventilation)

Displaced trachea (mediastinal shift)

Decreased or absent breath sounds on affected side

Hyperexpansion of affected side

Heimlich valve, that lets air and drainage escape but keeps atmospheric air from entering the chest cavity.

Recurring spontaneous pneumothorax may be treated initially with a flutter valve, as an alternative to surgery. Usually, it requires pleurodesis by intrapleural instillation of a chemical irritant (such as tetracycline, talc, or kaolin), or thoracotomy with pleural abrasion or pleurectomy. These procedures, sometimes performed as prophylaxis after even a single pneumothorax, prevent recurrence by causing the visceral and parietal pleurae to adhere. Another preventive measure is thoracotomy with plication, ligation, or excision of blebs.

Traumatic and tension pneumothoraces require chest tube drainage; traumatic pneumothorax may also require surgical repair. Chronic pneumothorax without a continuing air leak requires decortication. Hemopneumothorax, which is usually self-limiting, responds to chest tube drainage, but persistent bleeding requires thoracotomy.

Pleural effusion. Depending on the amount of fluid present, symptomatic effusion may require thoracentesis to remove fluid, or careful monitoring of the patient's spontaneous rate of reabsorption of the fluid. Hemothorax requires drainage with a thoracostomy tube placed in the sixth intercostal space (since gravity causes fluid to settle), and perhaps

decortication, to prevent fibrothorax formation. Associated hypoxia requires administration of oxygen. A pyogenic effusion requires chest tube insertion, antibiotics, and oxygen.

Empyema. Treatment includes insertion of one or more chest tubes after thoracentesis to allow drainage of purulent material, and possible decortication or rib resection to allow open drainage and lung reexpansion. It also requires antibiotics, to quell infection, and oxygen therapy to relieve associated dyspnea.

NURSING MANAGEMENT
Because pleural disorders usually complicate an existing abnormality, a complete history and physical examination can reveal the underlying cause in almost any body system. But if the patient suffers chest trauma, seems to have a tension pneumothorax, or is otherwise in acute respiratory distress, you won't have time for a complete assessment. You'll want to restrict the history and physical examination to baseline needs so treatment can begin promptly. Later, when the patient is breathing more easily, you can perform a more extensive examination.

Take patient history
Ask the patient to describe his chief complaint. Typically, he'll report pain and dyspnea, the most common symptoms of pleural disor-

der. He may be anxious, because of dyspnea, and afraid that sudden pain means myocardial infarction. As you probe his history, remember that pleural pain is sharp and stabbing; breathing and exertion aggravate it, and splinting relieves it. In contrast, myocardial pain doesn't worsen with breathing and exertion, radiates down the left arm and/or up into the neck, and is associated with diaphoresis as well as dyspnea.

Ask the patient to point to the location of his pain. Chest wall pain derives from the underlying chest wall pleura; posterior shoulder pain, from pleura over the diaphragm's midsection; and simultaneous pain in abdomen and lower ribs, from pleura over the diaphragm's costal area.

During the patient history, thoroughly investigate any symptoms or complaints that suggest an underlying cause. For example:
• Sharp, stabbing pain that increases on inspiration suggests inflammation.
• Dyspnea and sudden pleuritic or chest pain suggest pneumothorax. These symptoms also suggest pulmonary infarction if preceded by long-term immobility, recent surgery, thrombophlebitis, or pregnancy.
• Recent trauma suggests chylothorax or hemothorax.
• Abdominal pain suggests pulmonary complications of acute pancreatitis, which occur in up to 20% of patients with pancreatitis, or of cholecystitis.
• A history of fever, malaise, or purulent sputum suggests empyema or pleural effusion.
• Drug therapy with hydralazine, methysergide, nitrofurantoin, or procainamide may lead to effusion; with anticoagulants, to hemothorax; and with cytotoxic chemotherapy, to spontaneous pneumothorax.
• Preexisting cardiac, hepatic, or renal disease suggests pleural effusion.
• Previous malignancies, especially sarcomas, suggest pneumothorax from pleural or pulmonary metastasis, even though the chest X-ray may not confirm it.
• Previous radiation treatments suggest induced pleural or pulmonary fibrosis leading to a ruptured bleb and spontaneous pneumothorax.
• Catamenial onset of spontaneous pneumothorax, either initial or recurrent, in women of child-bearing age may be linked to menstrual cycle abnormalities.
• Cavitary or cystic pulmonary disorders may lead to spontaneous pneumothorax. These disorders include asthma, a metastasizing tumor, congenital cystic disease or cystic fibrosis, emphysema, fungal infection, lung abscess, sarcoidosis, and tuberculosis.
• Absence of previous pulmonary or other disease suggests spontaneous pneumothorax.
• Recent travel suggests exposure to endemic pathogens. For example, travel to the southwestern United States may lead to exposure to the bacterium *Coccidioides immitis.*
• Previously active tuberculosis, recent exposure to it, or positive skin tests suggest tuberculosis.
• Exposure, up to 30 years previously, to occupational or environmental respiratory carcinogens can cause pleural disorders. For example, exposure to asbestos may lead to malignant mesothelioma.

Perform a physical examination
Although pleural inflammation and pneumothorax usually produce characteristic and localized symptoms, pleural effusion may produce varied and widespread symptoms that reflect the underlying disorder. As a result, determining the cause of pleural disorders may require examination of all body systems. However, examination of the respiratory system often reveals these significant findings:

Inspection. If you find shallow, tentative breathing or tachypnea, suspect pleural inflammation. Dyspnea that's apparent only on exertion may indicate minimal lung collapse from pleural effusion or pneumothorax. Signs of acute respiratory distress—cyanosis and severe dyspnea; anxiety; diminished and delayed movement plus overexpansion and rigidity of one hemithorax, and tracheal deviation toward the other hemithorax—suggest extensive lung collapse. Additional signs of pallor, neck vein distention, hypotension, and tachycardia strongly suggest tension pneumothorax.

Palpation. If you feel coarse vibration over one hemithorax, suspect pleural inflammation. A crackling sensation under the skin of the chest, neck, or face suggests pneumothorax with subcutaneous emphysema. Decreased or absent tactile and vocal fremitus suggest decreased airflow from air or fluid accumulation. Tracheal displacement indicates mediastinal shift.

Percussion. If you hear a flat sound over the lungs, suspect atelectasis; a dull sound, consolidation. Hyperresonant or tympanic sound indicates pneumothorax, massive atelectasis, or large emphysematous blebs. Pronounced asymmetry in diaphragm level from left to

Positions for thoracentesis

Leaning over a table

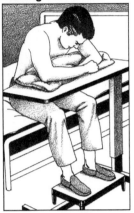

Straddling a chair

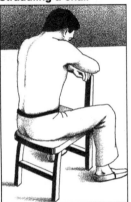

Sitting in bed in semi-Fowler's position

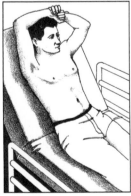

Examining pleural fluid

Appearance	Possible cause
Light straw-colored	• Normal
Purulent	• Empyema
Blood-tinged	• Hemothorax • Tuberculosis • Pulmonary infarction • Neoplastic disease • Accidental tissue damage from thoracentesis
Milky	• Chylothorax • Invasion of thoracic duct by a tumor, or an inflammatory process • Traumatic rupture of thoracic duct • Cellular debris or cholesterol crystals

right may indicate a neuromuscular disorder.

Auscultation. If you hear a localized pleural friction rub—a coarse, creaky sound heard during late inspiration and early expiration, often over the lower lateral chest wall—suspect pleural inflammation. Decreased or absent breath sounds indicate decreased airflow from air or fluid accumulation. Egobronchophony—a bleating vocal resonance—indicates lung tissue compressed by pleural effusion. Bilateral rales and gallop heart rhythms suggest heart failure—a frequent cause or companion of pleural effusion. Pericardial friction rub suggests Dressler's disease, which can cause pleural inflammation. When heard with a pleural friction rub, it suggests pleuropericarditis. Displaced heart sounds suggest pneumothorax with mediastinal shift. Crackling of subcutaneous emphysema is sometimes audible. Hamman's sign suggests pneumomediastinum.

Formulate nursing diagnoses

Once you've thoroughly examined the patient and assembled a detailed history that may indicate the cause of pleural disorder, you're ready to formulate nursing diagnoses and set appropriate care goals. In pleural disorders, these nursing diagnoses, goals, and interventions are commonly included:

Ineffective breathing pattern related to lung collapse or to pain on inspiration. Your goals are to promote adequate oxygenation, patient comfort, and lung reexpansion, if applicable.

Promote adequate oxygenation by raising the head of the patient's bed to a 45° angle, if

not contraindicated, to achieve more efficient ventilation. Watch for signs of oxygen deficiency, such as pallor or cyanosis, diaphoresis, confusion or change in level of consciousness, altered blood pressure, and increased heart and respiratory rates. To correct oxygen deficiency, administer humidified oxygen, as ordered, by face mask or cannula. In patients with hypercapnia due to COPD or other chronic respiratory insufficiency, maintain a flow rate below 2 liters/minute. As you know, in these patients the respiratory stimulus is a reduced blood oxygen level rather than an increased carbon dioxide level; high oxygen concentrations suppress this hypoxic drive and allow the accumulation of arterial carbon dioxide to fatal levels.

If the patient experiences pain from pleural inflammation, promote comfort by advising him to lie on the affected side as much as possible and to splint the painful area when coughing or breathing deeply. These actions reduce pain by restricting stretching of the inflamed pleura. Administer anti-inflammatory and analgesic drugs as ordered. Assess the resulting analgesia and notify the doctor if pain persists. Keep in mind that narcotics may diminish the cough reflex and respirations, so closely watch the patient receiving them. Call the doctor immediately if any sign of respiratory depression occurs.

In lung collapse from pleural effusion or pneumothorax, promote lung reexpansion and patient comfort by assisting with thoracentesis to remove fluid, or with chest tube insertion to remove fluid or air, as ordered.

Assist with thoracentesis. Explain the procedure to the patient and tell him to expect a stinging sensation from the local anesthetic and a feeling of pressure when the needle is inserted. Instruct him to report immediately any discomfort or breathing difficulty during the procedure. Place the patient in an appropriate position (see *Positions for thoracentesis*) if his condition permits. Reassure him during the procedure, and remind him to breathe normally and to avoid sudden movements, such as coughing or sighing. Watch closely for altered skin color, pulse, and breathing patterns, because a sudden change in thoracic pressure from overly rapid fluid removal can cause syncope, bradycardia, hypotension, pain, pulmonary edema, or even cardiac arrest. After thoracentesis, reassure the patient and allow him to rest for a few hours. Promptly send fluid specimens to the laboratory for analysis. Encourage deep breathing to promote lung reexpansion. Watch closely for complications, such as lung tissue damage or pneumothorax. To detect lung damage, check sputum for traces of blood. To detect pneumothorax, check the patient at least once every 30 minutes for any of these signs and symptoms: increased respiratory or pulse rate, blood pressure changes, pallor or cyanosis, asymmetric chest expansion, dyspnea, chest pain, and diminished or absent breath sounds on the affected side. If you suspect pneumothorax, call the doctor immediately and give oxygen as ordered. The doctor will probably order a chest X-ray.

Assist with chest tube insertion. Before insertion, explain the procedure to the patient and tell him to expect a needle prick and a feeling of pressure as the doctor administers the anesthetic, makes a small incision, and inserts the chest tube. Place the patient on his side with the area for chest tube insertion facing up, or place him upright or semiupright, as the doctor prefers. Reassure the patient during the procedure, and instruct him not to cough or move during insertion to ensure correct placement.

After insertion, connect the chest tube to a water-seal drainage system, with or without suction, as ordered. (See *Underwater-seal drainage systems* on page 114.) Allow him to assume any comfortable position not prohibited by the doctor. Tell him he may sit up or get out of bed, as long as he keeps the drainage bottles below chest level (to avoid fluid backflow into the chest), maintains the water seal, and keeps the tubing patent. Encourage him to sit semierect as much as possible when in bed, to permit accumulated air to rise, or fluid to settle, and escape through the chest tube. Encourage coughing and deep breathing to promote drainage and lung reexpansion, and teach range-of-motion exercises for the affected side. To relieve pain at the insertion site, teach or assist with splinting, and administer analgesics as ordered. Check the drainage color and consistency (see *Examining pleural fluid* on page 112) hourly for the first 24 hours after chest tube insertion, then once every 2 hours, each time marking the drainage level on the collection bottle with date and time. Although drainage is usually heaviest in the first 24 hours, call the doctor immediately if more than 100 ml of fluid/hour accumulates, since excessive fluid loss could cause shock. Watch for signs of shock: increased respiratory rate, hypotension, tachycardia, anxiety, and cold, clammy skin.

Check the rate and quality of the patient's respirations and auscultate the lungs periodically to assess air exchange in the affected lung. Diminished or absent breath sounds may indicate that the lung has not reexpanded. Tell the patient to report any breathing difficulty immediately. Notify the doctor immediately if the patient develops cyanosis, rapid shallow breathing, subcutaneous emphysema, chest pain, or excessive bleeding, since these may indicate tension pneumothorax, mediastinal shift, hemorrhage, pulmonary embolism, or cardiac tamponade.

Provide meticulous chest tube care, using aseptic technique for changing dressings around the insertion site, especially for the patient with empyema. If the chest tube and drainage tubing become disconnected, do not clamp the chest tube to avoid tension pneumothorax. Instead, quickly cleanse the ends of the tube with an antiseptic, such as povidone iodine, or clip off the contaminated ends, and then rejoin the tube with a fresh sterile connector. If the chest tube becomes dislodged from the chest, quickly apply a pressure dressing while the patient performs Valsalva's maneuver to promote lung expansion. Ask an assisting nurse to notify the doctor to insert a new chest tube. Meanwhile, remain with the patient and observe for signs of pneumothorax: increased respiratory and pulse rates, blood pressure or skin color changes, asymmetric chest expansion, dyspnea, chest pain, and diminished or absent breath sounds on the affected side.

Impaired gas exchange related to ventilation/perfusion mismatch from a collapsed lung. Your goals are to promote adequate oxygenation, to prevent complications of oxygen therapy, and to promote lung reexpansion.

To achieve these goals, observe the patient often for signs of hypoxia: increased respiratory and heart rates, altered blood pressure, cyanosis, change in level of consciousness, dysrhythmias, and cool extremities. Monitor arterial blood gases as needed, to detect developing hypoxia before signs and symptoms appear. A PO_2 below 80 mm Hg may indicate hypoxemia; a PO_2 below 60 mm Hg, minimal respiratory reserve; and a PCO_2 above 46 mm Hg, hypercapnia and hypoventilation. Give humidified oxygen by face mask or cannula, as ordered, to relieve dyspnea and improve oxygenation.

Prevent complications of oxygen therapy by first observing strict safety precautions to prevent combustion. Remember to give oxy-

Promoting an effective cough

Help your patient cough efficiently to mobilize secretions that otherwise would lead to atelectasis and pneumonia. Instruct or help him to:
• sit erect for maximum ventilation, or assume a position appropriate to his condition (see illustration)
• splint the affected area to reduce pain
• flex his knees to support abdominal muscles
• take a deep breath to increase cough pressure
• tighten his abdominal muscles as he coughs vigorously
• repeat the procedure at least hourly at first, then as needed.

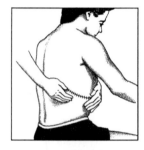

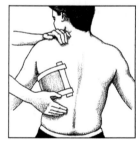

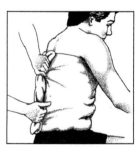

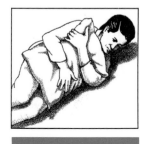

Monitoring drainage systems

• Look for fluid fluctuation of 2″ to 4″ (5 to 10 cm) in the water-seal straw or chamber as the patient breathes. With mechanical suction, fluctuation is minimal; with positive-pressure ventilation, the usual direction of fluctuation (inspiratory rise, expiratory fall) reverses. Fluctuation stops with tube obstruction, faulty suction, or lung reexpansion.

• Observe for intermittent bubbling in the water-seal bottle or chamber during expiration. Absence of bubbling indicates that evacuation is complete and pressure of the expanded lung has sealed the chest tube opening. Constant bubbling indicates a leak.

• Look for gentle bubbling in the suction control bottle or chamber, indicating a proper suction level. Vigorous bubbling increases the water evaporation rate.

• Check air vent patency. Occlusion increases pressure and can lead to tension pneumothorax.

• Milk the tubing as needed to keep it patent. Perform this procedure cautiously, since the temporary rebound pressure when tubing is released can exceed −400 cmH$_2$O (normal intrapleural pressure is −5 cmH$_2$O) and may cause tissue damage. Also, the average patient may not need it, as blood remaining in the pleural space for a few hours rarely clots, and serous drainage rarely causes obstruction.

• Clamp the tubing only to locate the source of a leak, or to replace a full or cracked collection bottle. Then clamp it only momentarily, since clamping halts air and fluid evacuation from the pleural space and can lead to tension pneumothorax. Preferable methods for changing bottles include having the able patient perform Valsalva's maneuver; and temporarily holding the tube's drainage end under water, sterile saline solution, or I.V. solution.

Underwater-seal drainage systems

One- and two-bottle drainage systems drain the pleural space with gravity's help. Three-bottle and commercial systems add mechanical suction to help manage a large fluid volume, pulmonary air leak, or small-lumen chest tube.

In the one-bottle system (1), the bottle acts as both collection container and water seal. The short straw acts as an air vent to equalize pressure between the bottle's air space and the atmosphere. The long straw connects to the patient's drainage tubing and extends about ¾″ (2 cm) under the water level. This water seal allows the expulsion of drainage but prevents air from reentering the chest during inspiration. Because water and drainage share the same bottle, continuous fluid accumulation eventually creates resistance to further drainage and increases the work of breathing.

In the two-bottle system (2), drainage falls through a short straw into the collection bottle, and air flows beyond it into the water-seal bottle. This bottle's long straw creates the water seal; its short straw functions as the air vent. This setup keeps the water seal at a fixed level, allowing more accurate observation of the volume and type of drainage. If ordered, suction may be connected to the air vent stem of the water-seal bottle.

The three-bottle system (3) adds a suction control bottle. Its long straw opens to the atmosphere at the upper end, providing another air vent, and creates a water seal at the lower end. The depth of the submerged control straw determines the approximate amount of suction that can be exerted on the drainage system.

Commercial chest drainage units resemble the bottle systems. The Pleur-evac (4) is a one-piece disposable, molded plastic unit with three chambers duplicating the three-bottle system. Special features include a positive pressure-release valve that prevents pressure buildup in the pleural space. The Argyle double-seal unit (5) is similar to the Pleur-evac unit, but adds a fourth chamber—an additional water seal that's vented to the atmosphere to prevent pressure buildup.

1. One-bottle system

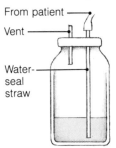

From patient —

Vent —

Water-seal straw

2. Two-bottle system

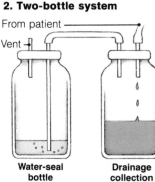

From patient —

Vent —

Water-seal bottle   **Drainage collection bottle**

3. Three-bottle system

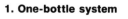
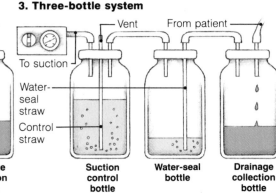

— Vent   From patient —

To suction

Water-seal straw

Control straw

Suction control bottle   **Water-seal bottle**   **Drainage collection bottle**

4. Pleur-evac system

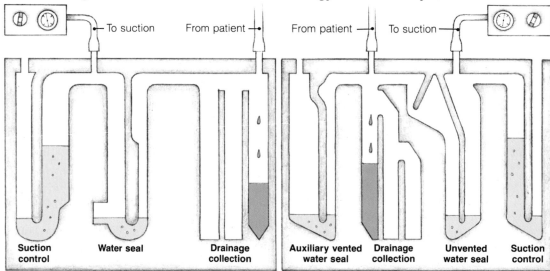

— To suction   From patient —

Suction control   **Water seal**   **Drainage collection**

5. Argyle double-seal system

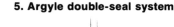

From patient —   To suction —

Auxiliary vented water seal   **Drainage collection**   **Unvented water seal**   **Suction control**

gen carefully to patients with chronic lung disorders, since flow rates above 2 liters/minute can suppress hypoxic respiratory drive. Continue to monitor ABG levels and immediately report any imbalance, such as persistent hypoxemia or sudden rise in PCO_2.

Promote lung reexpansion by assisting with thoracentesis or chest tube insertion. Encourage the patient to cough and breathe deeply at least hourly; if the doctor orders incentive spirometry, instruct the patient in its use. Assess lung sounds regularly to evaluate the effect of therapy.

Be prepared for emergency administration of oxygen to remedy insufficient gas exchange in case of sudden lung collapse. Regularly observe the patient for signs and symptoms of pneumothorax, since this complication can occur suddenly—during rest or exertion— and may lead rapidly to tension pneumothorax. If pneumothorax does occur, notify the doctor. Try to calm the patient to reduce anxiety and control dyspnea. Administer oxygen, as ordered, and help the patient sit up to improve ventilation. Assist with thoracentesis and/or chest tube insertion, as ordered. Monitor vital signs for indications of shock, increasing respiratory distress, and mediastinal shift.

Cough discomfort related to pain from pleural inflammation. Your goal is to promote patient comfort. Elevate the head of the bed or encourage the patient to sit up as much as possible; this position relaxes the chest and abdominal muscles and makes coughing less strenuous. Administer an analgesic as ordered, but be alert for oversedation that can inhibit the cough reflex and add to the effort of coughing. Administer antitussives as ordered. Show the patient how to splint the affected area during coughing to reduce pain. Increase daily fluid intake to 2,000 ml, if not contraindicated. Discourage smoking. Use a vaporizer, if necessary, to maintain room humidity.

Painful respirations related to movement of inflamed pleura. To promote comfort and rest, administer analgesic and anti-inflammatory drugs as ordered. Since pleuritic pain can range from mild discomfort during coughing or deep breathing to severe stabbing pain during inspiration, appropriate drugs range from aspirin to narcotics. For 1- to 10-hour relief of mild pain, the doctor may freeze the affected area with ethyl chloride spray; when narcotics fail to subdue severe pain, the doctor may inject procaine hydrochloride subcutaneously or as an intercostal nerve block.

Explain this procedure to the patient, and assist the doctor as needed.

In inflammation with pleural effusion, place the patient in a sitting position to allow optimal and least painful chest expansion. Have him change positions often and lie on the affected side to splint it. Also, apply heat to the affected area. Permit the patient as much uninterrupted rest as possible.

Anxiety related to fear of the unknown and interruption of normal respiratory function. To relieve anxiety and provide support, stay with the patient constantly during an acute episode. Since anxiety can further aggravate respiratory distress, try to calm the patient. To remove hidden anxiety, encourage him to ask questions and express his feelings. Keep him informed about his progress and care plan. Encourage interaction with family or friends.

Knowledge deficit about the disorder and its treatment. To increase the patient's understanding of his disorder and its treatment, explain all procedures to him before they're performed. Teach him to cough productively to prevent exhaustion and retention of secretions, which can lead to atelectasis and pneumonia.

For the patient with a chest tube, explain the positions that promote drainage and those that are contraindicated. Emphasize the importance of keeping the chest tube free of kinks and tension and the drainage system below chest level. Teach breathing exercises that promote muscle relaxation and relieve anxiety. Keep the patient informed about discharge plans, and prepare him for self-care at home.

If pleural effusion was a complication of pneumonia or influenza, advise prompt medical attention for any subsequent chest colds.

Evaluate your interventions
Consider your interventions successful if the patient shows indications of adequate gas exchange (absence of cyanosis, normal vital signs, and adequate ABG levels); pain-free respirations without dyspnea or shortness of breath; calm appearance; and a working knowledge of his disorder and its treatment.

A final word
Pleural disorders challenge all of your nursing skills. Accurate assessment, for example, can lead to early recognition and treatment—and prevention of life-threatening complications. Timely nursing interventions also help prevent complications and promote recovery.

Points to remember

• Pleural disorders may result from inflammation, increased pleural fluid pressure, or increased intrapleural gas pressure.
• Sharp, stabbing pain and dyspnea commonly occur in pleural disorders.
• Within minutes, spontaneous or traumatic pneumothorax can progress to a life-threatening tension pneumothorax.
• Major nursing goals in pleural disorders include restoring adequate oxygenation, promoting lung reexpansion, and preventing complications of treatment.
• Keeping the patient calm, comfortable, and informed are important in his care, since anxiety impairs respiration and the quality of gas exchange.

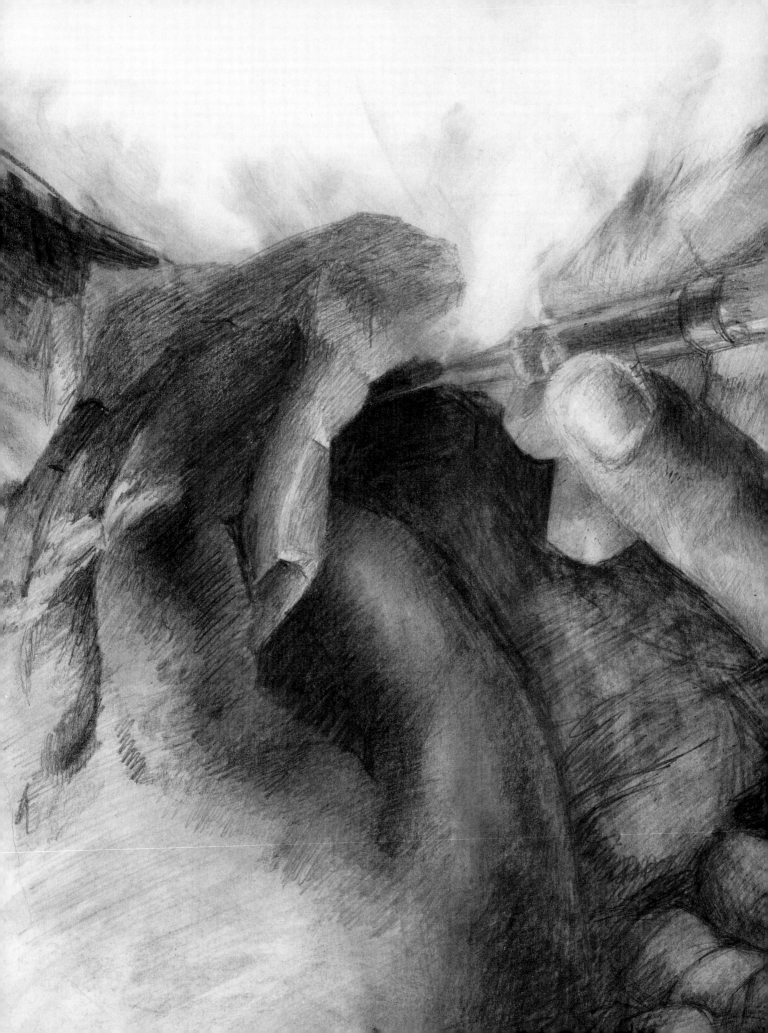

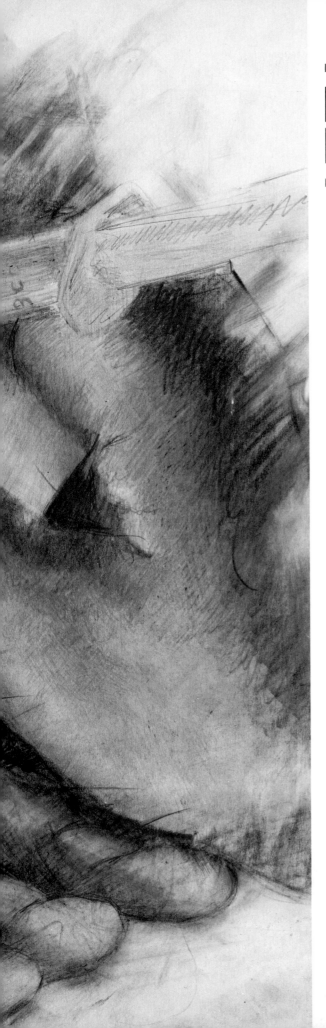

DISORDERS OF PERFUSION

8 TREATING VASCULAR DISORDERS

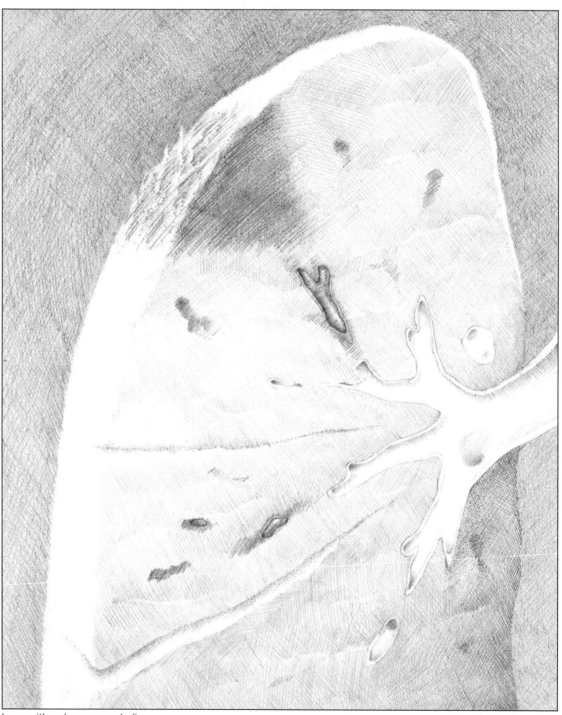

Lung with pulmonary emboli

Pulmonary vascular disorders rank among the most serious complications of cardiovascular or respiratory disease. These disorders include *pulmonary hypertension, pulmonary edema,* and *pulmonary vascular obstruction.* Pulmonary hypertension occurs in primary and secondary forms. Primary pulmonary hypertension is the only pulmonary vascular disorder that can't be attributed to preexisting cardiovascular or respiratory disease. Secondary pulmonary hypertension may result from congenital or acquired cardiovascular disease, as well as from obstructive or restrictive respiratory disease. Pulmonary edema usually stems from cardiac disease; pulmonary vascular obstruction may stem from embolism, from a tumor or neoplasm, or from vasculitis.

Untreated, these disorders cause severe lung damage that can drastically impair or threaten a patient's life-style. To promote prompt treatment that helps prevent irreversible complications, you must be able to identify patients at risk for developing these disorders. When dealing with patients who already have a pulmonary vascular disorder, to minimize permanent respiratory damage, you must know how to evaluate the effectiveness of prescribed therapy. In addition, you must be able to recognize significant and potentially life-threatening changes in the patient's condition.

PATHOPHYSIOLOGY
All pulmonary vascular disorders increase pulmonary vascular resistance. However, the pathophysiology of these disorders varies, depending on the underlying cardiovascular or respiratory disease.

Primary pulmonary hypertension
Primary pulmonary hypertension has a unique pathology. In this condition, the intima of the pulmonary arteries thickens for no apparent reason. This narrows the diameter and impairs distensibility of the arteries, increasing pulmonary vascular resistance. Most persons with primary pulmonary hypertension remain asymptomatic until lung damage becomes severe. Often, this disorder is not found until autopsy. While its cause is unknown, a hereditary defect appears likely, since this disorder tends to occur within families. Its incidence is higher among women.

Secondary pulmonary hypertension
Various pathology can lead to secondary pulmonary hypertension. Let's first consider preexisting cardiovascular disease, which can be congenital or acquired. Acyanotic congenital cardiac defects, such as patent ductus arteriosus and atrial and ventricular septal defects, allow left-to-right shunting of blood into the pulmonary artery. As a result, pulmonary blood flow in the fetus increases. This, in turn, prevents maturation of the pulmonary vasculature during the first week after birth. It also prevents pulmonary vascular resistance, which is normally elevated in the fetus, from decreasing to normal postnatally.

In acquired heart disease, the left ventricular failure diminishes the flow of oxygenated blood from the lungs. As a result, pulmonary vascular resistance increases, along with right ventricular pressure.

Secondary pulmonary hypertension can also result from obstructive or restrictive respiratory disease. Both forms of respiratory disease may destroy alveoli, causing the lungs to shunt incoming blood to the remaining healthy alveoli. As the number of these alveoli decreases, pulmonary vascular resistance rises, because more and more blood is being shunted to a progressively smaller area of the lungs. The hypoxemia resulting from this ventilation/perfusion mismatch also causes pulmonary vasoconstriction, further increasing pulmonary vascular resistance. If the underlying respiratory defect is chronic, the overwhelming work load on the right ventricle eventually causes it to become dilated and hypertrophic, resulting in cor pulmonale (see *Understanding cor pulmonale,* page 120).

Pulmonary edema
Preexisting cardiovascular disease, whether congenital or acquired, can also lead to pulmonary edema. Pulmonary edema damages ventricular walls and weakens contractility. Consequently, cardiac output also diminishes as blood pools in the pulmonary venous system. The accumulating blood increases pressure, disturbing the balance between hydrostatic pressure in the interstitium and oncotic pressure. This forces proteins and water to leak into the interstitium. If pressures rise high enough, ultrafiltrated plasma eventually leaks into the alveoli, causing alveoli to collapse.

Pulmonary vascular obstruction
This disorder can result from a tumor (such as an arterial myxoma), neoplastic invasion of the mediastinum, or vasculitis—all of which

Understanding cor pulmonale

Cor pulmonale, or right ventricular hypertrophy, is the end stage of chronic disorders that affect the function and/or structure of the lungs. Although prognosis is poor in cor pulmonale, treatment aims to reduce hypoxia, increase exercise tolerance, and, when possible, correct the underlying causes. These causes include:

• diseases affecting the airways, such as chronic obstructive pulmonary disease and bronchial asthma

• thoracic cage deformities, such as kyphoscoliosis and pectus excavatum

• disorders affecting pulmonary parenchyma, such as sarcoidosis, pulmonary fibrosis, pneumoconiosis, periarteritis nodosa, and tuberculosis

• chronic alveolar hypoventilation, which occurs in obese patients and those living at high altitudes

• pulmonary vascular diseases, such as vasculitis, pulmonary emboli or external vascular obstruction due to tumor or aneurysm

• neuromuscular disorders, such as muscular dystrophy and poliomyelitis.

Pathophysiology

In cor pulmonale, pulmonary hypertension increases cardiac work load. To compensate, the right ventricle hypertrophies to force blood through the lungs. However, this compensatory mechanism begins to fail, and larger amounts of blood remain in the right ventricle at the end of diastole, causing dilatation. In response to hypoxia, the bone marrow produces more red blood cells, resulting in polycythemia. Blood viscosity increases, further aggravating pulmonary hypertension, increasing the right ventricle's work load and causing failure.

Diagnosing cor pulmonale

Diagnosis is mainly based on the patient's history and the results of the physical examination and is supported by diagnostic tests. During the physical examination, you'll find displacement of the point of maximal impulse (PMI), indicative of right ventricular enlargement. You'll hear a gallop rhythm, a loud pulmonic sound, and, if tricuspid insufficiency is present, a pansystolic murmur at the left sternal border. You'll also detect distended neck veins, dependent edema, tachycardia, and an enlarged, tender liver from venous pooling; and weak pulse and hypotension from decreased cardiac output. Diagnostic tests, such as an echocardiogram, electrocardiogram, and chest X-ray, show right ventricular hypertrophy. Also, the complete blood count shows an elevated hematocrit reflecting erythrocytosis.

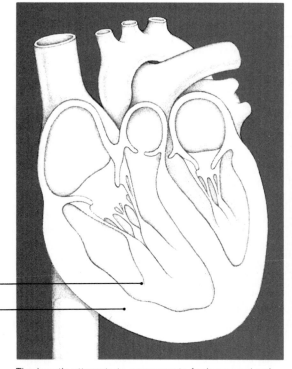

Dilated right ventricle

Hypertrophied ventricular wall

The heart's attempts to compensate for increased pulmonary vascular resistance cause hypertrophy of the ventricular wall and dilatation of the right ventricle.

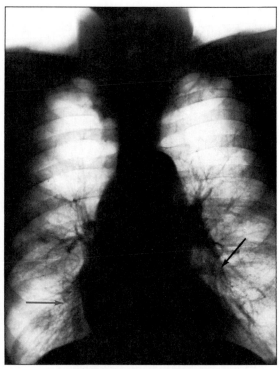

The chest X-ray above shows right ventricular enlargement (blue arrow) and prominent pulmonary arteries (black arrow), characteristic of cor pulmonale.

may obstruct the small or large pulmonary veins (see *Stages of pulmonary vascular obstruction*). The most common cause of pulmonary vascular obstruction, however, is embolism. An embolus can originate in the venous system, typically as a result of thrombophlebitis. Typically, such thrombi form in the veins of the legs. If the thrombi dislodge, they can pass through the vena cava and right heart and into the pulmonary arterial branches, where they may cause an occlusion. Such occlusion decreases blood flow to the area supplied by the vessel and creates alveolar dead space. Shunting of blood, with increased pulmonary vascular resistance, follows.

Similarly, tricuspid or pulmonic valve dysfunction can cause thrombi to form on the valve leaflets. If the thrombi dislodge, they too can enter the pulmonary vascular system, lodge in one of the smaller pulmonary arteries, and obstruct blood flow.

Nonthrombic emboli produce the same sequence of pathologic events from different points of origin.
• *Fat emboli* can result from excessive manipulation of long-bone fractures or even from long-bone, particularly compound, fractures themselves.
• *Septic emboli* can result from I.V. drug abuse.
• *Amniotic emboli* are associated with fluid leakage into the uterine veins as a result of uterine tears or vigorous contractions after membrane rupture.
• *Air emboli* can result from insertion of a central venous pressure (CVP) or neck vein catheter, chest trauma, tubal insufflation, pneumoperitoneum, or mechanical ventilation.

Compensatory mechanisms
The pressure required to propel blood through a healthy pulmonary vascular system is only about 10 mm Hg—roughly one tenth the average systemic intravascular pressure. In pulmonary vascular disorders, however, the increased vascular resistance means pressure within the pulmonary circulation must be great enough to overcome pulmonary vascular resistance to ensure adequate perfusion of the lungs. To compensate for this resistance, the body reacts with two mechanisms: tachycardia and tachypnea.

Tachycardia. Although tachycardia may help propel oxygenated blood through a resistive pulmonary vascular system, it may reduce cardiac output because of the concomitant decrease in ventricular filling pressure. As

a result, blood flow to the coronary arteries decreases, which, together with the heart's increased work load, can cause chest pain.

If pulmonary vascular resistance becomes chronic, right ventricular failure to adequately expel its contents during systole may eventually lead to right ventricular failure. Blood then accumulates in the venous system, causing jugular distention and liver engorgement. As right ventricular failure progresses, systemic venous pressure and hydrostatic pressure in peripheral veins rise. The result— peripheral edema.

Tachypnea. This second mechanism, coupled with an increase in the depth of respirations, attempts to compensate for decreased oxygenation. The body tries to take in more oxygen while expelling excess carbon dioxide. In chronic conditions, however, persistent tachypnea may result in overcompensation. Then, too much carbon dioxide is expelled, causing respiratory alkalosis.

MEDICAL MANAGEMENT
Effective treatment of a pulmonary vascular disorder can begin only after detection of its cause. This requires integration of diagnostic tests, with patient history and physical examination results. Careful analysis of all subjective and objective data gathered may also reveal the extent of the disease and the significant events in the patient's life that may have led to its development.

Diagnostic tests
A typical diagnostic workup for a patient with a suspected pulmonary vascular disorder includes *chest X-rays, lung scan, arterial blood gas (ABG) analysis, electrocardiography, complete blood cell count, sputum analysis,* and *pulmonary function tests.*

Chest X-rays. Obvious differences in the diameters of major vessels may reflect shunting of blood around alveolar dead space to areas supplied by the dilated vessels. Small pulmonary infiltrates may be seen in some alveoli. Secondary to decreased pulmonary blood flow or decreased ventilation and inadequate surfactant, such infiltrates reflect atelectasis. Usually, the infiltrates appear at the bases of the lungs.

Lung scan. This test may confirm pulmonary vascular obstruction by showing decreased or absent blood flow, most likely the result of an embolus. The scan doesn't show the actual obstruction but the affected areas beyond it.

Stages of pulmonary vascular obstruction

Normal pulmonary artery

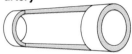

Hypertrophied pulmonary artery

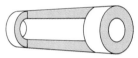

Thickened intimal layer with occlusion of pulmonary artery

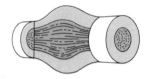

ABG analysis. Because fewer alveoli are available for gas exchange, a decreased PaO_2 level is a common finding in pulmonary vascular disorders. The $PaCO_2$ level usually decreases as well, but may rise in the early stages of a disorder, reflecting respiratory acidosis. In chronic disorders, overcompensation for respiratory acidosis may decrease the $PaCO_2$ level.

Electrocardiography. The results of this test may be normal or may show only tachycardia. However, if the right ventricle is being overworked, the pattern of the precordial leads may reflect right axis deviation and right ventricular hypertrophy.

Complete blood cell count. Rarely, leukocytosis, reflecting the inflammatory process beyond the point of a pulmonary infarction, may be present. Chronic hypoxemia may cause erythrocytosis, a result of the body's attempts to increase the oxygen-carrying capacity of the blood.

Sputum analysis. Because bacteria or viruses are usually absent, microscopic examination of sputum isn't necessary. Gross examination, however, may reveal small amounts of blood or a pinkish tinge, the result of capillaries bursting from increased vascular pressure. Pink-tinged and foamy sputum usually indicates pulmonary edema, and hemoptysis (bloody sputum) usually indicates pulmonary embolism.

Pulmonary function tests. These tests can show the extent of lung damage and the patient's pulmonary reserve, which may suggest appropriate forms of therapy and facilitate discharge planning.

Treatment: Oxygen, drugs, surgery

In pulmonary vascular disorders, treatment includes *oxygen therapy, drug therapy* (with digoxin, diuretics, morphine, bronchodilators, or heparin), and *surgery.*

Oxygen therapy. Initially, oxygen is administered by nasal cannula or face mask to improve arterial oxygenation. However, if the patient fails to maintain an acceptable PaO_2 level, or if he tires from persistent tachypnea, mechanical ventilation may be needed. With mechanical ventilation, oxygen concentration can be controlled better. Also, lung damage can be determined more accurately by observing the amount of pressure needed to deliver the preset tidal volume. If the amount of pressure must be increased, it may indicate increased pulmonary vascular pressure.

Positive end-expiratory pressure (PEEP)

may have to be applied if impaired alveolar functioning has markedly decreased the patient's functional residual capacity. PEEP may resolve this problem by forcing alveolar fluid to diffuse across the respiratory membrane and back into the intravascular spaces. Redistribution increases the number of alveoli available for gas exchange. However, because PEEP can stress the heart, the patient requires continual assessment.

Drug therapy. *Digoxin* decreases cardiac work load by improving myocardial contractility, thereby increasing cardiac output. As cardiac output increases, both cardiac and pulmonary perfusion and the ventilation/perfusion ratio improve.

Diuretics, such as furosemide and ethacrynic acid, are potent loop diuretics that act on the ascending loop of Henle. These diuretics can help shift accumulated interstitial fluid back into the intravascular spaces, where it can be transported to the kidneys for excretion. As a result, pulmonary capillary pressure decreases. Diuretics must be administered cautiously, however, to prevent fluid depletion. Such depletion decreases cardiac output, forcing the heart to work harder and possibly weakening the right ventricle.

Morphine may alleviate anxiety and promote blood flow from the pulmonary circulation to the periphery. However, because morphine can severely depress respiration, naloxone hydrochloride and intubation equipment must be readily available.

Increased pulmonary capillary pressure may cause bronchospasms in the terminal segments of the bronchi. If such bronchospasms occur, *bronchodilators,* such as aminophylline, may help open the bronchi and promote better aeration. Aminophylline must be administered slowly to prevent a sudden—and possibly fatal—drop in blood pressure. This drug also increases heart rate, causing tachydysrhythmias.

Heparin may be administered to a patient with diagnosed pulmonary emboli to prevent further clot formation. It may also be administered to a patient on extended bed rest, who is at risk for developing pulmonary emboli due to venous stasis.

Surgery. Of the three types of pulmonary vascular disorders, only pulmonary vascular obstruction caused by embolism may be relieved by surgery. Recurrent pulmonary emboli from thrombophlebitis may require surgery to prevent migration of emboli to the lungs. The most common procedures for managing emboli are vena cava ligation, insertion of an umbrella filter, and bronchoscopy.

Vena cava ligation may prevent migration of small recurrent emboli. The *vena cava umbrella* procedure involves insertion of an umbrella filter into the vena cava to trap emboli while allowing uninterrupted blood flow.

Bronchoscopy allows removal of a foreign object from the lungs. It also allows removal of accumulated secretions or fluid, which helps aerate functioning alveoli.

For nonthrombic emboli, prevention is the best treatment. Air emboli, for example, may be prevented by placing the patient in a head-down position during insertion of a CVP or neck vein catheter and during subsequent tubing changes. This position prevents air from entering the venous system. Having the patient hold his breath whenever the catheter is open to the air serves the same purpose. However, once an embolism has occurred, supportive measures must begin at once to prevent lethal complications (see *Treating air emboli,* page 124).

NURSING MANAGEMENT

Nursing management of the patient with a pulmonary vascular disorder begins with the taking of a thorough patient history, followed by systematic physical examination. These two steps provide the subjective and objective data you'll need to formulate nursing diagnoses, set care goals, and plan and evaluate interventions.

Take patient history

History taking aims to elicit details about the onset of the patient's illness, his home and work environments, and any drugs he's taking. Be sure to ask the following questions at the initial interview unless the patient is in acute distress. In such cases, postpone the complete history until a more opportune time or, if a family member is present, ask him to provide the necessary information.

Onset of illness. When did the patient's illness begin? Were there any possible precipitating factors, such as a bone fracture (especially in a leg) or a febrile illness? Does

Surgical techniques

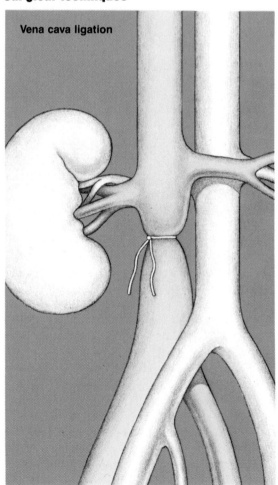

Vena cava ligation

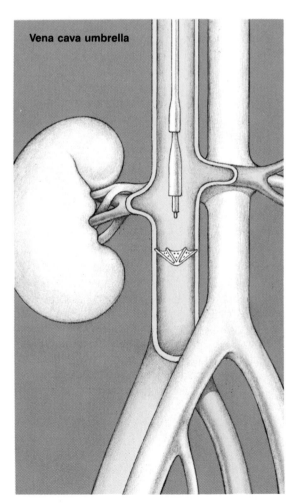

Vena cava umbrella

EMERGENCY MANAGEMENT

Treating air emboli

Air emboli can result from many causes, such as head and neck surgery, pneumoperitoneum, and insertion, removal, or routine care of central venous lines. If you suspect air emboli, prompt nursing intervention is essential to prevent lethal complications. Immediately turn the patient onto his left side, place him in a head-down position (see illustration), and notify the doctor. This position helps air bubbles float toward the right atrium and away from the pulmonary artery, preventing obstruction of the outflow tract and allowing blood to enter the lungs. Usually, the trapped air dissipates slowly through the pulmonary system. If not, the doctor may insert a catheter into the right atrium and attempt to remove the air.

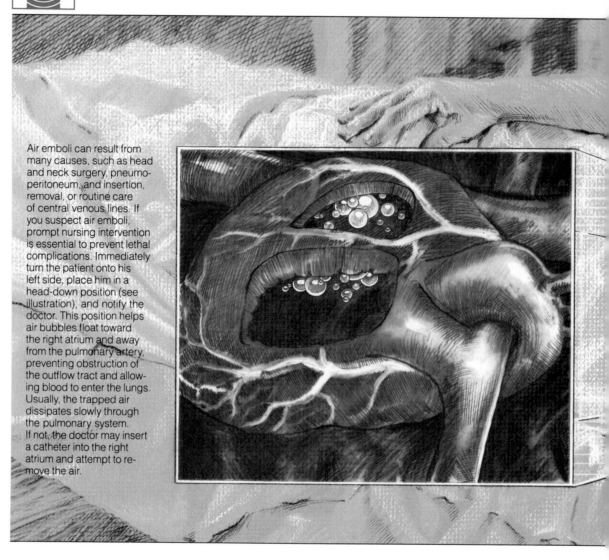

the patient have a history of cardiovascular or respiratory disease? Has he recently noticed a change in heart rhythm? Was a CVP or neck vein catheter inserted recently?

Environment. Ask the patient to describe his home and work environments. Is he exposed to toxic chemicals or excess carbon dioxide at work? Is his home adequately ventilated and free of dampness? (Poor ventilation or dampness may reduce the amount of oxygen available for gas exchange.) Remember that the patient's home environment has important implications for rehabilitation. You'll want to know how many steps he has in his house, for example.

Drugs. Ask the patient if he takes any prescribed drugs, such as narcotics, diuretics, or antiarrhythmics. If so, when does he take

them? Don't forget to ask about over-the-counter medications (such as sleeping pills, diet pills, or cough medicines), too. If the patient is a woman, ask about use of oral contraceptives. Some of the above drugs can contribute to the development of a pulmonary vascular disorder, and others can interfere with prescribed therapy.

Smoking. Ask the patient if he smokes. If so, obtain a smoking history in pack years.

Activities. What is the patient's current activity level? Is his life-style active or sedentary? Will he need to change his life-style?

Perform the physical examination

A modified systematic approach works best in conducting a physical examination of the patient with a suspected pulmonary vascular

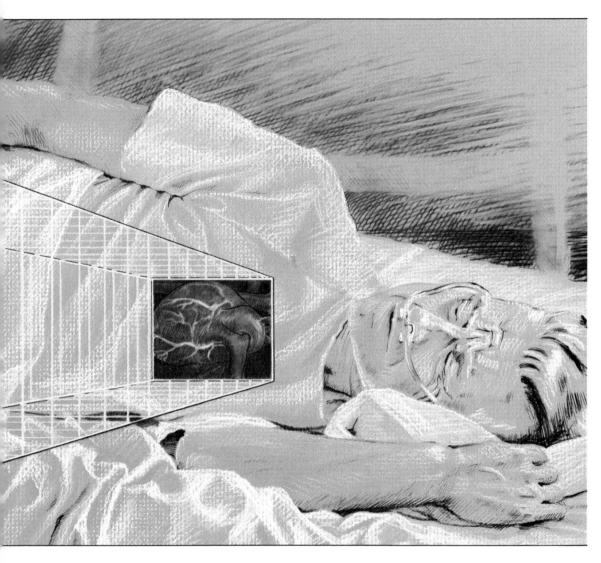

disorder. Start with a thorough assessment of the respiratory and cardiovascular systems, then assess the abdominal area before moving to the neurologic system.

Respiratory system. Begin by observing the patient's breathing pattern. Note whether his chest moves symmetrically during respiration. Look for guarding secondary to pain on inspiration, perhaps indicating the presence of a foreign object or embolus in the pulmonary vascular system. Also, look for the use of accessory muscles, such as the abdominal and intercostal muscles. Use of these muscles may reflect reduced alveolar function, which increases the work of breathing.

Other key findings on inspection include decreased diaphragmatic excursion, which may result from pulmonary fibrosis, and cya-

nosis or pallor, indicating decreased arterial oxygenation.

Next, palpate the chest. Be alert for decreased fremitus at the lung bases, which may reflect atelectasis or pleural effusion. Fluid-filled areas in the interstitium—a sign of pulmonary edema—produce increased fremitus. On percussion, listen for dull sounds at the lung bases, which may reflect atelectasis or pleural effusion.

Auscultate for rales, which you'll hear throughout the lungs if fluid has accumulated in the alveoli. Discontinuous rales, heard only at the end of inspiration, may result from the reopening of collapsed alveoli. Listen for rhonchi or wheezing, indicating partial obstruction of the airways by mucus, fluid, or bronchospasm. Listen, too, for a pleural friction rub, which can result from pulmonary infarction or pleurisy.

Cardiovascular system. During inspection, look for jugular vein distention, which reflects pooling of blood in the right ventricle because of increased pulmonary vascular resistance. If this condition becomes severe, you may also see edema in the legs or above the sacrum secondary to decreased venous return to the heart.

Now, palpate all pulses for rate, rhythm, and quality; bounding pulses may result from an increased blood supply. Next, find the point of maximal impulse (PMI) at the fifth intercostal space along the midclavicular line. A displaced PMI indicates right or left ventricular enlargement.

Check the patient's heart rhythm, since pulmonary vascular disorder predisposes the patient to atrial tachycardia and fibrillation. Any distention of the major airways disturbs atrial function, since the atria lie directly in front of them.

Auscultate for abnormal heart sounds. A pulmonic click can result from increased pulmonary artery pressure, which impairs pulmonic valve function. Mitral murmurs may occur secondary to mitral regurgitation, which forces cardiac output into the atria; a gallop

rhythm, secondary to myocardial failure and/or excessive fluid accumulation in the lungs.

Before assessing the neurologic system, gently palpate the upper right quadrant of the abdomen to check for pain or liver enlargement. Either finding could reflect liver engorgement secondary to increased right ventricular pressure. Check, too, for bowel sounds, since hypoxemia can diminish intestinal motility and lead to ileus.

Neurologic system. Because pulmonary vascular disorders usually decrease cerebral oxygenation, assess the patient's level of consciousness and orientation to time and place, which may reflect brain oxygenation. Also watch for restlessness or anxiety, which may follow hypoxemia and decreased cerebral perfusion. (See *Clinical findings in pulmonary vascular disorders and cor pulmonale.*)

Formulate nursing diagnoses

Using the subjective data from the patient history and the objective data from the physical examination, you're ready to form appropriate nursing diagnoses. In pulmonary vascular disorders, the most important nursing diagnoses are *ineffective breathing pattern, ineffective airway clearance, impaired gas exchange, decreased cardiac output,* and *alter-*

Clinical findings in pulmonary vascular disorders and cor pulmonale

Body system or area	Pulmonary hypertension	Pulmonary edema	Pulmonary vascular obstruction	Cor pulmonale
Respiratory system	Dyspnea Cyanosis Decreased breath sounds (with loud tubular sounds) Decreased diaphragmatic excursion and depth of respirations	Dyspnea Orthopnea Cyanosis Crepitant rales Dullness on percussion Possible wheezing	Tachypnea Cyanosis Decreased diaphragmatic excursion and depth of respirations Rales at lung bases Pleural friction rub	Tachypnea Shortness of breath with mild exertion Cyanosis Possible rales at lung bases
Cardiovascular system	Tachycardia Displaced point of maximal impulse (beyond the midclavicular line) Possible neck vein distention Widely split S_2; S_3 or S_4 Systolic ejection murmur	Tachycardia Neck vein distention Gallop rhythm Pulsus alternans	Tachycardia Widely split S_2; possible S_3 or S_4 Normal or bounding pulses (may be weaker in legs)	Tachycardia Displaced point of maximal impulse (beyond the midclavicular line) Gallop rhythm Neck vein distention Lower extremity and presacral edema
Neurologic system	Restlessness Decreased level of consciousness Confusion, memory loss	Restlessness Decreased level of consciousness Confusion, memory loss	Restlessness Decreased level of consciousness Confusion, memory loss	Restlessness Decreased level of consciousness Confusion, memory loss
Abdomen	Liver enlargement and/or tenderness	Liver enlargement and/or tenderness Possible use of abdominal muscles	Possible use of abdominal muscles	Liver enlargement and/or tenderness

ation in comfort. Each of these, in turn, carries a specific set of nursing goals and interventions.

Ineffective breathing pattern. This may occur secondary to pain or fluid accumulation in the lungs. Your nursing goals are to prevent respiratory arrest by recognizing its early signs and symptoms, and to find a comfortable position for the patient that will promote adequate aeration of the lungs without increasing the work of breathing.

Appropriate nursing intervention includes assessing the patient's respiratory status at least every 2 hours during the acute phase of his illness and every 4 hours after his condition has stabilized to ensure prompt recognition of respiratory distress. To provide for adequate lung expansion, keep the patient in semi-Fowler's or high Fowler's position, with his body properly aligned. Monitor ABGs for a decreased PaO_2 level.

Ineffective airway clearance. This may occur secondary to fatigue and weakness. Key nursing goals are to maintain a patent airway and to mobilize secretions.

To achieve these goals, administer intermittent positive pressure breathing or heated aerosol treatment, as ordered, to keep secretions loose. Then, perform chest physiotherapy to aid in the mobilization of secretions. Finally, to help remove secretions, have the patient cough and deep breathe. If the patient's cough is ineffective, suction him as needed.

Impaired gas exchange. With this diagnosis, your goals are to help maintain adequate oxygenation, find a comfortable position for the patient that promotes adequate lung expansion, maintain a patent airway, and mobilize secretions.

Appropriate nursing intervention includes making sure the oxygen-delivery system is properly applied and maintaining the prescribed oxygen concentration. Also, to help assess adequate oxygen delivery, monitor ABGs for a decreased PaO_2 level. To keep airway patent, perform suctioning, as necessary.

Decreased cardiac output. This may result from increased cardiac work load. Your nursing goals are to balance the patient's fluid intake and output and to prevent further deterioration in the patient's condition by recognizing early signs and symptoms of heart failure.

Your nursing intervention includes measuring the patient's output every hour and monitoring the amount of infused fluid. Restrict oral intake to no more than 800 ml every 24 hours. If the patient is receiving diuretics to reduce fluid accumulation in the lungs, monitor their effects carefully and watch for signs of electrolyte imbalance. Be alert for signs of digitalis toxicity, such as nausea, yellow-green halos around visual images, and agitation. Also watch for changes in heart rate or rhythm, such as atrial or ventricular dysrhythmias or heart block. Plan your care to allow the patient adequate rest.

Alteration in comfort. Usually pain occurs secondary to the increased work of breathing. Your primary nursing goal is to keep the patient free from pain and capable of breathing and moving about with the least amount of discomfort.

Relevant nursing intervention includes administering prescribed analgesics at the patient's request and before performing procedures that might cause him pain. Be especially cautious when administering narcotics, since they can depress the patient's respirations.

Teach the patient breathing techniques that minimize discomfort, such as splinting the chest with a pillow and maintaining a position that provides adequate aeration of the lungs. Instruct the patient to report any discomfort immediately.

Evaluate your care plan

You'll need to evaluate your care plan periodically to assess its effectiveness and modify it as the patient's condition changes. Look for signs of improved oxygenation, such as decreased cyanosis or pallor and reduced restlessness or anxiety. Observe the patient carefully to see if dyspnea or tachypnea has subsided.

If the patient is receiving drugs to alleviate breathing problems, determine their effects. Report any complications of drug therapy to the doctor—for example, an increase in heart rate after administration of a bronchodilator, signs of bleeding in a patient receiving heparin, or signs of toxicity in a patient receiving digoxin.

Above all, watch for signs of deterioration in the patient's condition, such as decreased level of consciousness. Remember that the prognosis for surviving a pulmonary vascular disorder depends not only on the severity of the acute episode, but also on the development of additional complications. Your ability to recognize such complications quickly and intervene correctly may well mean the difference between life and death.

Points to remember

• Except for primary pulmonary hypertension, all pulmonary vascular disorders result from preexisting cardiovascular or respiratory disease and cause increased pulmonary vascular resistance.
• The severity of an acute episode and the development of complications are the major factors in determining whether a pulmonary vascular disorder proves fatal.
• Without prompt treatment, pulmonary vascular disorders can cause severe lung damage that may permanently alter the patient's life-style and even threaten his life.
• Nursing management of pulmonary vascular disorders requires thorough history-taking and physical examination skills. It also requires formulation of nursing diagnoses that suggest realistic nursing goals and appropriate interventions.

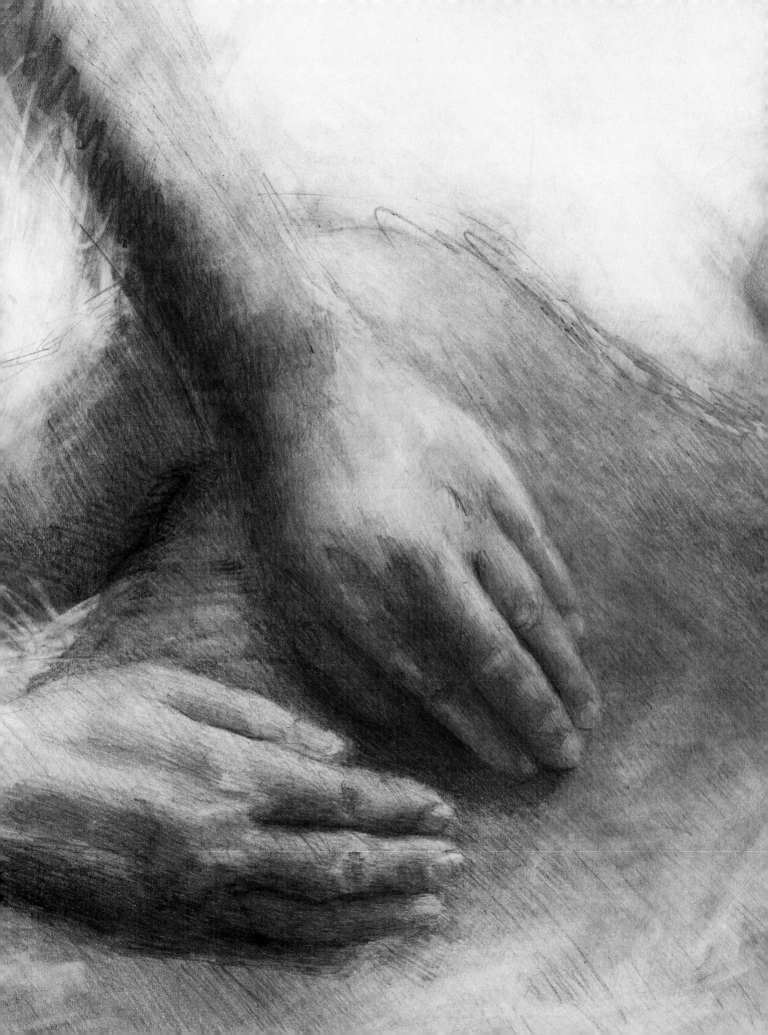

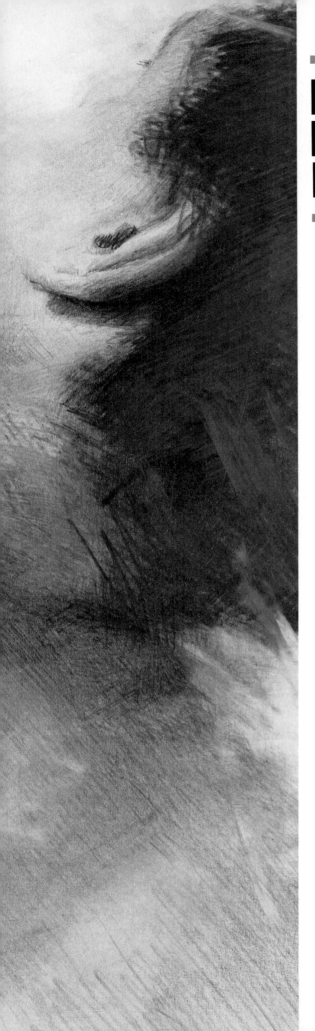

DISORDERS OF LUNG PARENCHYMA

9 PREVENTING ACUTE DISEASE

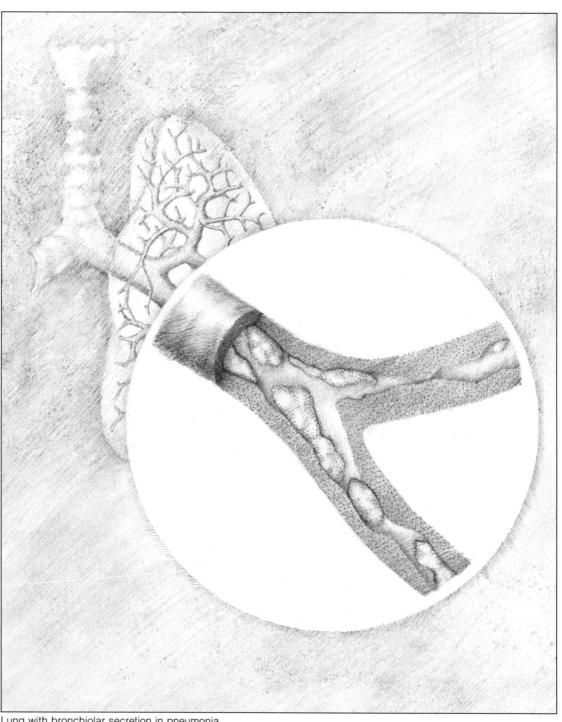

Lung with bronchiolar secretion in pneumonia

Lung parenchymal disease can range from mild, self-limiting influenza to severe, life-threatening viral pneumonia. However, the untreated common cold or other initially mild disease can progress to acute disease, such as pneumonia. In fact, pneumonia accounts for about 10% of all hospital admissions and 15% to 20% of all nosocomial infections.

Fortunately, nurses can do much to prevent acute parenchymal disease. In the hospital, you can reduce the incidence of parenchymal disease by strictly adhering to infection control measures. In the community, your involvement in health-teaching programs can promote early recognition of acute parenchymal disease, which may mean the difference between home care and hospitalization.

Who gets parenchymal disease—and when?

An estimated 3.2 million people develop respiratory infections every year. Most effectively combat these infections and experience only minor, short-lived symptoms. But some people, especially the young and the elderly, are highly susceptible to respiratory infections and require aggressive treatment to prevent serious parenchymal damage. Typically, the young have yet to acquire immunity to respiratory pathogens, whereas the elderly have exaggerated susceptibility because of age-related deterioration of respiratory function. Also, chronic cardiac, pulmonary, renal, and metabolic diseases and malnutrition can predispose respiratory infection. So can immunodeficiency disease, and treatment with corticosteroids or chemotherapeutic drugs by hindering effective antibody response to combat infection.

According to the U.S. Department of Health and Human Services, influenza and pneumonia taken together rank as the sixth leading cause of death. Although the mortality rate has declined over the past decade, these diseases still account for about 45,000 deaths annually. This mortality rate is higher in men than in women (except for women in their childbearing years) and in blacks than in whites.

Influenza may occur in endemics, epidemics, or pandemics. The catastrophic pandemic of 1918 caused roughly 20 million deaths. The most recent pandemics—in 1957, 1968, and 1977—began in mainland China. Typically, outbreaks of influenza occur during winter— presumably not the result of exposure to cold air but of increased indoor activities, promoting spread of infection. Outbreaks favor large population groups and are most commonly reported in large cities, military bases, schools, and other institutions. Influenza rarely progresses to pneumonia in the healthy individual, but in the compromised host it often does. Consequently, the incidence of pneumonia rises correspondingly during outbreaks of influenza.

A look at respiratory pathogens

Influenza results from infection by *Myxovirus influenzae,* a virus with a remarkable capacity for antigenic variation. As a result, new viral strains encounter little or no immunologic resistance in the affected population. The influenza virus is classified as Type A, B, or C. Type A, the most lethal, strikes every 2 to 3 years, with a major new strain occurring every 10 to 15 years. Type B strikes every 4 to 6 years, typically causing epidemics. Type C is endemic and causes only isolated cases.

Bacterial pneumonia results from a wide variety of pathogens. *Streptococcus pneumoniae* (also known as pneumococcus or *Diplococcus pneumoniae*) causes about 80% of community-acquired bacterial pneumonias. In fact, almost everyone has been a carrier of streptococcus at some time, and roughly 40% of the population are carriers at any given time.

Staphylococcus aureus is the second most common pathogen and usually causes a post-influenza pneumonia. Staphylococcal pneumonia is typically complicated by lung abscess and has a high mortality when viral pneumonia is superimposed.

Klebsiella pneumoniae, a relatively rare pathogen, appears in less than 4% of bacterial pneumonias but has a mortality of 20% to 50%. *Klebsiella* pneumonia is often associated with alcoholism and complicated by lung abscess. A characteristic sign of this pneumonia is hemoptysis, or sputum resembling red currant jelly. *Hemophilus influenzae,* another rare pathogen, appears most often superimposed on other bacterial pneumonias or chronic bronchitis.

Legionella pneumophilia, a relatively uncommon gram-negative bacillus, was first isolated in water samples after an outbreak of bacterial pneumonia at an American Legion convention in 1976. *Legionella* pneumonia may cause fatal shock or respiratory failure.

Four routes of infection

Pathogens can reach the lungs by inhalation, aspiration, circulation, or direct contact. *Inhalation* of microbes suspended in the air is the most common route of infection. Coughing and sneezing release a mist of microbe-laden droplets into the air, which can remain airborne and infectious for an hour or more. The influenza virus is usually spread by this route.

Bacteria usually reach the lungs by *aspiration* of oropharyngeal secretions, which are normally rich in flora. For this reason, aspiration of even small amounts of these secretions can lead to bacterial pneumonia. Also, aspiration of foreign substances, such as acidic gastric secretions and hydrocarbons (found in gasoline, insect sprays, and cleaning supplies), can cause parenchymal damage.

The *circulatory system* can carry bacteria and viruses to the lungs from primary infection sites, such as the small intestine, heart, urinary tract, or the skin of burn victims.

Direct contact with a nearby subdiaphragmatic abscess or penetrating chest trauma, such as a stab wound, may also spread pathogens to the lungs.

Safeguards against infection

Fortunately, the respiratory system has several defenses against infection, beginning in the nasal passages and extending down the tracheobronchial tree into the alveoli. Maintaining these defenses is critical to ensure pulmonary hygiene and combat infection.

Upper airways: First line of defense. The nasal passages humidify and warm inspired air, which keeps secretions moist and loose. Nasal hairs trap dust and large particles; mucus traps finer particles, which the cilia move to the oropharynx for swallowing. Sneezing and nose blowing also clear irritating particles. Reflexive bending of the epiglottis closes off the larynx to swallowed substances, preventing aspiration of foreign material into the trachea and lungs. Elicited by touching the soft palate or posterior pharynx, the gag reflex also helps prevent aspiration. The cough reflex, another essential protective mechanism, clears secretions that might otherwise provide an excellent medium for bacterial growth. It's induced by vagal stimulation from the trachea and carina and, consequently, also helps prevent aspiration of foreign material. Effective cough involves a deep inspiratory breath, a pause, tight closure of the glottis, contraction of the accessory abdominal muscles of expiration (which raises intrathoracic pressure), and forceful expiration of air through a partially closed glottis.

Lower airways: Second line of defense. Some smaller particles may breach upper airway defenses and enter the trachea. Here, the mucociliary transport system acts as the major defense mechanism. The cilia—tiny filaments arising from epithelial cells—beat about 1,000 times/minute. Mucus, secreted by goblet cells and submucosal glands, lies in two layers over the cilia: a thin, inner layer composed mainly of water and a thick, patchy outer layer of gellike consistency. The cilia and mucus form a protective blanket that traps foreign particles and transports them up the tracheobronchial tree for swallowing or expectoration. However, the number of cilia and mucus-secreting cells gradually declines toward the bronchiolar level. Particles reaching this level are engulfed by alveolar macrophages (see *Phagocytosis: Alveolar defense against infection,* page 135).

Prophylactic drug therapy: A boost for natural defenses

Vaccines and antiviral drugs can boost the body's natural defenses against infection. Pneumococcal vaccine combats the 23 most common strains of pneumococcus, giving it an overall effectiveness of 90% in preventing pneumococcal pneumonia. This vaccine, administered subcutaneously or intramuscularly in a single dose of 0.5 ml, can produce local tenderness and erythema, but rarely causes more serious effects. After vaccination, detectable antibody levels remain for at least 5 years. Generally, vaccination is indicated for debilitated or elderly persons who risk serious illness or death from pneumonia. It's contraindicated in febrile respiratory illness or active infection, pregnancy, and children younger than 2 years old.

Before discussing influenza virus vaccine, recall that *Myxovirus influenzae* has a remarkable capacity for antigenic variation. Consequently, influenza virus vaccine changes yearly, with its composition based on the previous year's influenza activity. Influenza virus vaccine is available in whole or split virus preparations. Split virus vaccines cause somewhat fewer side effects than whole virus in children. For adults and youths older than 13, this vaccine is administered intramuscularly in a single dose of 0.5 ml whole or split virus. For children ages 3 to 12 years, the dose is 0.5 ml split virus intramuscularly; for children ages 6 to 35 months, 0.25 ml split virus intramuscularly. One or two doses are needed for

Common bacterial pathogens in respiratory infection

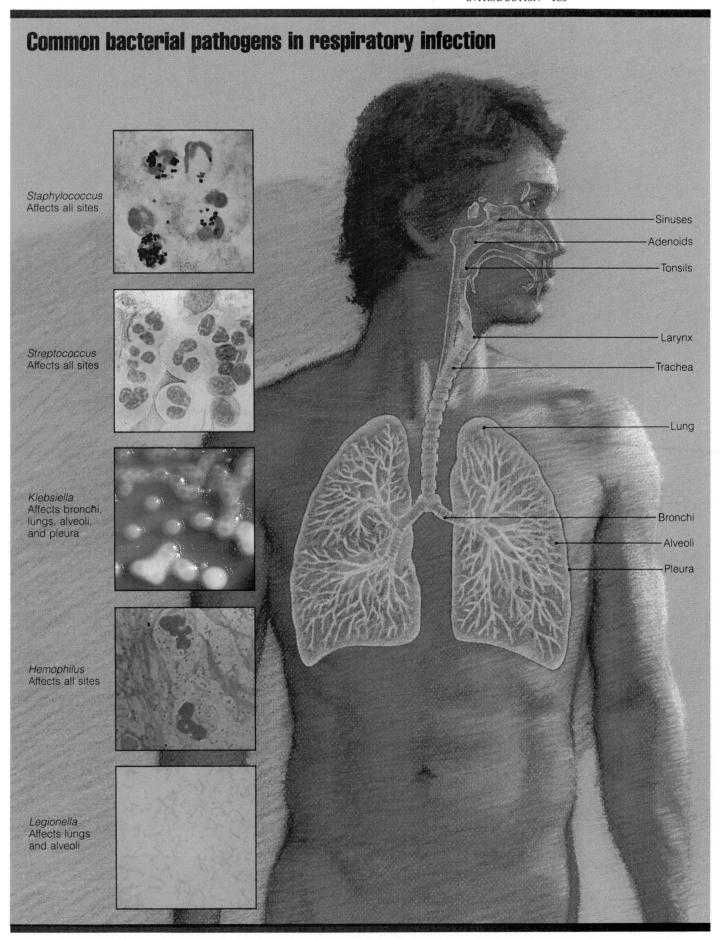

Staphylococcus
Affects all sites

Streptococcus
Affects all sites

Klebsiella
Affects bronchi,
lungs, alveoli,
and pleura

Hemophilus
Affects all sites

Legionella
Affects lungs
and alveoli

Sinuses
Adenoids
Tonsils

Larynx
Trachea

Lung

Bronchi
Alveoli
Pleura

Upper airway defenses against infection

The upper airways form the front line in defending the body from infection. Nasal hairs trap dust and large particles in inspired air. Mucus then traps finer particles, which the cilia move to the oropharynx for swallowing. At the same time, turbinates—bony structures that project into the nasal cavity—humidify and warm inspired air, which keeps secretions moist and loose. In the pharynx, the soft palate and epiglottis separate air and food preventing aspiration. The gag and cough reflexes also prevent aspiration, and the cough reflex clears secretions that might provide a medium for bacterial growth.

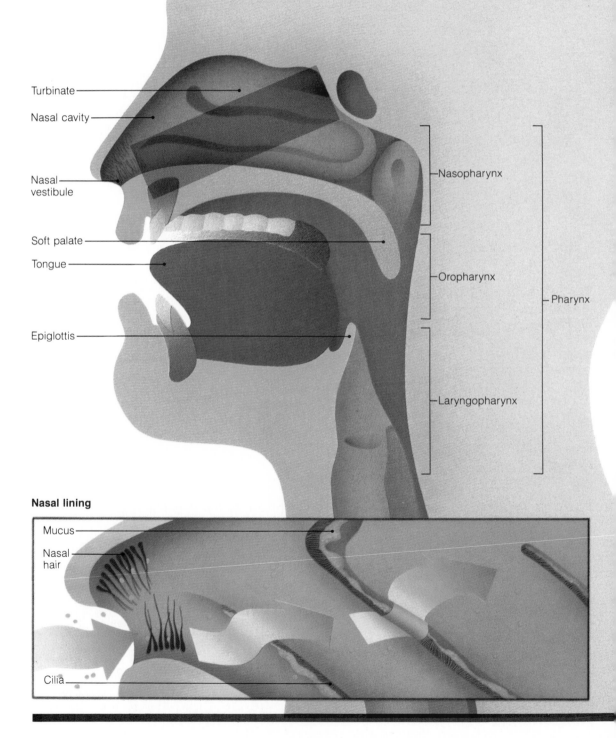

Turbinate

Nasal cavity

Nasal vestibule

Soft palate

Tongue

Epiglottis

Nasopharynx

Oropharynx

Laryngopharynx

Pharynx

Nasal lining

Mucus

Nasal hair

Cilia

the last two age groups. For maximum effectiveness, the dose must be repeated in 4 weeks unless the child received one dose of influenza vaccine from 1978-9 to 1982-3. Like pneumococcal vaccine, influenza virus vaccine can produce local tenderness and erythema, but rarely causes more serious effects. It's contraindicated in patients with egg allergy.

Although vaccination is preferred for influenza A, the antiviral drug amantadine is 70% effective. Recommended when vaccine is unavailable or contraindicated, amantadine is administered by mouth in daily doses of 200 mg. Typically, it's administered for at least 10 days after known exposure to influenza A or for the duration of an epidemic.

PATHOPHYSIOLOGY

Various factors can compromise natural defense mechanisms and, without the backup of vaccination, can trigger parenchymal infection. For example, decreased level of consciousness compromises upper airway defenses by impairing the cough and gag reflexes. This, in turn, tends to promote aspiration of foreign material. Decreased level of consciousness can result from drug overdose, central nervous system disorders, alcohol ingestion, and head injury. Impaired cough and gag reflexes can also result from prolonged use of a nasogastric or endotracheal tube. Both restrictive and obstructive lung disease can impair deep breathing and cause a nonproductive cough.

Factors that compromise the mucociliary transport system do so primarily by drying mucus secretions or by decreasing ciliary action. For example, chronic mouth breathers bypass the normal filtering and humidification system of the nose. This poorly humidified inspired air dries the mucociliary blanket, causing the cilia to become brittle and the mucus thick and tenacious. Dehydration may produce the same effect, as water vapor in inspired air is drawn into the vascular system. Atropine, commonly used preoperatively, also decreases ciliary action by drying the mucociliary blanket. Cigarette smoking, alcohol ingestion, and inhaled drugs such as cocaine directly depress ciliary action.

At the alveolar level, any factor that compromises macrophage function can impair lung defenses. Steroids, alcohol, uremia, cigarette smoking, and environmental pollutants such as ozone diminish the bactericidal effect of the macrophages.

Phagocytosis: Alveolar defense against infection

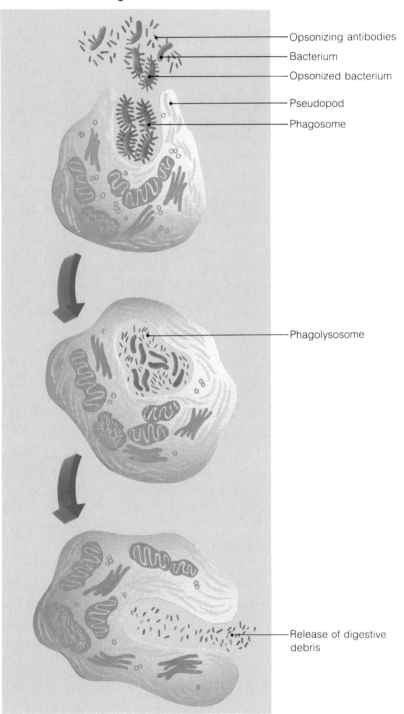

Bacteria and foreign particles that bypass upper airway defenses and reach the alveoli are greeted by macrophages—specialized reticuloendothelial cells that carry out phagocytosis. First, bacteria attach to the cell surface, initiating opsonization—an antibody coating of the bacteria that enables phagocytosis. Then, macrophages surround the bacteria by forming pseudopods—footlike extensions. Phagosomes digest the bacteria and merge with lysosomes to form phagolysosomes, which release enzymes that help iodine, bromide, and chloride bind to the cell wall to destroy the bacteria. Finally, macrophages release digestive debris, so they can continue to fight infection.

Understanding atelectasis

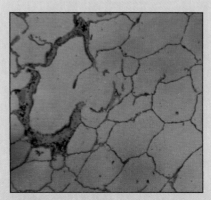

This tissue section shows normal lung tissue with clearly defined alveoli bounded by capillaries.

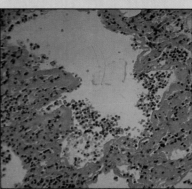

Initial inflammatory changes in parenchymal infection appear. Formation of microemboli and fibrin within the alveoli and a decreased number of alveoli mark the beginning of consolidation.

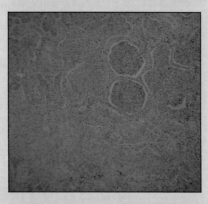

Fibrin, blood, and cellular debris eventually fill the alveoli as pneumonia progresses.

Total alveolar collapse occurs with hyaline membrane formation, represented by the heavy lines. This advanced stage of infection is known as ARDS.

Atelectasis—the collapse of clusters of alveoli—may trigger respiratory infection or be its end result. In fact, atelectasis is one of the more common precursors of nosocomial respiratory infection. It reduces the surface area available for effective gas exchange, causing intrapulmonary shunting and, ultimately, hypoxemia.

How atelectasis develops

Understanding how atelectasis develops is the first step toward proper treatment or, at best, prevention.

Ineffective ventilation is the most common cause of postoperative atelectasis. Shallow breathing to avoid incisional pain, common after abdominal surgery, decreases airflow to the alveoli and contributes to pooling of secretions. External compression of the alveoli by tumor, abscess, or pleural effusion can also reduce airflow.

Airway obstruction by a mucous plug or foreign body causes pooling of secretions and absorption atelectasis. In absorption atelectasis, trapped air distal to the obstruction diffuses into the pulmonary circulation, without being replaced by newly inspired air. Then, alveoli shrink and collapse.

Insufficient surfactant can also play a role in atelectasis. Before considering the effect of insufficient surfactant, recall that surfactant coats the lining of the alveoli, lowering surface tension and preventing alveolar collapse during exhalation. Decreased production or inactivation of surfactant may thus contribute to alveolar collapse. But whether insufficient surfactant is a cause or an effect of atelectasis is still unclear.

In severe viral or bacterial infection, atelectasis is the end result of *inflammatory changes* in the alveoli, capillaries, and interstitium. The slides shown at left depict these progressive changes associated with increasingly severe hypoxemia.

When one airway defense is impaired, the others rally to combat infection. However, when more than one defense falters, parenchymal infection usually follows.

How inflammation develops and spreads

Depending on the type of parenchymal infection, inflammation may develop first in the airways, the interstitium, or the alveoli.

Influenza. The influenza virus primarily attacks the epithelial cells of the upper airways, causing inflammation and desquamation. Proliferation of the virus destroys large numbers of cilia, crippling the mucociliary transport system.

Pneumonia. When caused by bacterial infection, pneumonia may involve the distal airways and alveoli (bronchopneumonia), part of a lobe (lobular pneumonia), or an entire lobe (lobar pneumonia). Bacterial infection initially triggers alveolar inflammation and edema. The capillaries become engorged with blood and white blood cells, causing stasis. As the alveolar-capillary membrane breaks down, the alveoli fill with blood and exudate, resulting in atelectasis. In severe bacterial infection, the lungs assume the heavy, liver-like appearance characteristic in acute respiratory distress syndrome (ARDS).

Viral infection, which typically causes diffuse pneumonia, first attacks the epithelial cells in the bronchioles, causing interstitial inflammation and desquamation. It then spreads to the alveoli, which fill with blood and fluid. In advanced infection hyaline membrane formation may be evident. As in bacterial infection, severe viral infection may present a clinical picture resembling ARDS.

Aspiration of gastric juices or hydrocarbons can cause marked inflammatory changes. Aspiration occurs most often into the right lung because the right bronchus is more in line with the trachea than the left. Acidic gastric juices may directly damage the airways and alveoli, causing mucosal damage, pulmonary edema, hemorrhage, and alveolar flooding. Generally, more acidic fluid (pH of less than 2.5) produces the most damage. Particles within the aspirated gastric juices may also obstruct the airways and reduce airflow. This, in turn, leads to pooling of secretions and atelectasis, which predisposes secondary bacterial pneumonia.

Aspirated hydrocarbons trigger similar inflammatory changes and also inactivate surfactant over a large alveolar area; decreased surfactant leads to alveolar collapse.

Lung abscess—a pus-filled cavity within the parenchyma—is a common sequela of aspiration pneumonia. Suppuration typically occurs at the site of aspiration damage and may be associated with anaerobic or aerobic organisms. Lung abscess is usually surrounded by a wall of fibrous granulated tissue. When the abscess communicates with a bronchus, pus drains into the trachea, producing purulent sputum.

Clinical course

Except for bacterial pneumonia, parenchymal infection typically has an insidious onset, usually beginning with systemic symptoms. Characteristically, pulmonary symptoms follow within 6 to 36 hours (see *Recognizing acute parenchymal disease,* pages 138 and 139).

Hypoxemia, a characteristic systemic sign, results from impaired gas exchange. Pneumonia stiffens the lungs, causing increased work of breathing and rapid, shallow respirations which, in turn, cause ventilation-perfusion mismatch. Localized or patchy atelectasis causes intrapulmonary shunting, which also impairs gas exchange.

Hypoxemia initially triggers a compensatory increase in heart rate and cardiac output to pump more blood past the remaining functional alveoli and thus maintain tissue oxygenation. But prolonged hypoxemia eventually causes cardiac function to deteriorate, and heart failure may follow. Tissue hypoxia is the final outcome.

MEDICAL MANAGEMENT

Management of parenchymal disease hinges on accurate differential diagnosis and careful evaluation of the severity of disease. This involves distinguishing between bacterial and viral infection, determining respiratory tract involvement, and detecting complications, especially lung abscess. The patient history and physical examination often provide valuable baseline data. Various diagnostic tests can then supplement or confirm this data (see *Differential diagnosis of acute parenchymal disease,* page 142).

Diagnostic tests

Typically, diagnosis of mild influenza follows from the presenting symptoms alone. But prolonged or unusually severe symptoms may signal secondary infection or other complications and require these diagnostic tests:

Chest X-ray. This test helps identify the type of infection, the extent of parenchymal

Nosocomial respiratory infections

Respiratory infections account for 15% to 20% of all nosocomial infections, and most commonly result from *Pseudomonas aeruginosa, Klebsiella, E. coli,* and *Staphylococcus aureus.* Poor hand-washing technique and contaminated respiratory care equipment are the major culprits in spreading respiratory infection. To prevent such infection, observe these precautions:
• Wash your hands thoroughly before and after each patient contact.
• Maintain sterile technique for suctioning.
• Change sterile solutions and tubing used with humidifiers and nebulizers every 24 hours. Write the date on opened solution bottles to avoid using old solutions.
• Observe isolation precautions as indicated.

involvement, and the presence of complications. Viral and bacterial infections are often characterized by diffuse or localized parenchymal involvement.

Cultures. Although useless in viral infection, sputum cultures can isolate a bacterial pathogen, thereby directing antibiotic therapy. Blood cultures also help detect bacterial infection and determine its severity. Positive blood culture indicates systemic infection, which carries a poor prognosis.

Serologic tests. These tests can confirm diagnosis of viral infection retrospectively, since antibody titers typically increase fourfold during convalescence.

Arterial blood gases. ABG analysis reveals the severity of impaired gas exchange, which corresponds to the severity of parenchymal disease. Initially, ABG levels are usually normal. However, as such disease progresses, decreasing PO_2 and increasing PCO_2 signal deterioration of respiratory function.

Treatment: At home or in the hospital?
Whether parenchymal disease is treated at home or in the hospital obviously depends on its type and severity. Treatment of mild influenza is typically symptomatic and easily managed at home. However, treatment of bacterial or viral pneumonia usually demands hospitalization.

Bed rest and adequate fluid intake are key measures for treating mild influenza. Fluid replacement corrects loss of body fluids from fever and rapid breathing. Adequate fluid balance also loosens secretions, facilitating their removal through coughing. An expectorant helps relieve nonproductive coughing, and aspirin relieves fever and muscle pain. Amantadine hydrochloride may reduce the duration of signs and symptoms for Type A influenza, if given within 24 hours of onset.

In pneumonia, adequate fluid intake is also important to maintain perfusion of vital organs and to reduce the heart's work load brought on by hypoxemia. If anemia is present, transfusion of whole blood may be needed to enhance the blood's oxygen-carrying capacity. Analgesics are usually needed to relieve pleuritic pain, which may be severe enough to require a narcotic such as morphine sulfate. Watch for respiratory depression with administration of morphine sulfate. Bronchodilators may ease discomfort by relaxing smooth muscle fibers in the tracheobronchial tree, which reduces airway resistance and improves airflow. As a result, the patient breathes easier and expectorates sputum with less difficulty.

Administration of humidified oxygen aims to correct hypoxemia. Low flow rates of 4 to 6 liters per minute by nasal cannula or of 40% oxygen by mask usually restore adequate oxygenation. However, in the patient with chronic lung disease, oxygen therapy requires lower flow rates of 1 to 2 liters per minute

Recognizing acute parenchymal disease

Characteristics	Influenza	Acute bronchitis	Bacterial pneumonia	Viral pneumonia
Onset	Insidious	Insidious (develops as complication of other pulmonary illness)	Abrupt	Insidious
Early signs and symptoms	Low fever, malaise, headache, and, possibly, nonproductive cough	Chest tightness; wheezing; hacking, productive cough; purulent, blood-tinged sputum	High fever; shaking, chills; pleuritic pain; productive cough with purulent, rusty sputum; hyperventilation; fever blisters	Cold or influenza symptoms: fever, malaise, nonproductive cough
Late signs and symptoms	High fever, anorexia, persistent cough	Fever, cyanosis, dyspnea	Increased severity of early symptoms	High fever, dyspnea, purulent cough, blood-streaked sputum, cyanosis, respiratory failure
Complicating disorders and diagnostic difficulties	Secondary bacterial or viral pneumonia may follow.		May present first as upper respiratory infection, with minor symptoms for a week.	Localized form produces fewer symptoms. Diffuse form may produce severe symptoms and be complicated by bacterial pneumonia.

and careful monitoring to ensure that it doesn't dampen the hypoxic drive to breathe. If hypoxemia is unresponsive to oxygen delivered by nasal cannula or mask (common in severe pneumonia), ventilator therapy with positive end-expiratory pressure (PEEP) is necessary. PEEP increases the alveolar surface area and helps open collapsed alveoli, thereby improving gas exchange.

Antimicrobial therapy varies with the causative pathogen and typically begins directly after collection of sputum samples, before culture results are known. Pneumococcal pneumonias respond to penicillin, the drug of choice, or to erythromycin and chloramphenicol. Klebsiella pneumonia usually responds to gentamycin and tobramycin or to alternative drugs including cephalosporins, chloramphenicol, and amikasin. Staphylococcal pneumonia responds to oxacillin; Legionella pneumonia, to erythromycin. Lung abscess requires high doses of penicillin or, if the abscess fails to resolve after antibiotic therapy, manual aspiration and thoracotomy with chest tube drainage. Nosocomial bacterial pneumonia, which often results from antibiotic-resistant strains of bacteria, requires sensitivity studies to help tailor antibiotic therapy to the current hospital flora.

Unfortunately, viral pneumonias don't respond to antibiotic therapy. But if bacterial infection is superimposed, erythromycin or tetracycline may relieve some symptoms.

Similarly, aspiration pneumonia doesn't respond to antibiotic therapy unless the aspirate contained bacteria. Then, penicillin or other antimicrobial drugs may prove helpful, depending on the pathogen. Administration of high-dose steroids, a controversial therapy, may help minimize lung damage when instituted within 24 hours of aspiration. Other supportive measures for treating pneumonias include airway management and chest physiotherapy with postural drainage.

The above treatment measures, if begun promptly, help ensure the patient a smooth recovery. Of course, convalescence and return to normal activities vary with the patient's age, health history, and the severity of parenchymal infection. Mild infection can resolve in 3 to 5 days; severe infection can take up to 6 weeks.

NURSING MANAGEMENT

Effective nursing management of acute parenchymal disease begins with reliable respiratory assessment based on a skillful patient interview and a thorough physical examination.

The patient interview

Anxiety is characteristic in acute parenchymal disease because of the patient's fear of breathlessness or pleuritic pain. Because anxiety can color or even obscure assessment findings, it's important to evaluate the patient's level of anxiety first (see *Anxiety affects assessment findings*). Is the patient too anxious to respond appropriately to your questions? Is pain or dyspnea increasing his anxiety? Is the patient's family contributing to or reducing anxiety?

Remember that a thorough patient interview and physical examination may only heighten the patient's anxiety, thereby increasing the work of breathing and oxygen consumption. Consequently, do not attempt a complete admission assessment for the patient with obvious distress. Instead, restrict the initial interview to a few "yes or no" questions. And aim to reduce the patient's anxiety by asking questions like "Where is the chest pain?" or "Do you always have trouble breathing, or only when you lie down?" Obtain additional information from the patient's family if possible. Otherwise, wait to complete assessment. Continue the interview and physical examination after the patient receives oxygen and pain medication, and has rested for at least 8, but preferably 24, hours.

Aspiration pneumonia	Lung abscess
Insidious (latent period before onset, except in aspiration of large amounts of gastric juice or hydrocarbons)	Insidious (symptoms of superimposed disease, such as bacterial infection, may be present)
Productive cough, perhaps containing gastric juice or food particles	Malaise, low-grade fever, chills, mild pleuritic pain
Hemoptysis, copious secretions, superimposed bacterial pneumonia	High fever, pleurisy, dyspnea, cyanosis, purulent cough when abscess drains
Chronic aspiration may be asymptomatic until abscess formation.	May be mistaken for pneumonia until abscess drains.

Anxiety affects assessment findings

Because anxiety can affect assessment findings, evaluate the patient's level of anxiety before performing a complete physical examination. Watch for these signs.

Appearance

Muscular tension (rigidity)
Pale, clammy skin
Fatigue
Increased small motor activity (restlessness)

Conversation

Asks many questions
Shifts topic of conversation
Describes fears with sense of helplessness
Avoids focusing on feelings

Behavior

Shortened attention span
Inability to follow directions
Increased acting out

Physiologic signs

Increased heart and respiratory rate
Extreme shifts in body temperature, blood pressure, and menstrual flow
Diarrhea, urinary urgency
Loss of appetite
Increased perspiration
Dilation of pupils

Positions for postural drainage

As the term implies, postural drainage is the use of various positions to drain specific segments of the lungs and bronchi by gravity. Chest physiotherapy assists in drainage, and coughing or suctioning then removes secretions from the trachea. Because retained secretions provide an excellent medium for bacterial growth, postural drainage can do much toward preventing respiratory infection.

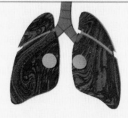

To drain *the posterior basal segments of the lower lobes,* elevate the foot of the bed 30°. Instruct the patient to lie on his abdomen with his head lowered. Then, position pillows as shown here. Percuss the lower ribs on both sides of the spine.

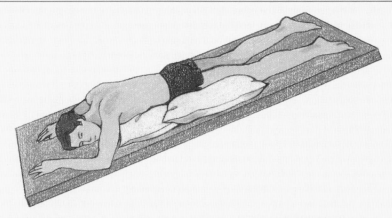

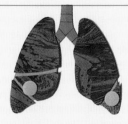

To drain *the lateral basal segments of the lower lobes,* elevate the foot of the bed 30°. Instruct the patient to lie on his abdomen with his head lowered and his upper leg flexed over a pillow for support. Then have him rotate a quarter turn upward. Percuss the lower ribs on the uppermost portion of the lateral chest wall.

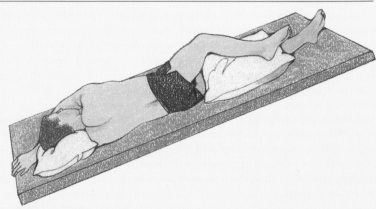

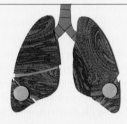

To drain *the anterior basal segments of the lower lobes,* elevate the foot of the bed 30°. Instruct the patient to lie on his side with his head lowered. Then, place pillows as shown here. Percuss with a slightly cupped hand over the lower ribs just beneath the axilla.
Note: If an acutely ill patient experiences breathing difficulty in this position, adjust the angle of the bed to one he can tolerate. Then, begin percussion.

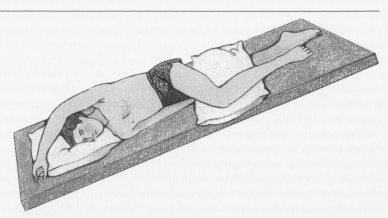

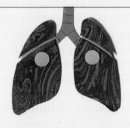

To drain *the superior segments of the lower lobes,* make sure the bed is flat. Then, instruct the patient to lie on his abdomen, and place two pillows under his hips. Percuss on both sides of his spine at the lower tip of the scapulae.

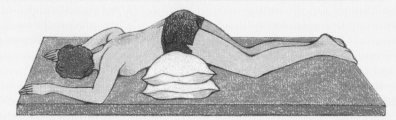

In the patient with acute parenchymal disease, copious secretions or ineffective secretion clearance indicates that postural drainage is needed. Auscultation first pinpoints congested segments of the lungs requiring drainage. Use of one or more of the positions illustrated below then drains affected segments. After postural drainage, describe the color, odor, amount, and consistency of sputum produced.

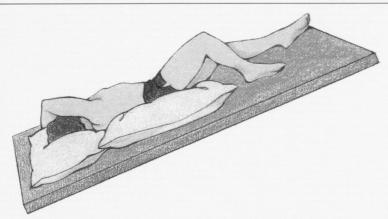

To drain *the medial and lateral segments of the right middle lobe,* elevate the foot of the bed 15°. Instruct the patient to lie on the left side with his head lowered and his knees flexed. Then, have him rotate a quarter turn backward. Place a pillow beneath him, as shown here. Percuss with your hand moderately cupped over the right nipple. In females, cup your hand so its heel is under the armpit and your fingers extend forward beneath the breast.

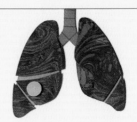

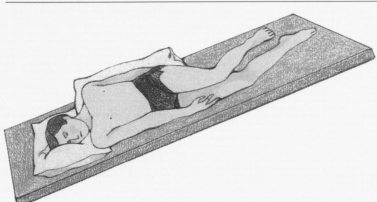

To drain *the superior and inferior segments of the lingular portion of the left upper lobe,* elevate the foot of the bed 15°. Have patient lie on his right side with his head lowered and knees flexed. Then have him rotate a quarter turn backward. Place a pillow behind him, from shoulders to hips. Percuss with your hand moderately cupped over the left nipple. In females, cup your hand so its heel is beneath the armpit and your fingers extend forward beneath the breast.

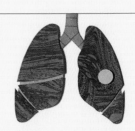

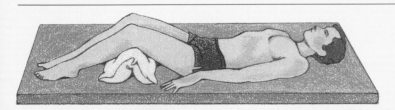

To drain *the anterior segments of the upper lobes,* make sure the bed is flat. Instruct the patient to lie on his back with a pillow folded under his knees. Then, have him rotate slightly away from the side being drained. Percuss between the clavicle and nipple.

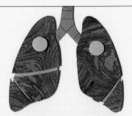

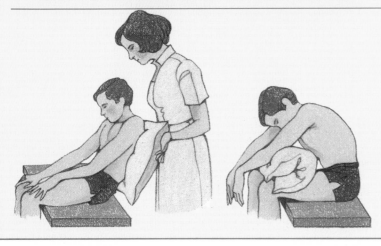

To drain *the apical segment of right upper lobe and apical subsegment of apical-posterior segment of left upper lobe,* keep the bed flat. Have the patient lean back on a pillow at a 30° angle against you. Percuss with your hand cupped between the clavicle and the top of each scapula.

To drain *the posterior segment of the right upper lobe and the posterior subsegment of apical-posterior segment of the left upper lobe,* keep bed flat. Have the patient lean over folded pillow at 30° angle. Stand behind him; percuss and clap the upper back on each side.

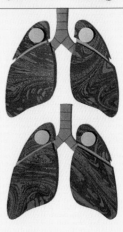

Differential diagnosis of acute parenchymal disease

Clinical findings	Bacterial pneumonia	Postinfluenza viral pneumonia	Aspiration pneumonia
History	Often preceded by viral infection, such as influenza; concomitant family or community involvement is rare due to long incubation period (up to 14 days); pleuritic chest pain	Epidemic or family involvement common because of short incubation period and highly contagious infection	Recent vomiting after anesthesia, recent dental or mouth infection, or history of chronic alcoholism or neurologic disorder; bronchospasm, pleuritic chest pain
Physical exam	Localized, bronchial breath sounds; dullness on percussion; impaired chest movement due to pleuritic pain	Minimal signs at influenza stage, uniformly decreased breath sounds and crepitus at pneumonia stage	Decreased breath sounds over affected area
Chest X-ray	Localized, well-defined hazy shadow; airspace consolidation	May be negative initially; as disease progresses, diffuse, patchy consolidation appears, followed by the "white lung" appearance of ARDS in severe cases	Small-volume aspiration resembles bacterial pneumonia; large-volume aspiration may produce diffuse atelectasis, pulmonary edema, and massive consolidation
White blood cell (WBC) count	Elevated, usually above 15,000 mm³	Normal	Elevated in aspiration of oral secretions with anaerobic bacteria
Sputum culture and sensitivity	Abundant bacteria and WBCs	No bacteria, some epithelial debris, few WBCs	Gram-negative bacilli with anaerobic and aerobic bacteria
Blood culture	Positive in 25% to 40% of cases	Negative	Negative
Serologic tests	Not significant	Increased viral antibody titers	Not significant

Explore the history of present illness

This part of the patient interview provides valuable information about the onset, duration, and characteristics of parenchymal infection. Ask the patient with suspected bacterial or viral pneumonia these questions:

• Did your illness begin with symptoms of influenza—malaise, low fever, headache, or nonproductive cough? Do any family members have similar symptoms?

• How many windows are in your home? Is there good cross ventilation? How many people live in your home? Then focus on the patient's workplace. Is it poorly ventilated or overcrowded?

• Do you smoke? If so, for how long and how much?

• Do you have a history of chronic lung disease? If so, when were you last hospitalized?

Ask the patient with suspected aspiration pneumonia these questions:

• Have you had anesthesia recently? Have you had a recent oral or dental infection?

• Do you drink alcohol often? How much? Has it ever caused you to lose consciousness?

The patient's answers to these questions may pinpoint problem areas that will help you formulate nursing diagnoses. For example, the patient who lives or works in a poorly ventilated, crowded environment may not realize how this contributes to the spread of influenza. For this patient, the nursing diagnosis "knowledge deficit about disease" readily follows, with health teaching your appropriate intervention.

Evaluate the patient's knowledge

Besides evaluating the patient's ability to identify environmental risk factors, find out if he can describe early signs and symptoms that require treatment. The patient without this knowledge may face repeated hospitalizations for severe infection that could have been treated at home in an earlier, mild stage.

Evaluate the patient's understanding of the medical and nursing regimen. For instance, does he know the purpose of diagnostic tests? Does he understand the importance of coughing, deep breathing, and postural drainage? Remember, a well-informed patient is most likely to follow prescribed treatment.

Assess respiratory status

Begin the physical examination by observing the rate and depth of respirations. Is the patient dyspneic or hyperventilating? Is this due to oxygen deprivation or anxiety? Determine if the patient experiences nocturnal dyspnea or orthopnea. Does the patient need several pillows to breathe more easily during sleep?

Next, instruct the patient to take a deep breath and cough, if possible. Is the cough productive? Describe the color, odor, amount, and consistency of sputum.

Now, auscultate the lungs for abnormal or adventitious breath sounds. Abnormal bronchial breath sounds over one area indicate bacterial pneumonia, while decreased or absent breath sounds over one area indicate lung abscess or aspiration pneumonia. Uniformly decreased breath sounds point to viral pneumonia. Rales and rhonchi indicate increased secretions, and wheezing indicates bronchitis or bronchospasm.

Observe skin condition

The skin provides clues to tissue oxygenation as well as body temperature. Look for cyanosis—a sign of hypoxemia—in the lips, the nail beds, the tip of the nose, the ear helices, and the underside of the tongue. Uniformly pale skin may point to anemia—the result of reduced hemoglobin levels. Diaphoresis may accompany fever or anxiety.

Assess cardiovascular status

Take the patient's pulse and blood pressure. Hypoxemia typically increases heart rate and cardiac output—a compensatory response to improve tissue perfusion. However, prolonged uncorrected hypoxemia eventually causes deterioration of cardiac function.

Evaluate nutritional status

This is especially important since malnutrition can predispose the patient to acute parenchymal infection. Acute infection, in turn, can cause loss of appetite because of associated dyspnea or malaise.

Observe the patient for poor skin turgor, muscle wasting, and lethargy. Ask about recent weight loss to detect malnutrition. Find out the patient's normal daily caloric intake and meal pattern. Determine if loss of appetite or dyspnea limits his caloric intake. Ask about food preferences and allergies to help plan an appropriate diet.

Formulate nursing diagnoses

After completing the patient interview and physical examination, you're ready to correlate their findings and formulate nursing diagnoses. In acute parenchymal disease, these diagnoses typically address emotional, physical, and cognitive problems.

Anxiety related to fear of breathlessness. After formulating this diagnosis, your goal is to reduce anxiety. First, carefully assess the patient's level of anxiety. Then, explain how respiratory infection causes symptoms and treatment measures relieve them. Encourage the patient and his family to ask questions and express their fears or concerns. Then, involve them in your care plan. Report the patient's anxiety level to the doctor. Also, document his response to teaching, his questions, and any stated fears or concerns.

Consider your nursing interventions successful if the patient and his family can describe the symptoms, causes, and treatments of respiratory infection; and if the patient reports reduced breathlessness and complies with the treatment regimen.

Alteration in comfort related to pain. To promote comfort, first locate the pain. Then, apply warm compresses to the area and administer analgesics, as ordered. Splint the patient's chest during coughing to avoid undue pleuritic pain. Allow the patient to rest between procedures to avoid fatigue, which can magnify pain.

Consider your interventions successful if the patient is free of pain and can breathe deeply without discomfort.

Impaired gas exchange related to inflammation of the lung parenchyma. As you'll recall, alveolar changes can cause ventilation-perfusion mismatch, which impairs gas exchange. To maintain adequate oxygenation, administer the prescribed volume of oxygen by face mask or nasal cannula. Monitor serial ABG levels to evaluate effectiveness of oxygen therapy. To minimize oxygen demand, provide frequent rest periods and take measures to reduce fever and anxiety. Monitor vital signs and observe for signs of hypoxemia—restlessness, decreased level of consciousness, lethargy, tachypnea, tachycardia, and cyanosis. Because of the brain's sensitivity to oxygen deprivation, expect cerebral signs (restless-

Evaluating common oxygen delivery systems

Oxygen delivery system	Advantages	Disadvantages	Nursing considerations
Nasal cannula (Low-flow system) 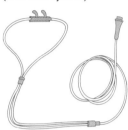	• Safe and simple • Comfortable; easily tolerated • Nasal prongs can be shaped to fit facial contour • Effective for delivering low oxygen concentrations • Allows freedom of movement; doesn't impede eating or talking • Inexpensive; disposable • Can provide continuous positive airway pressure (CPAP) for infants and children	• Contraindicated in complete nasal obstruction; for example, mucosal edema or polyps • May cause headaches or dry mucous membranes if flow rate exceeds 6 liters per minute • Can dislodge easily • Strap may pinch chin if adjusted too tightly • Patient must be alert and cooperative to help keep cannula in place	• Remove and clean cannula every 8 hours with a wet cloth. Give good mouth and nose care. • If patient is restless, explore other methods of oxygen delivery. • Check for reddened areas under nose and over ears. Apply gauze padding, if necessary. • Moisten lips and nose with water-soluble jelly, but avoid occluding the cannula.
Simple face mask (Low-flow system) 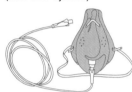	• Effectively delivers high oxygen concentrations • Humidification can be enhanced by using large-bore tubing and aerosol mask • Doesn't dry mucous membranes of nose and mouth	• Hot and confining; may irritate skin • Tight seal, necessary to ensure accurate oxygen concentration, may cause discomfort • Interferes with eating and talking • Can't deliver less than 40% oxygen • Impractical for long-term therapy	• Place pads between mask and bony facial parts. • Periodically massage face with fingertips. Wash and dry face every 2 hours. • For adequate flush, maintain flow rate of 5 liters per minute. • Don't adjust strap too tightly. • Remove and clean mask every 8 hours with a wet cloth.
Partial rebreather mask (Low-flow system) 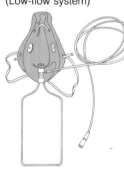	• Oxygen reservoir bag lets patient rebreathe exhaled air from such passages as the trachea and bronchi, where no gas exchange occurs, so it's high in oxygen content. This increases his fraction of inspired oxygen concentration (FIO_2). • Safety valve allows inhalation of room air if oxygen source fails • Effectively delivers high oxygen concentrations (35% to 60%) • Easily humidifies oxygen • Doesn't dry mucous membranes • Insertion of a rubber flange over the reservoir bag usually allows conversion to nonrebreather mask.	• Hot and confining; may irritate skin • Tight seal, necessary to ensure accurate oxygen concentration, may cause discomfort • Interferes with eating and talking • Bag may twist or kink • Impractical for long-term therapy	• Never let bag totally deflate during inhalation. Increase liter flow, if necessary. • Avoid twisting bag. • Keep mask snug to prevent inhalation of room air. • To initially fill bag, apply mask during exhalation.
Nonrebreather mask (Low-flow system) 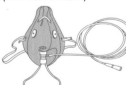	• Delivers the highest possible oxygen concentration (60% to 90%) short of intubation and mechanical ventilation • Effective for short-term therapy • Doesn't dry mucous membranes • Can be converted to a partial rebreathing mask, if necessary	• Requires a tight seal, which may be difficult to maintain; may cause discomfort • May irritate skin • Impractical for long-term therapy	• Never let bag totally deflate. • Avoid twisting bag. • Keep mask snug to prevent inhalation of room air. • Make sure that all rubber flaps remain in place. • Watch patient closely for signs of oxygen toxicity.
Venturi mask (High-flow system) 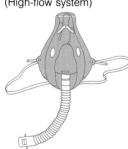	• Delivers exact oxygen concentration despite patient's respiratory pattern • Diluter jets can be changed, or dial-turned, to change oxygen concentration • Doesn't dry mucous membranes • Can be used to deliver humidity or aerosol therapy • Never delivers more than the prescribed oxygen concentration, even if knob on flowmeter is accidentally bumped and liter flow is increased	• Hot and confining; mask may irritate skin • FIO_2 may be lowered if mask doesn't fit snugly, if tubing's kinked, if oxygen intake ports are blocked, or if less than recommended liter flow is used. • Interferes with eating and talking • Condensation may collect and drain on patient if humidification is being used	• Check arterial blood gas measurements frequently. • Soften skin around mouth with petrolatum to prevent irritation. • Remove and clean mask every 8 hours with a wet cloth.

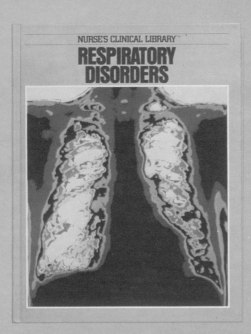

NURSE'S CLINICAL LIBRARY
RESPIRATORY DISORDERS

This is your order card. Send no money.

YES! Please send me *Respiratory Disorders* and enter my subscription to the NURSE'S CLINICAL LIBRARY. If I decide to keep *Respiratory Disorders*, I will pay just $17.95 (a savings of $2.00 off the single-volume price), plus shipping and handling. I understand that I will receive a new NURSE'S CLINICAL LIBRARY book every 2 to 3 months on the same 10-day, free-examination basis. There is no minimum number of books I must buy, and I may cancel my subscription at any time by notifying you.   CB5S

Please send me *Respiratory Disorders,* but do not enter my subscription to the NURSE'S CLINICAL LIBRARY. I will pay $19.95, plus shipping and handling, for each copy. Please send _____copies and bill me later.   5CB

Name _____
Address _____
City _____ State _____ Zip _____

Offer valid in U.S. only. Prices subject to change without notice.

Respiratory Disorders is a comprehensive book. Every bit of information you need to care for your respiratory patients with skill and confidence is included. This one source gives you concise facts on these vital topics:

● **Assessment** How to correctly identify lung sounds, how to differentiate between rales and rhonchi, tips on history taking, inspection, auscultation...and more.
● **Symptoms** Complete review of common signs, symptoms, and complaints, how to relate subtle symptoms to a possible acute process...and much more.
● **Diagnostics** How to use test results to develop more effective nursing goals.
● **Therapy** How to use the very latest advancements in respiratory therapy delivery systems...and more.
● **Management** Tips on managing a patient on a ventilator, how and when to use postive end-expiratory pressure (PEEP), how to set obtainable goals and manage a successful weaning.
● **Drugs** Complete list of respiratory drugs, highlighting indications, dosages, and adverse effects, interactions, and nursing considerations.
● **Patient teaching** Valuable pages you can photocopy and give to patients on how to manage a long-term life-support system, effects of smoking and air pollution, and more.
● **Prognosis** Learn the impact of effective infection-control programs on nosocomial infections, and more.

10-DAY FREE TRIAL

USE THE ABOVE CARD TWO WAYS.

1. Pass it along to a colleague who might want to subscribe to the NURSE'S CLINICAL LIBRARY...saving your friend $2.00 off the single-copy price of every book in the series.

or

2. Use the above card to order additional copies of *Respiratory Disorders* without subscribing to the series.

Either way, you (or your colleagues) may examine *Respiratory Disorders* for 10 days...free!

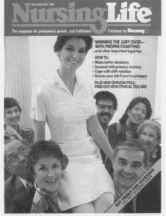

Keep your professional expertise growing with *NursingLife.*®

Mail the postage-paid card at right. ▶

Use this card to order *NursingLife.*®
The fastest growing nursing journal in the world.

Subscribe for 2 years for only $15.95. Mail this card today and receive an added bonus issue at no cost!

☐ Yes! Please send me the next issue of *NursingLife* and enter my 2-year trial subscription. Add the bonus issue to my subscription at no cost for ordering promptly.

Name _____
Address _____
City _____ State _____ Zip _____

NursingLife is published bimonthly. The single-copy price is $3, $18 per year.   RCLS-X

BUSINESS REPLY CARD

FIRST CLASS PERMIT NO. 2307 HICKSVILLE, N.Y.

POSTAGE WILL BE PAID BY ADDRESSEE

 Springhouse Book Company

6 Commercial Street
Hicksville, N.Y. 11801

NO POSTAGE
NECESSARY
IF MAILED
IN THE
UNITED STATES

Introduce yourself to the new NURSE'S CLINICAL LIBRARY™ series.

A comprehensive book for each specific body system disorder. That's what makes this set of books so valuable to nurses. No longer will you have to go to one book for drug information, then another for pathophysiology, and still another for diagnostics. Each book in the NURSE'S CLINICAL LIBRARY is a complete source for each body system disorder. And as a subscriber to the series, you'll save $2.00 off the single-copy price of each book. Act now. Send the postage-paid card above today!

© 1983 Springhouse Corporation

BUSINESS REPLY CARD

FIRST CLASS PERMIT NO. 635, MARION, OHIO 43306

POSTAGE WILL BE PAID BY ADDRESSEE

NursingLife®

10 Health Care Circle
P.O. Box 1961
Marion, Ohio 43306

NO POSTAGE
NECESSARY
IF MAILED
IN THE
UNITED STATES

Mail the card at left to get your trial copy of *NursingLife.*

Send no money now. Just mail the card at left and we'll send you a trial copy of *NursingLife,* the fastest growing nursing journal in the world. You'll discover how to avoid malpractice suits, answer touchy ethical questions, get along better with doctors and other nurses, work better under pressure, and much more. Send for yours today!

ness, decreased level of consciousness) to appear first. Remember that cyanosis is a relatively *late* sign of hypoxemia.

Watch for a change in the color, odor, amount, and consistency of sputum. Blood-streaked, green sputum of increased viscosity may indicate worsening infection. Sudden expectoration of pus may indicate rupture of a lung abscess.

Administer antibiotics, as ordered, to treat infection; bronchodilators, to decrease inflammation and prevent bronchospasm. Turn the patient every 2 hours to promote lung expansion. Before sleep, elevate the patient's head with two or three pillows to facilitate breathing. If the patient's on bed rest, perform or encourage leg exercises to reduce the risk of thrombophlebitis. Encourage early ambulation to promote lung expansion and help mobilize secretions.

Consider your interventions successful if the patient's ABG levels and breathing return to normal and signs of hypoxemia disappear.

Ineffective airway clearance related to increased viscosity of secretions. To promote adequate removal of secretions, humidify inspired air to loosen them and administer mucolytic agents, if ordered. Instruct the patient to cough and deep-breathe at least four times every hour to mobilize secretions. If the patient watches television, help him to remember by suggesting that he cough and deep-breathe at every commercial break.

Assess lung sounds to determine areas of consolidation. Then position the patient appropriately to drain these areas (see *Positions for postural drainage,* pages 140 and 141). Since chest physiotherapy typically accompanies postural drainage, remember to administer pain medication 30 minutes beforehand to reduce inspiratory pain. Suction secretions, as necessary. Avoid repositioning the patient before suctioning to prevent secretions from draining back into the lungs. Reassess lung sounds to evaluate the effectiveness of therapy. Provide mouth care after therapy to promote patient comfort.

Consider your interventions effective if the patient coughs effectively and expectorates sputum, and if auscultation reveals no abnormal or adventitious breath sounds.

Alteration in nutrition related to dyspnea. After evaluating the patient's nutritional status, consult the doctor and dietician to determine required caloric intake. Next, find out the patient's food preferences and usual meal pattern. Then, integrating this information, pro-

vide small frequent meals, as necessary, to ensure a well-balanced diet. To encourage the anorexic patient, allow home-prepared meals within the prescribed dietary restrictions. Provide high-calorie supplemental feeding if the patient can't tolerate food by mouth. Record all intake for a total daily calorie count and weigh the patient daily.

Consider your interventions effective if the patient's appetite improves as dyspnea decreases, and his weight stabilizes or increases.

Knowledge deficit related to the disease, tests, or therapy. Of the many nursing goals in acute parenchymal disease, health teaching is one of the most important—and its success requires knowledge, skill, and patience. First, select an appropriate time for health teaching. Don't approach the anxious, dyspneic patient; the patient who's concerned about his next breath won't be receptive. Instead, wait until the patient is relaxed and comfortable, and encourage his family to be present.

Once you've established the appropriate climate for health teaching, consider the patient's cognitive ability and use terms he can readily understand. Explain the symptoms and effects of respiratory infection and measures to control them. Review the signs and symptoms of early infection—cough, sore throat, fever—that require immediate medical attention. Carefully outline discharge instructions, including activity and dietary restrictions and the drug regimen. Be sure the patient understands the dosage, route, schedule, and side effects of prescribed drugs. If appropriate, encourage the patient to stop smoking. Describe environmental factors that aggravate or cause respiratory infection. Emphasize the importance of adequate indoor ventilation and of avoiding areas of high air pollution. Document your teaching and the patient's response.

Consider your interventions effective if the patient and his family understand the disease, reportable signs and symptoms, drug regimen, and environmental hazards.

A final word
More than any other aspect of nursing care, skillful health teaching can influence both the development and outcome of acute parenchymal disease. Health teaching promotes early detection of disease, which can eliminate or shorten hospitalization. It can prevent acute parenchymal disease from complicating the recovery of the hospitalized patient. And it can help prevent recurrent disease.

Points to remember

• Acute parenchymal disease results from viral or bacterial infection, and usually has an insidious onset.
• Early recognition of acute parenchymal disease can mean the difference between home care and hospitalization.
• Inflammation of the airways, interstitium, or alveoli may accompany bacterial or viral infection.
• Inflammatory changes ultimately impair gas exchange, causing hypoxemia.
• Treatment aims to correct hypoxemia with oxygen therapy and combat infection with antibiotic or antiviral drugs.
• Nursing care includes airway management, maintenance of adequate nutrition, and, most important, health teaching.

10 MANAGING CHRONIC DISEASE

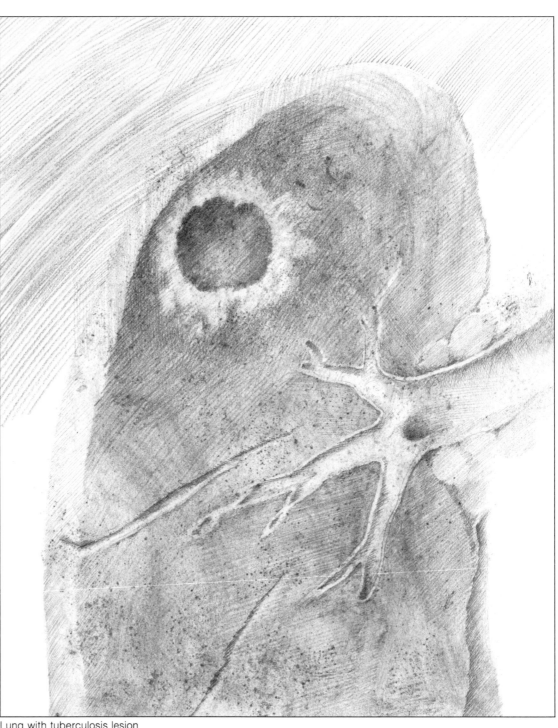

Lung with tuberculosis lesion

Chronic parenchymal diseases comprise fungal infections—histoplasmosis, coccidioidomycosis, blastomycosis, and aspergillosis—and mycobacterial infections—tuberculosis and nontubercular (or atypical) mycobacterial infections. These diseases are becoming more common as expanded use of immunosuppressive drugs and widened opportunities for travel expose persons to these diseases for which they have little or no immunity. Specific predisposing factors for developing fungal or mycobacterial infections of the lung include immunosuppression from high-dose steroid therapy, chemotherapy, radiation therapy, or acquired immune deficiency syndrome (AIDS); advanced age with inadequate nutrition and substandard living conditions; debilitation from diabetes, alcoholism, and chronic obstructive pulmonary disease (COPD), including emphysema, chronic bronchitis, and asthma; and in endemic areas, exposure to contaminated soil. To help limit the spread of these diseases in the community, you should be aware of their changing patterns of incidence. And to prevent life-threatening progression, you should know the pathophysiology of these infections; learn their clinical characteristics so you can recognize them in their early, most treatable stages; and know the current methods of effective management.

Fungal and mycobacterial infections: What they have in common

Fungal and mycobacterial diseases have similar signs and symptoms, similar clinical courses, and similar prognoses. Most are primary and self-limiting if the patient's immune system is intact. Typically, they cause no symptoms or only symptoms of mild upper respiratory infection, such as fever, cough, and malaise. In patients with such infections, the lungs' defense systems commonly deal with the primary infection so that chest X-rays may not show residual lesions; generally, only positive skin tests can confirm them.

The course of fungal and mycobacterial infections depends on the number and virulence of the infecting organisms and on the effectiveness of the patient's immune mechanisms. Prognosis is better for patients who can contain the infection in the lung. In progressive lung infections, such signs and symptoms as cavitary lesions in the lung, fever, dry or productive cough, hemoptysis, and empyema, may persist for years after the initial infection. In disseminated infections, the blood and lymph carry organisms to all parts of the body, where they cause complications such as hepatomegaly, splenomegaly, lymphadenopathy, endocarditis, and pericarditis.

PATHOPHYSIOLOGY

Phagocytosis and cell-mediated immunity represent two defenses against fungal and mycobacterial infections. Phagocytosis is a nonspecific inflammatory response. It's initiated when inhaled foreign organisms lodge in the bronchioles and alveoli, stimulating neutrophils and macrophages to attack and destroy. Macrophages—more powerful phagocytes than neutrophils—can engulf five times as many particles as neutrophils and can remove larger fungal and mycobacterial cells as well as necrotic tissue from infected areas.

After a foreign particle has been phagocytized by tissue-fixed macrophages in the alveolar walls, proteolytic enzymes in the macrophage digest this foreign matter and release digested products into the lymph, so the cell can continue phagocytizing other foreign particles. However, tubercle bacilli and fungi are not easily digested, so the macrophage forms a characteristic "giant cell" after encapsulating these organisms (see *How a tubercle forms*, page 150). This walling-off process is the prototype of granuloma formation, an effect of chronic inflammation common in many fungal infections, such as histoplasmosis and coccidioidomycosis. In this way, the infection may be halted, minimized for long periods, or progress, depending on the strength of the defense mechanisms.

After neutrophils and macrophages digest infected tissue, suppuration—the formation of pus—occurs. Pus, which is composed of necrotic tissue and dead neutrophils and macrophages, accumulates in cavities formed in the inflamed tissues. In many fungal and mycobacterial infections, caseation necrosis accompanies suppuration. Caseation, a destructive process, converts necrotic tissue into a white or yellow, cheeselike, crumbly material. Calcification and fibrosis of lung tissue are common to most chronic parenchymal infections, and in many cases, combine with pre-existing pulmonary disease to cause diffuse ventilatory defects in the lung.

Cell-mediated immunity, the major specific host defense against mycobacterial and fungal invasion, is a highly specific response. It occurs when T cells recognize the organism

How fungi and bacteria differ

Fungi and bacteria differ structurally, although they cause diseases with a similar clinical presentation. In a fungus, a membrane surrounds the nucleus, separating deoxyribonucleic acid (DNA) from cytoplasm, and the cytoplasm contains organelles that carry on cellular functions. Typical fungi consist of single filaments called hyphae that grow together to form compact woolly tufts called mycelia. The mycelia produce asexual or sexual spores, depending on the structures from which the spores originate. Some fungi reproduce from the asexual spores; others, such as *Aspergillus*, reproduce from sexual spores.

Fungi that infect man exist in two forms: In nature, they're saprophytic, absorbing nutrients directly through the cell membrane from decomposing animal or plant material. However, during infection these fungi become parasitic and potentially lethal.

Mycobacteria, or funguslike bacteria, have more primitive structures than fungi. Their single, long strand of DNA has no surrounding membrane, and the cytoplasm lacks the specialized organelles seen in fungi. They multiply by binary fission, an asexual process. Spherical bacteria are called *cocci*; spiral-shaped, *spirilla*; and rod-shaped, *bacilli*. Mycobacteria, such as *Mycobacterium tuberculosis,* are acid-fast bacilli—aerobic organisms that fail to respond to the usual staining methods used to identify bacteria, but yield to a special acid-fast stain.

Common fungal and mycobacterial diseases of the lungs

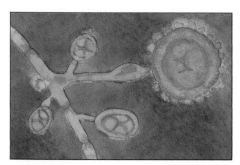

Histoplasmosis
Histoplasma capsulatum
• Found in most countries; endemic to the Ohio and Mississippi Valleys, where more than 50% of population have positive skin tests.
• Can occur at any age, but dissemination most common in infants and the elderly.

Source and method of infection
• Soil contaminated by droppings of chickens, birds, or bats.
• Inhalation of airborne spores results in lesions in lungs and hilar nodes, leading to granulomas, caseation necrosis, fibrosis, and calcification. Most infections don't reactivate.

Signs and symptoms
• *Asymptomatic* (in endemic areas): no respiratory symptoms, positive skin test.
• *Acute disseminated* (in children): fever, prostration, mediastinitis, lymphadenopathy, hepatosplenomegaly, pericarditis.
• *Chronic cavitary pulmonary* (most common): acute onset, malaise, fatigue, cough, chest pain, purulent sputum, hemoptysis, weight loss, pulmonary infiltrates and fibrosis, chronic obstructive pulmonary disease (COPD).
• *Progressive disseminated* (in infants, children, and immunosuppressed adults): hepatosplenomegaly, lymphadenopathy, chronic meningitis, GI tract ulcerations, granulomatous hepatitis, Addison's disease, endocarditis, peritonitis, chronic mucosal lesions on mouth and larynx, anemia, azotemia, abnormal liver function tests.

Treatment
• *Acute:* self-limiting; no treatment required.
• *Chronic cavitary and disseminated:* amphotericin B. Surgery to resect cavitary lesions, enlarged nodes, single pulmonary nodules; relieve constrictive pericarditis; and treat severe hemoptysis.

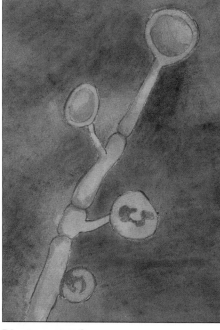

Blastomycosis
Ajellomyces dermatitidis (Blastomyces dermatitidis)
• Found in Canada, Africa, and South America; most common in middle and southeastern United States.
• Most often infects males aged 30 to 50, in contact with soil.

Source and method of infection
• Inhalation of spore dust results in dissemination, leading to pulmonary infiltrates, hilar adenopathy, absent or extensive granulomas with caseation necrosis, and possible pyogenic and ulcerated skin lesions.

Signs and symptoms
• *Systemic* (most common form): flulike symptoms, productive sputum, pleuritic pain, hilar adenopathy, pneumothorax, skin lesions, fungal osteomyelitis, erosion of vertebral bodies, destruction of vertebral disks, indurated prostate, pyuria, perineal discomfort.

Treatment
• Drug therapy with amphotericin B and 2-hydroxystilbamidine isethionate. Surgery to resect cavitary lesions (rare).

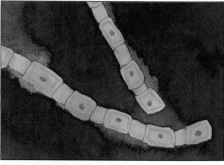

Coccidioidomycosis
Coccidioides immitis
• Endemic to southwestern United States, Mexico, and Central America.
• Primary, pulmonary form usually self-limiting. Rare, progressive form more prevalent in males, blacks, immunocompromised patients, and pregnant women.

Source and method of infection
• Soil, products, and clothes contaminated by coccidioidal spores; coccidioidal cultures.
• Inhalation of airborne spores results in rapid growth of fungi on alveoli. Spherules, with hundreds of endospores, form in the lung. Released when mature, each endospore develops a new spherule with hundreds more endospores. Leads to hilar and mediastinal node adenopathy, granuloma formation with caseation necrosis and chronic fibrotic cavities or nodules, and pulmonary tissue necrosis (calcification less common than in tuberculosis [TB]).

Signs and symptoms
• *Primary:* flulike symptoms and erythema nodosum, pleural effusion, infiltrates, pneumonia, lymphadenopathy, dissemination (rare).
• *Chronic* (develops from unresolved acute pneumonia, most often in immunosuppressed adults): bronchiectasis, bronchopleural fistula, hemoptysis, productive cough, weight loss, chronic pulmonary disease, cavitation.

Treatment
• *Primary:* usually resolves spontaneously. Possible drug therapy with amphotericin B.
• *Chronic, disseminated:* drug therapy with ketoconazole and amphotericin B. Surgery to resect chronic pulmonary cavitations, drain abscesses, treat recurrent hemoptysis, and repair bronchopleural fistulas.

engulfed by the macrophage and generate sensitized T cells that are specific to the invading antigen. Some of these sensitized T cells migrate to the infected lung, where they identify the sensitizing organism and secrete chemicals called lymphokines that destroy the antigen. Other sensitized T cells circulate as memory cells, which can rapidly release lymphokines as a protective response to reinfection.

MEDICAL MANAGEMENT
Early diagnosis and treatment may prevent progressive, life-threatening dissemination of fungal and mycobacterial infections. Unfortunately, early, precise diagnosis is difficult to achieve since many of these infections have similar clinical features and often mimic other diseases, such as rheumatologic disorders and malignant lymphomas. Consequently, a combination of chest X-rays and laboratory

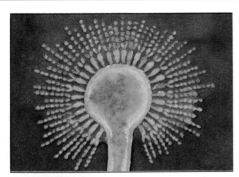

Aspergillosis
Aspergillus fumigatus
• Found worldwide.
• Most common in immunosuppressed patients. Occasionally occurs in nonimmunosuppressed patients with liver and lung disease.

Source and method of infection
• Widespread in environment. Grows on stored grain, decaying vegetation, soil, and dung. May be colonized in lung for years until immunosuppression allows activation of infection.
• Inhalation of airborne spores results in noninvasive *endobronchial aspergillosis*, a colonized form, which produces a nonspecific inflammatory response and a fungus ball in old pulmonary cavities due to other causes; or *invasive aspergillosis*, in which hyphae penetrate bronchi and bronchioles, cause thrombosis, and disseminate to brain, heart, and liver, leading to fibrosing granulomas with giant cells.

Signs and symptoms
• *Allergic bronchopulmonary* (in patients with asthma): pulmonary infiltrates, bronchiectasis, pulmonary hyperinflation.
• *Acute* (in immunosuppressed patients): high fever; pneumonia; consolidation on chest X-ray; dissemination to brain, heart, or liver; cerebral infarctions.
• *Chronic* (in patients with preexisting lung disease): hemoptysis, bronchopleural fistulas, fungus balls in old cavities, dissemination to pleura and thoracic vertebral bodies.

Treatment
• *Bronchopulmonary:* desensitization.
• *Acute:* amphotericin B and flucytosine; lobectomy.
• *Chronic:* amphotericin B through endobronchial catheter into a fungus ball, or resection.

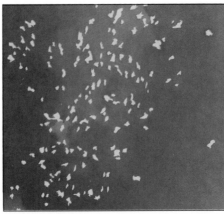

Tuberculosis
Mycobacterium tuberculosis
• Highest incidence in underdeveloped countries; lower incidence persists in developed countries. In areas of the United States with a large population of recent immigrants, incidence has risen to the same levels as the countries of origin.

Source and method of infection
• Infected persons who cough or sneeze.
• Inhalation of droplet nuclei contaminated with tubercle bacilli or direct inoculation through skin or mucous membrane results in implantation in lung, causing inflammation. Engulfed by macrophages, bacilli continue to multiply, spreading infection to lymph nodes and extrapulmonary sites. Formation of tubercules results in pulmonary and tracheobronchial lymph node calcification. Over several weeks, activated cell-mediated immunity prevents further spread of bacilli. Occasionally, chronic reinfection disease develops later.

Signs and symptoms
• *Exposure* (no evidence of infection): possible negative TB test.
• *Infection without disease:* positive TB test, no symptoms.
• *Active infection:* fever, malaise, weight loss, headache (especially at night), palpitations on exertion, possible progressive dissemination to extrapulmonary viscera.

Treatment
• Drug therapy with isoniazid, rifampin, ethambutol, and streptomycin.

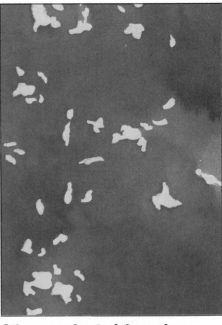

Other mycobacterial species
Mycobacterium avium intracellulare and *Mycobacterium kansasii* (most common forms)
• Incidence is unknown, as these diseases are not reportable and diagnosis is frequently unclear.

Source and method of infection
• Soil, dust, animals, water. No person-to-person transmission. In *Mycobacterium ulcerans,* grasses carrying the mycobacterium penetrate the skin.
• Method of transmission uncertain. Inhalation of organisms into alveoli can cause ventilatory defects and lead to granulomatous or suppurative skin lesions. Many grow more slowly but some more rapidly than *M. tuberculosis.*

Signs and symptoms
• Often no specific findings. Possible flulike symptoms, pneumonia, pneumothorax (rare), cavitations, preexisting COPD.

Treatment
• Drug therapy, including isoniazid, rifampin, streptomycin, cycloserine. Drugs are used in combination; selection is based on drug sensitivity tests. Surgery to resect diseased lung.

---

and skin tests is required to differentiate these diseases. Since you will probably administer the skin tests and may be asked to collect sputum specimens, you should be able to recognize abnormal results in all these tests.

Chest X-rays can demonstrate hilar adenopathy, pulmonary infiltration, cavitation, bronchopleural fistulas, and pleural effusion in fungal infections; findings vary with acute or chronic infection. In tuberculosis, chest X-rays typically show homogenous infiltrates, bronchogenic dissemination, and lesions in apical and/or posterior segments of upper lobes.

Cultures can identify *Histoplasma capsulatum*, which causes histoplasmosis, and *Blastomyces dermatitidis*, which causes blastomycosis. They can also confirm diagnosis of tuberculosis and nontubercular mycobacterial infections. Sputum cultures confirm the presence of pulmonary infections, while cultures

How a tubercle forms

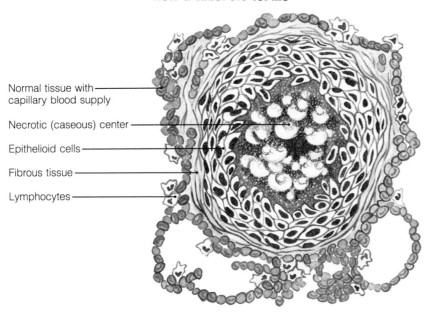

Normal tissue with capillary blood supply

Necrotic (caseous) center

Epithelioid cells

Fibrous tissue

Lymphocytes

The tubercle is the hallmark of tuberculosis. When an infected person coughs or sneezes, airborne droplets containing *Mycobacterium tuberculosis* are inhaled by a new host into the pulmonary alveoli. Here the host's immunologic defense system usually controls the tubercle bacillus by killing it or walling it up in a tiny nodule, a tubercle.

The tubercle forms as macrophages invade the infected area and fuse to form giant cells that engulf the bacillus. A layer of epithelioid cells covers this core, which, in turn, is covered by a layer of fibroblasts and lymphocytes.

If this walling-off process fails, tuberculosis bacilli spread throughout the lungs, causing destruction and fibrosis that reduces the amount of functional lung tissue. Destruction occurs as bacilli continue to multiply, enlarging the tubercle and killing the tissue in the tubercle's center. Caseation converts necrotic tissue into white or yellow, cheeselike material, which may localize and undergo fibrosis, or soften and liquefy, forming cavities as liquid drains from the necrotic center. Liquefaction can lead to destruction of bronchial walls and dissemination of the bacilli to other organs.

of urine, lymph nodes, skin lesions, and cerebrospinal fluid may verify suspected dissemination. Cultures identify coccidioidomycosis, but test results may be confusing. Therefore, infection is confirmed only when laboratory animals inoculated with the culture specimen develop endosporulating spherules. Recently, special media have been used to confirm diagnosis. Because *Aspergillus fumigatus* is widespread in the environment, cultures cannot easily confirm aspergillosis; a positive aspergillosis culture may be due to environmental contamination.

Histology, the microscopic examination of affected tissue, can help diagnose fungal and mycobacterial infections. However, many patients with such infections may be too ill to undergo the invasive procedures required to obtain tissue samples, such as bronchoscopy, transtracheal aspiration, or open-lung biopsy.

Serology demonstrates the presence of fungal infections, although not conclusively, due to frequent false-positive and false-negative readings. The study of the body's antigen-antibody response, serology measures complement fixation and the presence of immunoglobulins. High complement fixation titers occur in histoplasmosis, coccidioidomycosis, and blastomycosis. Immunoglobulins, large proteins secreted by plasma cells in response to specific antigens, function as specific antibodies. Serum antibody levels reflect recent infection, rising 2 to 5 weeks after infection, particularly in coccidioidomycosis.

Skin tests are used in combination with

other tests to diagnose fungal and mycobacterial infections. When specific antigens are injected intradermally, a positive skin reaction indicates a sensitized host.

Treatment aims to limit progression

Treatment for fungal infections—antifungal drugs, surgery, or both—depends on the infecting fungi and the stage of the disease. Amphotericin B, the most common antifungal, may produce severe side effects and complications and is recommended only in virulent infections after diagnosis is confirmed. Other drugs include 2-hydroxystilbamidine isethionate, ketoconazole, and miconazole. Surgery may be required to resect cavitary lesions and enlarged lymph nodes, drain empyema, close bronchopleural fistulas, and prevent cardiac tamponade due to restrictive pericarditis.

Antitubercular drugs usually control tuberculosis. However, certain factors influence treatment: bacilli must be susceptible to the drugs chosen; at least two drugs should be used to discourage development of drug-resistant organisms; bactericidal drugs are preferred over bacteriostatic drugs; if treatment fails over a few weeks, new combination therapy should be given; therapy is most effective when drugs are given in a single daily dose before breakfast; and treatment must continue until bacilli are eradicated (in 9 to 12 months when two bactericidal drugs are used and response is rapid; in 18 to 24 months when one of two drugs is bacteriostatic).

The preferred treatment combines isoniazid (INH) with rifampin (RIF), administered for 9 months or more. Traditional treatment combines INH, ethambutol, and streptomycin (SM) for 18 to 24 months. If resistance or toxicity develops, other antitubercular drugs may be combined. Corticosteroids may be administered in certain patients with life-threatening tuberculosis. However, their efficacy is doubtful, and they are hazardous if the organisms are drug-resistant.

Treatment for the most common nontubercular mycobacterial organisms causing chronic parenchymal disease in the lung—*M. kansasii* and *M. avium-intracellulare*—is based on identification of the pathogen and determination of its drug sensitivities. Treatment of *M. kansasii* usually consists of INH and RIF for 18 to 24 months. In some patients, SM may be administered initially and discontinued after the disease has stabilized.

Treatment of *M. avium-intracellulare* involves a combination of four to six drugs, selected according to the results of drug-sensitivity tests, since this organism is resistant to most drugs; the combination usually includes cycloserine. Treatment may also include resection of the diseased lung after a trial period of drug therapy.

NURSING MANAGEMENT
Effective nursing management of fungal and mycobacterial infections begins with suspecting them in a patient who may or may not have symptoms. For example, a routine chest X-ray of an asymptomatic patient may reveal calcified nodules seen in tuberculosis. Or a patient's general complaints of malaise, headache, and weight loss (often associated with stress or overwork) may indicate a fungal infection. Remember, too, you'll see these diseases in settings other than endemic areas.

Begin with a complete history
Note the patient's complaints, especially fever, weight loss, fatigue, anorexia, nausea, cough, and hemoptysis, which are common signs of fungal and mycobacterial infections. Ask males about pyuria, diffuse perineal pain, and testicular swelling (specific to blastomycosis).

Ask the patient where he lives, if he's recently traveled, and if he's aware of any exposure to infected persons. Travel to parts of South America, Honduras, and Guatemala, associated with typical signs and symptoms, may suggest coccidioidomycosis. Ask about activities that heighten susceptibility to infection, such as working with high-risk populations (Peace Corps or military personnel), performing cultures (laboratory personnel, who might inhale organisms), traveling in dust storms, or working with damp, moldy hay (farmers). Contact with chickens may suggest histoplasmosis, since *H. capsulatum* multiplies in chicken droppings. Living in crowded conditions with one infected family member suggests the transmission of tuberculosis to another family member who complains of fatigue, cough, and fever.

Ask the patient about any medical history of lung disease or other debilitating conditions, such as cancer or diabetes. Remember, too, that patients whose immune systems have been impaired by radiation therapy, cancer chemotherapy, organ transplants, steroid therapy, or AIDS are vulnerable to such infections. In AIDS, for example, a defect in the T cells that are responsible for cell-mediated immunity causes increased susceptibility to fungal and mycobacterial infections.

Also, ask about a smoking history and COPD. Most nontubercular mycobacterial infections coexist with COPD; productive purulent sputum can be associated with histoplasmosis and coccidioidomycosis. A history of asthma may indicate allergic pulmonary aspergillosis when associated with fever, malaise, and recurring respiratory distress.

Also, ask the patient about medications. Is he taking digoxin, steroids, antibiotics, or anticoagulants? Has he been unable to complete a regimen of antitubercular drugs?

Be sure to evaluate the patient's response to the diagnosis and his ability to comply with long-term drug therapy. The patient who is unable to complete a full course of drug therapy risks developing secondary infections with resistant strains. Also, consider his receptiveness to teaching and his occupational, financial, and family situations. Chronic, debilitating infections can financially and psychologically devastate a family, and you may need to refer the patient to community support agencies. Knowing the patient's role in the family and the support systems available to him will help you plan nursing care.

Next, perform a physical examination
First, note the patient's rate and depth of respirations. Are they easy or labored, effective or ineffective? Are sternal retractions present? What muscles are used for respiration—diaphragm, intercostal, or accessory muscles? Check for cyanosis in the lips and nail beds, a late sign of hypoxia. Is the patient complaining of dyspnea? Note the type of sputum produced and the presence of hemoptysis. Coughing and sputum production may be signs of preexisting COPD, infection, or both. Sputum cultures help diagnose and monitor the course of infection, so suction the patient with an unproductive cough or ask him to produce sputum by inhaling aerosols.

Auscultate the lungs for decreased ventilation and potential problems. Check for diminished or absent breath sounds due to pleural effusion, atelectasis, or pneumothorax. Decreased breath sounds on exhalation and crepitant rales at end inspiration suggest preexisting COPD. Rhonchi that improve with coughing or suctioning suggest secretions in the larger airways. Document breath sounds to help track the progression of infection and the effectiveness of therapy.

Listen to the heart for pericardial friction rub, murmur, or irregular rhythm, since disseminated infections may cause pericarditis

Preventing tuberculosis

Although mortality from tuberculosis (TB) has declined since 1900, worldwide statistics show 4 million new cases and 1 million deaths each year. You can help identify those at risk for TB and teach them about its causes, transmission, signs and symptoms, and treatment.

Also, you can inform high-risk patients and those who cannot avoid exposure, such as some military and Peace Corps personnel, about Bacillus Calmette-Guérin (BCG), an immune prophylactic vaccine considered inappropriate for the general population.

BCG moderates illness

BCG, a live, attenuated strain of *Mycobacterium bovis*, provides active immunity against tuberculosis. The drug doesn't prevent infection, but reduces clinical manifestations by about 80%.

Although the drug has few side effects, it may cause local ulcers and, less commonly, lymph node abscesses or suppuration.

BCG is administered intradermally to individuals with negative tuberculin skin tests who are not actively infected with tuberculosis.

Note that BCG changes the tuberculin skin test from negative to positive for varying lengths of time, therefore interfering with the test's usefulness.

or endocarditis. Palpitations are possible in tuberculosis and cor pulmonale and congestive heart failure in severe lung infections, so listen for an S_3 or S_4 gallop.

Check diet preferences, bowel sounds, and the type and amount of stool. Test stools and emesis for blood. Intestinal tract ulcerations are related to disseminated histoplasmosis.

Check for cutaneous lesions: subcutaneous nodules and wartlike granulomas in blastomycosis and pustules or draining ulcers in coccidioidomycosis.

Check for indurated prostate, pyuria, and deep perineal pain (blastomycosis) and for azotemia (histoplasmosis).

Obtain baseline information on urine output, specific gravity, creatinine clearance, and serum blood urea nitrogen and creatinine levels to monitor possible renal toxicity if the patient is treated with amphotericin B, rifampin, and streptomycin.

Plan goal-directed care

Use information from your patient assessment to develop nursing diagnoses and plan your care. Patients with fungal or mycobacterial infections may also have underlying diseases, such as leukemia or AIDS, so focus your care on this disease as well as on the infection's symptoms. Anticipate patient problems with nursing diagnoses similar to the following:

Potential for discomfort and fatigue related to flulike symptoms of fever, aches, and pains. To ensure rest and promote recovery, restrict visitors during patient naps and provide rest periods. Also, encourage exercise within limits. Reposition the patient to ease his discomfort, and give pain medication and cool baths (to decrease fever), when indicated.

Alteration of nutritional intake related to anorexia and vomiting. To counteract dehydration and meet increased metabolic demands, consult the dietitian for a diet high in carbohydrates and protein; force fluids, unless contraindicated. Also, check your patient's food preferences and help him fill out menus, or encourage his family to bring food from home. If indicated, supply needed fluids and vitamins intravenously.

Risk of developing side effects from antifungal and antitubercular drugs. To minimize side effects, carefully administer and monitor drug therapy. In fungal infections, nephrotoxicity occurs in more than 80% of patients treated with amphotericin B. Mild to severe anaphylaxis may occur with infusion; give a test dose and monitor vital signs for up to 4

hours before giving prescribed dose. Infuse this drug over 6 hours, and add hydrocortisone to solution to limit chills and tremors. Another antifungal drug, miconazole, may induce tachydysrhythmias, cardiorespiratory arrest, hyponatremia, and severe itching during infusion. Dilute miconazole and administer over 30 to (preferably) 60 minutes. Before infusing amphotericin B or miconazole, give antiemetics to combat severe vomiting and add heparin to the infusion, as ordered, to prevent phlebitis at the infusion site. Administration of INH, RIF, and SM in tuberculosis may be associated with nausea, vomiting, rash, and fever and more serious drug toxicities, such as hepatic toxicity, especially when INH and RIF are administered together. Also, closely observe the patient for peripheral neuropathy from INH and for ototoxicity from SM.

Anxiety related to lack of knowledge about thoracic surgery. To relieve anxiety, provide preoperative teaching and include a family member. Answer any questions and reinforce the doctor's explanation of the procedure. To give the patient some control over his situation, emphasize his participation in his recovery. Discuss what happens in the postoperative period: demonstrate chest physiotherapy, coughing, and deep breathing, and explain their purpose. Tell the patient these procedures are required every hour for the first 24 hours after surgery, but reassure him that their frequency decreases, perhaps to every 4 hours, as he recovers. Describe the equipment that will be present postoperatively (chest tube and underwater seal drainage system, intravenous lines, and ventilators). Before surgery, teach the patient how to perform respiratory exercises, such as incentive spirometry, to promote effective pulmonary function; leg exercises, to prevent thrombus formation; and arm and shoulder range-of-motion (ROM) exercises on the affected side. Encourage the patient to ask for pain medication and personal assistance when needed. If mechanical ventilation is anticipated, describe alternative methods of communication. Evaluate how well the patient understood your teaching, and clarify areas needing reinforcement. Encourage the patient and his family to express their concerns.

Potential for postoperative complications. After surgery, forestall complications by maintaining adequate ventilation and tissue perfusion. Remember, skillful nursing care promotes patient participation and recovery. Assess the patient continually, document your findings, and intervene quickly, when needed.

After he regains consciousness and vital signs stabilize, place the patient in semi-Fowler's position. This facilitates lung expansion, ventilation, and chest catheter drainage. Find out if the patient is allowed to be positioned on the operative side; then turn him every 1 to 2 hours to promote drainage and prevent thrombus formation. Be sure that chest drainage tubes remain patent. If the patient is on mechanical ventilation, maintain endotracheal tube patency, assist with communication, and provide support.

When possible, give pain medication 30 minutes before any respiratory treatment (chest physiotherapy, coughing, deep breathing, and suctioning) to allow maximum compliance. Provide rest periods during treatment. Perform passive and active ROM exercises to arms and legs every 4 hours, or as ordered.

Observe for signs of infection (fever, purulent drainage, or inflammation at the incision site) and hemorrhage (tachycardia, hypotension, continued bloody drainage from chest tube or dressing).

Administer drugs, as ordered, to assist in arresting the infection, and notify the doctor if signs indicate a worsening condition (altered mental status, respiratory distress) or ineffectiveness of medical regimen (continued purulent sputum, fever, complications).

Record intake and output and administer fluids carefully to prevent pulmonary edema. Monitor pulmonary arterial and central venous pressures, blood gas values, and electrolytes. Be alert to signs of increasing respiratory distress, such as dyspnea and deteriorating blood gas values.

Potential spread of tuberculosis due to airborne transmission of the tubercle bacillus. To prevent the spread of infection, help the patient comply with treatment. In suspected tuberculosis or positive tuberculosis sputum smears, also follow respiratory precautions: a private room; use of masks by anyone entering the room and use of gloves when in contact with the patient's sputum, such as during suctioning; and thorough hand washing on entering and leaving the room. Double-bag and sterilize linen and articles contaminated with sputum. Have an infected patient wear a mask whenever he leaves his room. Isolate patients with fungal infections only if cutaneous lesions are open and draining.

Potential for ineffective patient coping and distress among family members related to prolonged therapy, chronic infection, and fear of death. To help the patient and his family deal with chronic disease and long-term drug therapy regimens, provide emotional support and encourage them to voice their concerns. A patient who is immunocompromised due to a recent kidney transplant may be concerned about treatment with amphotericin B. Remember that lengthy treatment, loss of income, and changes in family roles add stress to the family unit. Help the patient and his family through the grieving process in life-threatening infections and death. (Fungal or mycobacterial infections hasten death for many debilitated patients, especially those with acute aspergillosis.) Make referrals to appropriate agencies if needed.

Insufficient knowledge about follow-up and therapy after discharge. To prepare the patient for discharge, begin comprehensive teaching upon admission and reinforce it before discharge. Alert him to the need for medical follow-up, and make appropriate referrals to public health agencies, a community clinic, or a nurse practitioner. If necessary, arrange to administer amphotericin B on an outpatient basis; when compliance may be a problem, refer the patient to a public health agency. Explain the chronic nature of the disease. Encourage the patient to exercise within individual limits, and instruct him about good nutrition. Teach the family how to control these infections and, in tuberculosis, begin prophylactic drug therapy, if ordered.

During the course of your nursing care, enlist the help of your patient and his family in evaluating and altering your care plan, as needed. Evaluate your intervention by asking: Is the patient comfortable, pain free, and eating an adequate diet? Have complications been prevented or treated immediately if they developed? Also, can the patient and his family discuss medication dosage schedules and side effects? Do they know how the disease is contracted and transmitted, so reinfection or spread of the disease can be diagnosed and treated early? Finally, did you help the terminal patient die in a peaceful environment with the support of family members?

A final word
Improved management of fungal and mycobacterial infections depends, in part, on early diagnosis, prompt action, and firm follow-up care. Your careful assessment, skillful intervention, and effective patient teaching directly help contain these infections and ensure patient recovery.

Points to remember

• Fungal and mycobacterial infections insidiously invade the lungs and usually produce asymptomatic, slow-growing lesions.
• In acute and chronic forms of these diseases, some infections heal without treatment while others progressively disseminate throughout the body, producing persistent destruction or causing death.
• The course of these infections depends on the quantity and virulence of the organisms and the patient's ability to combat infection.
• Increased travel and expanded use of immunosuppressives make individuals more susceptible to such infections than in the past.
• Unfamiliarity with these diseases can lead to delayed diagnosis and mismanagement.

11 PROVIDING SUPPORT IN CANCER

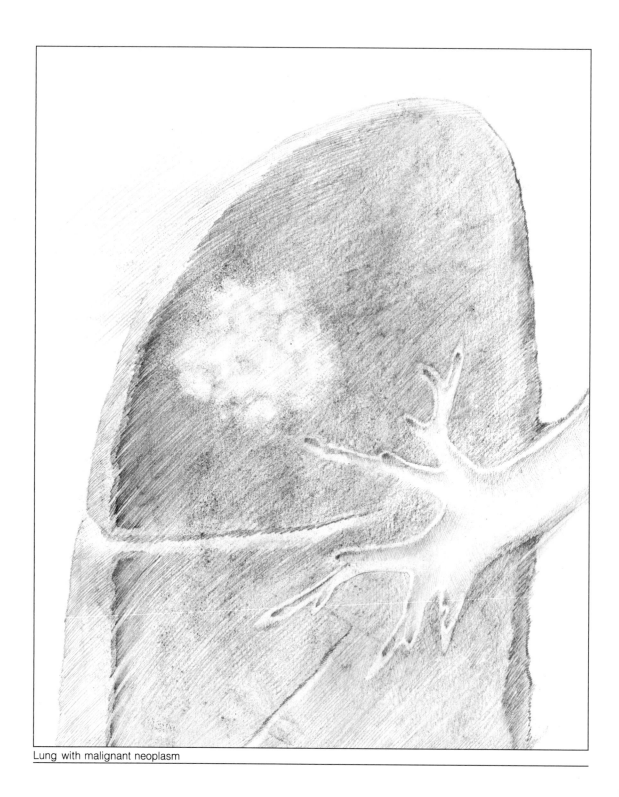

Lung with malignant neoplasm

Lung cancer is now the leading cause of cancer death in American men and is rapidly assuming similar status in women. Since the 1930s, the incidence of this once uncommon disease has risen dramatically in close correlation with a similar increase in the prevalence of smoking. While lung cancer has been clearly linked to various respiratory carcinogens, its major cause is indisputable: cigarette smoking. In fact, 80% of those with the disease are smokers. (See *How smoking affects lung cancer death rates,* pages 156 and 157.) Cigarette smoking also multiplies the risk of lung cancer when combined with exposure to occupational respiratory carcinogens such as asbestos (see *Smoking exaggerates risk of asbestos-related lung cancer,* page 159). Prognosis is poor because lung cancer is usually not detected until it's in an advanced stage. The average 5-year survival rate for men is only 8%; for women, 12%.

As a nurse, you're well qualified to become an activist in preventing lung cancer. You can help educate young people so that they don't start to smoke, promote the use of smoking withdrawal clinics, and support efforts to screen smokers for early lung cancer detection. You can warn workers who are exposed to occupational respiratory carcinogens of the need for protection on the job and of the dangerous synergistic effects of combining such occupational exposure with smoking.

You can also play an important role in helping patients and their families cope with the physical and emotional stress of lung cancer once it's been diagnosed. Performing your double role well requires an understanding of lung cancer's insidious development and current treatment.

PATHOPHYSIOLOGY
The term *lung cancer* actually refers to several types of cancer, four of which are the most common: epidermoid (squamous-cell) carcinoma, small-cell (including intermediate cell and lymphocytic or oat cell) carcinoma, adenocarcinoma, and large-cell anaplastic carcinoma.

Histologic classification of these cancers was developed in 1958 and revised in 1967 by the World Health Organization (WHO). In 1972, the Pathology Panel for the Working Party for Therapy of Lung Cancer (WP-L) modified the WHO classification. (See *Chief histologic classifications of lung tumors.*)

What causes lung cancer?
Recent data implicates smoking as *the* most significant factor for *all* cell types of lung cancer, even though occupational respiratory carcinogens also contribute to its rising incidence. Evidence is growing that even passive smoking—inhaling the smoke of cigarettes smoked by others—may promote development of this disease. Of course, not everyone who smokes develops lung cancer; several other etiologic factors are under current investigation, including the role of vitamin A, arylhydrocarbon hydroxylase (AHH), and constituents of tobacco smoke. Also, in adenocarcinoma, a predisposing scar from an earlier lung injury has been suggested as a possible etiologic factor.

Genetic factors may explain why only 12% to 15% of smokers develop lung cancer. In fact, smokers related to lung cancer patients have about an 11 times greater risk of developing the disease than smokers with no family history of the disease.

Is prevention possible?
Before lung cancer becomes clinically apparent, years of progressive metaplasia and dysplasia have already occurred (see *Clinical impact of tumor doubling time,* page 162). These cell changes occur in people exposed to respiratory carcinogens and are also associated with vitamin A deficiency. Thus, by administering vitamin A and eliminating exposure to smoking and other carcinogens, this disease could perhaps be checked before it progresses to carcinoma in situ. However, because of the slow growth pattern of these tumors, the incidence of lung cancer among ex-smokers does not approach that among nonsmokers until 5 to 10 years after smoking ceases. Clearly, today, the best form of prevention is the avoidance of carcinogens before any cell damage occurs.

Early diagnosis can also improve prognosis. An approach currently being evaluated is yearly chest X-ray and cytologic examination of sputum as a routine screening measure for cigarette smokers over age 45. In this type of screening, chest X-ray can detect peripheral cancers (those in the alveoli and smaller airways), while sputum cytology can detect central cancers (those in the bronchi and hilum). However, such screening is costly and its use is not yet widespread. A future approach to early diagnosis might employ monoclonal antibodies that are specific for lung cancer and tagged with radioisotopes.

Chief histologic classifications of lung tumors

World Health Organization (WHO)

Epidermoid carcinoma

Small-cell carcinoma
Fusiform
Polygonal
Lymphocyte-like (oat cell)
Others

Adenocarcinoma
Bronchogenic
Acinar
Papillary
Bronchoalveolar

Large-cell carcinoma
Solid tumor with mucin
Solid tumor without mucin
Giant cell
Clear cell

Working Party for Therapy of Lung Cancer (WP-L)

Epidermoid carcinoma
Well differentiated
Moderately differentiated
Poorly differentiated

Small-cell carcinoma
Lymphocyte-like (oat cell)
Intermediate cell

Adenocarcinoma
Well differentiated
Moderately differentiated
Poorly differentiated
Bronchopapillary

Large-cell carcinoma
With stratification
Giant cell
With mucin formation
Clear cell

How smoking affects lung cancer death rates

The rise in lung cancer deaths in this century has lagged 20 to 30 years behind the rise in smoking, as the graphs show. This lag is typical of other chemically induced neoplasms.

Lung cancer death rates for men may eventually level off, because of the sharp decline in male smoking habits after 1955. Any decline in death rates for women will be delayed and less pronounced, since the decline in female smoking habits began 5 years later and was less sharp.

In 1960, about 6 male deaths occurred for each female death. Now, however, the ratio is 3.5 to 1. If current trends continue, the death rates will be equal by the year 2000.

Key

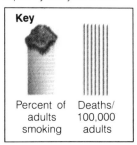

Percent of adults smoking

Deaths/ 100,000 adults

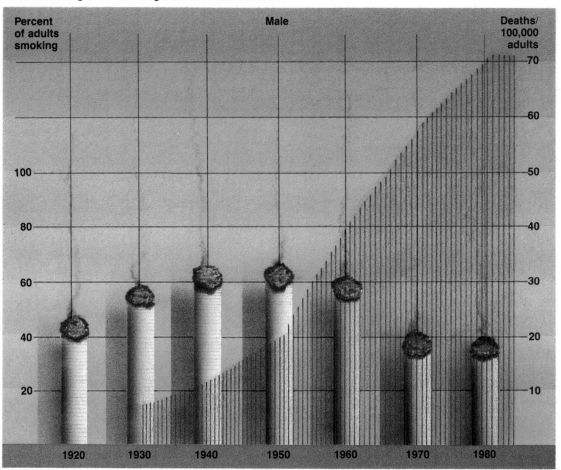

Lung cancer growth patterns

All of the common lung cancers originate in the bronchial epithelium (bronchogenic carcinomas). Once the initial cell changes progress to carcinoma in situ and, eventually, to invasive cancer, growth patterns can vary. (See *How lung cancer develops and spreads,* pages 160 and 161.)

Lung tumors may exhibit different growth characteristics according to their individual histologic classification.

Squamous-cell carcinoma and small-cell carcinoma. These tumors tend to grow centrally within the bronchial lumen. As they grow, they form large, polypoid, friable lesions that tend to obstruct the lumen and to bleed easily. Because of bronchial obstruction, patients with these types of cancer frequently have shortness of breath due to lung collapse and are prone to pneumonia. These friable tumors tend to shed malignant cells into bronchial secretions, which are coughed up to yield positive results on cytologic sputum examination. Squamous-cell and small-cell carcinomas tend to grow to a larger size

within the pulmonary parenchyma than adenocarcinoma and large-cell anaplastic carcinoma. As squamous-cell carcinoma enlarges, it may outgrow its blood supply. This results in central necrosis, which appears as a thick-walled abscess cavity on a chest X-ray. Squamous-cell carcinomas sometimes form apical tumors (Pancoast's tumors), which may eventually invade nearby structures. Small-cell carcinomas, in particular, metastasize early to involve many different organ systems.

Adenocarcinoma and large-cell anaplastic carcinoma. These tumors usually grow peripherally in the smaller airways and alveoli, and thus may interfere with ventilation and perfusion. Located near the pleura, they may also interfere mechanically with the expansion and contraction of the lungs by causing pleuritic pain on inspiration that limits lung expansion. Because they grow in the bronchial submucosa, they don't shed cells into the bronchial tree. These cancers rarely cause Pancoast's tumor. Usually, their local growth within the pulmonary parenchyma causes involvement of adjacent intrathoracic struc-

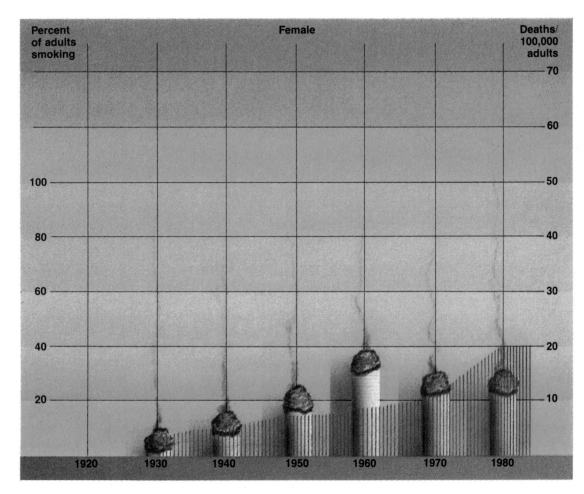

Percent of adults smoking / Female / Deaths/100,000 adults

1920 1930 1940 1950 1960 1970 1980

tures, such as the pleura and pericardium, and regional lymphatic spread to hilar and mediastinal lymph nodes.

Lung cancer symptoms. Symptoms are related to the location of the primary tumor, locations of metastases, paraneoplastic syndromes, and ectopic hormone production.

Central tumors. These tumors often cause increased cough, dyspnea, or diffuse chest pain that can involve the chest, shoulder blades, and back. The pain is the result of peribronchial or perivascular nerve involvement. In many patients, squamous-cell and small-cell tumors also cause hemoptysis and fecal breath odor, a result of secondary infection within a necrotic tumor mass. Central tumors also commonly cause postobstructive pneumonia, the result of infection behind an occluded airway. Its symptoms are cough, fever, chills, malaise, and anorexia, which often become chronic because antibiotics are relatively ineffective without drainage. After treatment shrinks the tumor enough to allow drainage, the infection subsides.

These tumors, particularly the small-cell

type, occasionally extend to the pericardium, causing pericardial effusion and tamponade. In cardiac tamponade, circulation becomes progressively inefficient and the body compensates through peripheral vasoconstriction and diversion of its limited blood supply to the vital organs. Resulting signs and symptoms are the sudden onset of dysrhythmia (sinus tachycardia or atrial fibrillation), paradoxical pulse, distant heart sounds, weakness, anxiety, dyspnea, and shock.

Apical (superior sulcus or Pancoast's) tumors. These tumors, most often squamous-cell tumors and less often adenocarcinomas, usually do not cause symptoms while confined to the pulmonary parenchyma. They can extend into surrounding structures and frequently involve the first thoracic and the eighth cervical nerves within the brachial plexus. This produces neuritic pain in the arm and shoulder on the affected side and atrophy of the muscles of the arm and hand. Further local tumor growth may erode the first and second ribs and the vertebrae, causing bone pain, and may also involve the sympathetic nerve

Industrial respiratory carcinogens and specific populations at risk

Radioisotopes (small-cell undifferentiated tumors)
Uranium miners
Iron ore miners
Hard rock miners
Nuclear waste workers

Mustard gas (squamous-cell tumors)
Research workers
WWI veterans

Asbestos (all cell types but especially adenocarcinoma)
Miners
Millers
Insulation workers
Textile workers
Shipyard workers
Cement workers

Polycyclic aromatic hydrocarbons: coal dust and carbonization products
Gas workers
Steel workers
Coal miners
Roofers

Halo ethers (small-cell tumors)
Chloromethyl ether production workers

Nickel
Nickel ore processors

Chromium
Chromium ore processors
Pigment workers

Inorganic arsenic
Metallurgic workers
Insecticide applicators
Copper smelters
Sheep dip workers
Gold miners
Crop dusters

Iron ore
Hematite miners
Steel workers

Vinyl chloride
Rubber workers
Chemical workers

Community pollution by industry

Combined exposure

ganglia, which are located paravertebrally. Involvement of the sympathetic nerve ganglia leads to Horner's syndrome. Apical tumors usually don't extend to regional nodes or metastasize to distant sites.

Peripheral tumors. These tumors are more often asymptomatic at diagnosis than central tumors. An exception may be the bronchoalveolar variant of adenocarcinoma, in which distal bronchial and alveolar involvement causes a productive cough.

These tumors may extend through the visceral and parietal pleura to the chest wall, irritating local nerves and causing pleuritic pain. Such pain tends to be localized and sharp and increases upon inspiration, unlike the dull, diffuse pain associated with central tumors. Restriction of lung expansion results from pain or the accumulation of pleural fluid.

Metastases to hilar and mediastinal lymph nodes. Extension of the tumor to the hilar lymph nodes alone is usually asymptomatic. Mediastinal lymph node involvement, however, is responsible for a variety of signs and symptoms, any one of which may indicate that surgery is no longer an option. Vocal cord paralysis, caused by entrapment of the recurrent laryngeal nerve, leads to hoarseness. Both vocal cords are rarely involved, but if they are, a tracheostomy to facilitate breathing is essential. Compression of the recurrent laryngeal nerve may also cause dysphagia. Compression of the phrenic nerve causes paralysis of the diaphragm on the affected side, which causes dyspnea. In a patient with compression of the phrenic nerve, a physical examination or fluoroscopy may reveal decreased, absent, or paradoxical excursion of the diaphragm (the diaphragm moves counter to normal during respiration).

Mediastinal node involvement may also cause superior vena cava syndrome, a result of vena caval compression by enlarged nodes. If the obstruction occurs distal to the junction of the superior vena cava and the azygous vein, it causes distention of arm and neck veins; suffusion and/or edema of the face, neck, and arms; and the appearance of tortuous collateral vessels on the upper chest and back. Obstruction of the superior vena cava proximal to the junction leads to the development of extensive collateral circulation along the anterior and posterior abdominal walls and, possibly, to venous stasis with secondary thrombus formation.

Enlarged mediastinal lymph nodes can compress the esophagus, causing dysphagia;

they can also directly invade and erode the esophagus and lead to bronchoesophageal fistula and recurrent aspiration pneumonia. Extensive mediastinal lymphatic obstruction can cause stasis of lymphatic flow through the affected lumen, with resultant pleural effusion.

Distant metastatic extension. Recognizing metastasis promptly can allow treatment that may prevent major complications and measurably prolong productive life.

Central nervous system (CNS) involvement. About 10% of all patients with lung cancer have CNS involvement at diagnosis; those who don't risk developing it eventually. Such involvement is most common in patients with small-cell carcinoma and adenocarcinoma, and the brain is the most common site. The major symptoms of brain metastasis result from increased intracranial pressure and include headache, nausea, vomiting, malaise, anorexia, weakness, and alterations in mentation. Less common symptoms include seizures, hemiparesis, cranial nerve abnormalities, cerebellar abnormalities, and aphasia.

Meningeal involvement (carcinomatous meningitis). Such metastasis is uncommon at diagnosis but often occurs later in the course of the illness, especially in patients with small-cell carcinoma. In addition to signs and symptoms similar to those of brain metastasis, meningeal involvement produces focal neurologic abnormalities, especially those involving cranial nerves and spinal roots.

Spinal cord involvement. Cord compression may result from direct invasion or from metastatic tumor growth in structures surrounding the spinal cord, causing diminished blood supply to the cord. Whatever the cause, the signs and symptoms of compression are the same. The patient first complains of back pain, which is either localized or radicular. This progresses to weakness and loss of sensation in the legs and, unless treated, irreversible paralysis in areas below the site of involvement. As epidural spinal cord compression intensifies, bowel and bladder incontinence results. Epidural cord compression is most common in small-cell carcinoma, least common in squamous-cell carcinoma.

Long-bone involvement. Metastasis to the weight-bearing long bones is common. Its primary signs and symptoms are bone pain and a tendency toward fractures.

Further complications. Two syndromes, whose mechanisms are poorly understood, may complicate the management of lung can-

Smoking exaggerates risk of asbestos-related lung cancer

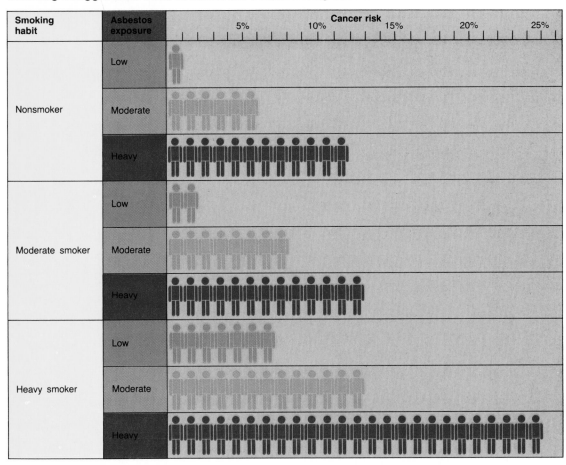

Smoking habit	Asbestos exposure	Cancer risk
Nonsmoker	Low	
	Moderate	
	Heavy	
Moderate smoker	Low	
	Moderate	
	Heavy	
Heavy smoker	Low	
	Moderate	
	Heavy	

Smoking compounds the risk of lung cancer for the person who's exposed to asbestos or other respiratory carcinogens. Conversely, reducing the smoking habit (and/or controlling exposure to known carcinogens, such as by wearing a protective mask on the job) lessens the cancer risk.

For example, the heavy smoker who sustains heavy exposure to asbestos has a 25% chance of developing lung cancer, compared with a 12% chance for the nonsmoker with similar exposure. The heavy smoker with minimal asbestos exposure still has a 7% chance of developing cancer, compared to only a 1% chance for his nonsmoking counterpart.

cer. While not related to metastasis, they produce signs and symptoms that mimic metastatic involvement.

Paraneoplastic syndromes. These syndromes occur in up to 20% of all patients with lung cancer. Their most typical signs and symptoms are skin rash; clubbing of the fingers; pigmentation disorders; arthralgias; thrombophlebitis; and muscle weakness, especially of the pelvic girdle. Such symptoms usually become apparent near the time of diagnosis and usually disappear when the disease is cured or in remission.

Ectopic hormone production. This complication produces symptoms that may suggest central nervous system metastasis. Symptoms range from gynecomastia to mental changes.

MEDICAL MANAGEMENT

When lung cancer is strongly suspected—usually because of a shadow on a chest X-ray and sometimes because of a persistent cough—physical examination and patient history may provide further clues. However, confirmation and staging require a series of special tests.

Histologic tests essential

Chest X-ray is the most important method of initially detecting lung cancer, but only a comprehensive series of diagnostic tests can confirm the diagnosis and describe the extent of the disease (see *Diagnostic tests for lung cancer,* page 163). Histologic diagnosis involves microscopic examination of a sample of tumor tissue or of shed tumor cells obtained from sputum, bronchoscopic washings, or fluid collected through thoracentesis. Fiber-optic bronchoscopy, mediastinoscopy, mediastinotomy, needle biopsy, and thoracotomy can all provide tumor tissue for histologic analysis. The last two procedures are used only when other diagnostic tests fail to provide accurate diagnosis: needle biopsy carries a slight risk of seeding tumor cells along the needle track; thoracotomy is a major surgical procedure.

While sputum cytology is an important diagnostic tool, it's not always specific for lung cancer, as head and neck malignancies may also produce a positive cytology for squamous-cell cancer.

Tests to detect metastasis include liver

How lung cancer develops and spreads

Once lung tumor cells grow through the basement membrane of the bronchial epithelium (see below), they spread locally, regionally, and metastatically.

Local growth. Local growth refers to growth within the lung and to direct extension of the primary tumor into nearby intrathoracic structures. The tumor may spread endobronchially via the submucosal lymphatics within the walls of the bronchial tree, or it may spread transbronchially by growing directly through the bronchial walls and thus to the peribronchial lymphatics and connective tissue. Both transbronchial and endobronchial extension of the primary tumor usually follow a centripetal course, in the direction of the mediastinum. However, if lymphatics become blocked by the tumor, the lymphatic flow is reversed and a centrifugal course toward the chest wall results. Local growth of the tumor may also extend to intrathoracic organs, such as the heart and pleura, if the primary tumor is located nearby.

Regional growth. This refers to extension of the tumor into hilar and mediastinal lymph nodes. As with local tumor growth, malignant cells reach hilar and mediastinal nodes via either submucosal or peribronchial lymphatics. Once tumor cells are established in a lymph node, they may extend through the node capsule to involve adjacent mediastinal structures.

Metastatic tumor growth. Metastasis occurs when the cancer spreads beyond the involved lung and mediastinal lymph nodes. Cancer cells may travel via the circulatory or lymphatic systems to any organ in the body. The most common metastatic sites are the brain, liver, bone, contralateral lung, and extrathoracic lymph nodes.

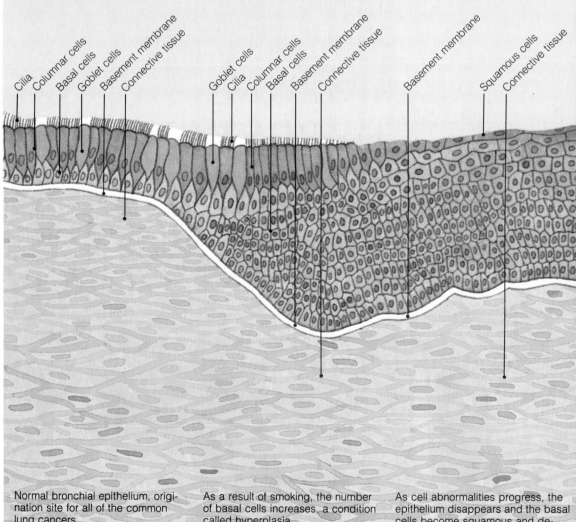

Normal bronchial epithelium, origination site for all of the common lung cancers.

As a result of smoking, the number of basal cells increases, a condition called hyperplasia.

As cell abnormalities progress, the epithelium disappears and the basal cells become squamous and develop darkened nuclei.

Lung cancer prognosis by cell type

Characteristic	Epidermoid (squamous)	Adeno-carcinoma	Large-cell	Small-cell
Approximate incidence	25% to 30%	30% to 35%	15% to 20%	20% to 25%
5-year survival	16% to 18%	10% to 12%	10% to 12%	4%
Operability	43% to 50%	35%	35% to 43%	Rare
Doubling time: mean/range (days)	88 days 7 to 381 days	161 days 17 to 590 days	92 days 48 to 112 days	29 days 17 to 71 days
Potential for metastasis	Low to moderate	Moderate	Moderate	High
Location in lung field	Central	Peripheral	Peripheral	Central
Response rate to systemic treatment	Low	Low	Low	Moderate

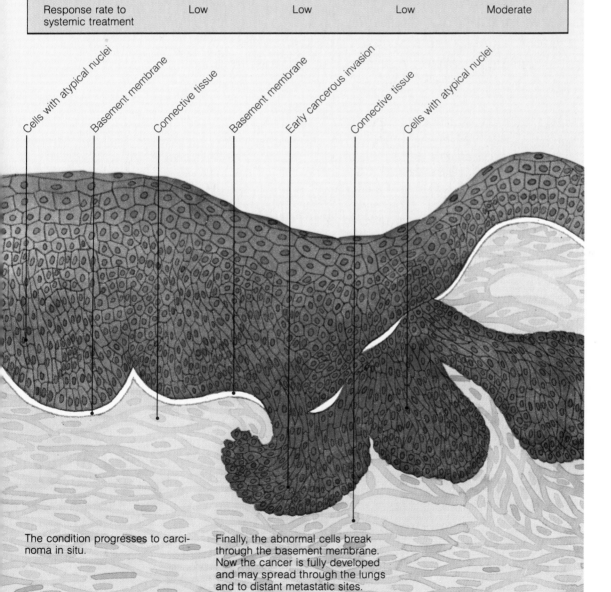

Cells with atypical nuclei

Basement membrane

Connective tissue

Basement membrane

Early cancerous invasion

Connective tissue

Cells with atypical nuclei

The condition progresses to carcinoma in situ.

Finally, the abnormal cells break through the basement membrane. Now the cancer is fully developed and may spread through the lungs and to distant metastatic sites.

Clinical impact of tumor doubling time

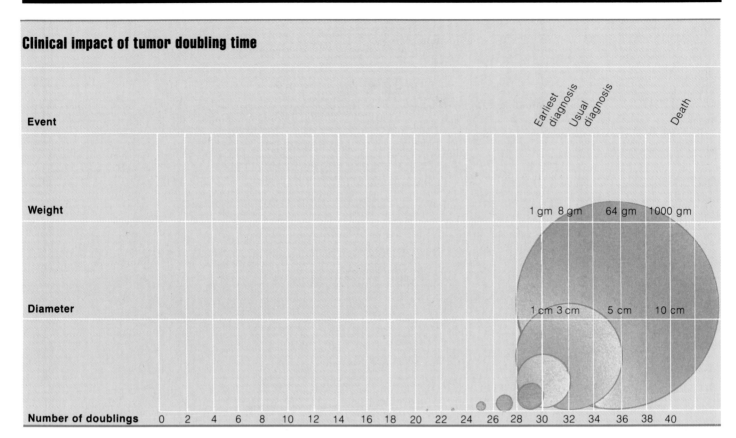

Event

Earliest diagnosis   Usual diagnosis   Death

Weight

1 gm   8 gm   64 gm   1000 gm

Diameter

1 cm   3 cm   5 cm   10 cm

Number of doublings   0   2   4   6   8   10   12   14   16   18   20   22   24   26   28   30   32   34   36   38   40

Doubling time, the time a tumor takes to double in size, determines the elapsed time before lung cancer becomes clinically apparent. This doubling time may be measured in terms of weight, diameter, or number of tumor cells. Mean doubling time is 29 days for small-cell tumors, 88 days for squamous-cell tumors, 92 days for large-cell tumors, and 161 days for adenocarcinomas.

Lung tumors usually are undetected until they've reached 1 to 3 cm in diameter. A random chest X-ray may reveal their existence before signs appear. For adenocarcinomas, diagnosis usually comes 13.2 to 15.4 years after the initial malignant change in a single cell (onset), with death occurring at 17.6 years. But for fast-doubling small-cell tumors, diagnosis comes 2.4 to 2.8 years after onset, with death occurring at 3.2 years.

Once detectable, tumors rapidly progress to lethal size (10 cm). A lethal tumor burden usually exists after 40 doublings, but most of that life span remains subclinical.

function studies; liver biopsy; bone scan; bone marrow biopsy; mediastinoscopy; skull X-ray; CT scan of the brain, thorax, and abdomen; and radionuclide scan of bone, spleen, liver, and adrenal glands.

Results of examination and diagnostic tests establish a diagnosis, help stage the disease (see *Staging lung cancer,* page 164), and determine operability (the patient's ability to withstand surgery and the prospects for complete surgical removal of the cancer) and the course of treatment.

Treatment

Because the disease is usually advanced at diagnosis, treatment tends to be palliative—designed to improve prognosis and extend life—rather than curative, although surgical cures are possible in limited disease. Current nonsurgical treatment uses combinations of radiation, chemotherapy, and immunotherapy. Most patients achieve at least 50% tumor shrinkage, while in others the tumor disappears. Unfortunately, this response to treatment is almost always transient.

Surgery. When a tumor is resectable, surgical removal is the treatment of choice for all lung cancers. A tumor may be resectable (capable of being completely removed in surgery) if it's well contained, with no appar-

ent metastasis, and the patient isn't limited by cardiac disease, chronic obstructive pulmonary disease, or other debilitating condition. Surgery ranges from wedge and segmental resections through lobectomy to pneumonectomy with removal of involved lymph nodes. Surgery may be feasible for selected cases of small-cell carcinoma, although this cancer usually escapes detection until after metastasis.

Radiation. An alternative when surgery is contraindicated, radiation is most effective against radio-sensitive tumors, such as small-cell and epidermoid carcinomas. The major role for radiation therapy today is for relief of tumor symptoms. In this role, it can offer weeks to months of relief from cough; dyspnea; hemoptysis; and bone, chest, and liver pain. Some experimental evidence also suggests that prophylactic brain radiation may reduce the incidence of CNS metastasis in some cell types.

Chemotherapy. Chemotherapy is indicated when lung cancer is extensive and surgery and high-dose radiation are unfeasible. In particular, it has improved the formerly poor prognosis for small-cell carcinoma, providing a 65% remission rate when used in tandem with other forms of treatment. However, long-term prognosis with chemotherapy remains poor. The most effective drugs, used singly or in combination, include adriamycin, lomustine (CCNU), cyclophosphamide, methotrexate, mechlorethamine (nitrogen mustard), and vincristine. Chemotherapy also relieves cancer symptoms, chiefly pain and pressure, and helps control metastasis.

Immunotherapy. Still experimental, immunotherapy may prolong survival rates by counteracting the immunosuppression that accompanies lung cancer. Administrations of live vaccine, such as BCG (bacille Calmette-Guérin) or C parvum (*Corynebacterium parvulum*), are used in an attempt to stimulate the immune system to destroy residual tumor cells after surgery.

Laser therapy. This new method for local tumor destruction uses laser energy directed through a bronchoscope. Still largely experimental, it may help treat tumors that can be directly visualized.

NURSING MANAGEMENT
Patients with lung cancer face an uncertain future, one that will more than likely be filled with physical difficulties, extensive medical treatment, and emotional changes. Your nursing assessment plays a critical role in developing the nursing care plan that will provide patient support.

Compile a nursing history
Begin by exploring the patient's chief complaint. In most instances the patient will complain of the following problems:

Productive or nonproductive cough. Find out when the cough occurs. For instance, is it more common in the morning? After exercise? Not related to activity? Present all the time? Is the cough dry and hacking or congested? When did it first start? Has it gotten progressively worse? If the cough is productive, how much sputum is usually produced? Is it bloody? Does it have a foul odor?

Dyspnea. If the patient complains of dyspnea, find out when it started, if it's gotten worse, and what types of activities, if any, precipitate it. Is the dyspnea associated with any other symptoms, such as diaphoresis?

Pain. The pain varies with the type of tumor and the extent of the disease, so try to determine the type and exact location of pain. Is it dull or sharp? Diffuse or localized?

Signs of metastasis. Other symptoms (see *Lung cancer growth patterns*, page 156) are related to tumor extension and metastasis, so investigate them thoroughly.

Diagnostic tests for lung cancer

Test	Purpose
Chest X-ray	Locate tumor, pneumonia, or pleural effusion (not diagnostic)
Sputum analysis	Search for cancer cells to diagnose lung, head/neck cancer
Bronchoscopy	Locate central tumor and biopsy for tissue, brush and wash suspect area for peripheral tumor, diagnose cell type
Computerized tomography (CT scan)	Locate tumor, determine extent of disease (not diagnostic), plan surgical strategy, determine radiation port
Radionuclide scans	Determine extent of brain, liver, or bone metastasis and adrenal gland involvement after confirmed diagnosis
Mediastinoscopy	Diagnose metastasis from right lung or left lower lobe tumor, determine operability
Mediastinotomy	Diagnose metastasis from left upper lobe or left hilar tumor, determine operability
Thoracentesis	Diagnose pleural effusion, determine operability
Needle biopsy of pleura	Diagnose tumor involvement of pleura
Needle biopsy of tumor	Diagnose tumor in selected cases
Thoracotomy	Diagnose tumor when other methods fail or in selected patients with peripheral nodules

Other important points. Keep in mind that the primary factors that put people at high risk for developing lung cancer are a history of smoking cigarettes, exposure to occupational respiratory carcinogens, and a family history of the disease. Ask the patient about all three possibilities. Also, try to determine the patient's socioeconomic situation, since this will have an impact on the availability of services to maintain him at home as long as possible.

Perform a physical assessment
After completing a history, begin your physical assessment (see *Assessment findings in lung cancer,* pages 165 through 167). First, give the patient an overall inspection. What is his general respiratory status? Does he look dyspneic or anxious? What's his mental status?

Staging lung cancer

T refers to the primary tumor, N to nodal involvement, and M to metastasis. Numerical subscripts refer to different categories, lower numbers offering better prognosis.

T_1 A tumor 1¼" (3 cm) or less in diameter, confined to one lobe, and surrounded by normal tissue.

T_2 A tumor over 1¼" (3 cm) in diameter and at least ¾" (2 cm) from the carina. Any atelectasis or obstructive pneumonitis involves less than the whole lung.

T_3 A tumor of any size that extends into neighboring structures, such as the chest wall or mediastinum, or that's less than ¾" (2 cm) from the carina.

N_0 No lymph node involvement

N_1 Ipsilateral hilar lymph node involvement

N_2 Mediastinal lymph node involvement

M_0 No metastasis

M_1 Distant metastasis

Stage I
(potentially operable)

T_1 N_0 M_0

T_1 N_1 M_0

T_2 N_0 M_0

Stage II
(potentially operable)

T_2 N_1 M_0

Stage III
(inoperable)

T_3 with any N or M

N_2 with any T or M

M_1 with any T or N

Inoperable disease is divided into two prognostic categories. *Limited disease* includes disease limited to one hemithorax, mediastinum, and ipsilateral supraclavicular area. *Extensive disease* includes all other extensions and metastases.

Can he communicate and understand? Is he oriented to time and place?

Next, inspect the skin for central or peripheral cyanosis, ecchymosis, petechiae, and hyperpigmentation. Also be alert for digital clubbing from chronic hypoxia, neck vein distention from right ventricular failure or superior vena caval obstruction, and fecal breath odor from tumor necrosis.

Palpate over bony areas and ask if this causes any pain. Look for decreased diaphragmatic excursion, indicating phrenic nerve involvement, and decreased or absent tactile fremitus, which will occur over areas of tumors or lung compression.

Perform percussion and auscultation. When you percuss, listen for any dull sound that will indicate an area of tumor growth. When you auscultate, listen for decreased or absent breath sounds, indicating areas of consolidation, tumor growth, atelectasis, or pleural effusion. Also listen for rales, a sign of fluid in the alveoli or reexpansion of collapsed alveoli.

Plan your nursing care

Once you've completed your assessment, you can begin to determine goals and a nursing care plan that best meets the patient's needs. In setting up your nursing care plan, you will need to consider both the nursing responsibilities important for collaboration with the doctor in providing medical and surgical treatment and the nursing diagnoses necessary to identify and resolve the patient's adverse responses to his disease or treatment.

An important nursing aspect of the medical treatment of the patient with lung cancer is the need to observe for signs that may indicate tumor extension or metastasis. You'll be alert for evidence of complications, such as airway obstruction by tumor, superior vena cava syndrome, cardiac tamponade, infection in necrotic lung tissue, laryngeal nerve involvement, phrenic nerve paralysis, Horner's syndrome, esophageal compression, esophageal invasion resulting in bronchoesophageal fistula, aspiration pneumonia resulting from bronchoesophageal fistula, brain metastasis, carcinomatous meningitis, spinal cord compression, and paraneoplastic syndromes.

Your nursing interventions for these complications will include identifying their signs, reporting them to the doctor, and collaborating with the doctor on medical treatment. Such collaboration may involve assisting with diagnostic studies and administering any or-

dered treatments.

You'll continually be assessing the patient to identify problems. Your nursing diagnoses and the interventions you implement can have a significant impact on the quality of the patient's life. Nursing diagnoses often used in lung cancer include the following:

Anxiety related to fear of death, pain, inability to breathe, or impact of the disease on the patient's family or life-style. Your goals include encouraging the patient to express the reasons for his anxiety, helping him understand and learn to cope with conditions he can't change, and getting him to help himself and accept the help of others in improving conditions within his control.

To relieve the patient's anxiety, contact members of the health-care team who can best resolve the causes of his anxiety. Help him understand the nature of his disease and the planned treatment, side effects, and expectations of treatment. Aid the patient by being approachable, becoming involved in his most integral concerns, remaining with him during periods of acute anxiety, and assuring him of continued support by other members of the nursing team. Work with the doctor in creating the best plan for relieving physical and mental symptoms that nurture anxiety. Then, continue to intervene in your patient's behalf if the plan needs modification. Also, teach the patient relaxation exercises.

You'll know you're succeeding when your patient appears relaxed, more readily expresses his concerns or physical discomfort, shows signs of trusting the health-care team, and is able to explain his illness and details of treatment; when any pain is relieved by medication or treatment; and when the patient is making realistic short- and long-term plans.

Partial or complete obstruction of large or small segments of the bronchial tree related to tumor growth, excess secretion production, or both. Your goal is to attempt to maintain oxygen to all body cells by helping the patient gain maximum benefit from respirations, decreasing the amount of secretions blocking the airways, and/or promoting tumor shrinkage by implementing the treatment plan.

To meet these goals, provide oxygen as ordered and elevate the head of the bed for maximum thoracic excursion. Instruct the patient in breathing and coughing exercises, initiate pulmonary physical therapy or postural drainage, and suction the patient as ordered. Also administer and monitor antibiotic and antineoplastic drugs as ordered.

Assessment findings in lung cancer

Type of tumor, involved structures	History findings	Physical findings
Within the pulmonary parenchyma		
Central tumors		
Airway obstruction	Dyspnea; cough; fever, chills, malaise, anorexia (if pneumonia results)	Dullness on percussion; decreased to absent breath sounds, tactile and vocal fremitus; wheezing
Nerve involvement (peribronchial, perivascular)	Dull, diffuse pain in chest, shoulders, or back	None
Tumor friability	Hemoptysis	None
Tumor necrosis (secondary infection)	Foul-smelling sputum	Fecal breath odor
Peripheral tumors		
Tumor in distal bronchi and/or alveoli	Cough (sometimes productive)	None from bronchial tumor; rales with alveolar extension
Apical tumors	Usually asymptomatic	Dullness on percussion, possible increased tactile and vocal fremitus
Extension beyond pulmonary parenchyma		
Central		
Pericardial tumor involvement	Dyspnea	Tachycardia, neck vein distention, decreased blood pressure, increased cardiac diameter, distant heart sounds, pulsus paradoxus
Peripheral		
Pleural and/or chest wall involvement	Pleuritic pain—sharp, localized, increased upon inspiration; dyspnea	Signs of pleural effusion—dullness on percussion, usually at lung base; breath sounds, tactile and vocal fremitus decreased below effusion, increased above
Apical (Pancoast's)		
Nerve involvement (C-8, T-1)	Shoulder and arm pain in area of ulnar nerve innervation	Usually none
Sympathetic nerve ganglia involvement	Droopy eyelid, decreased sweating on involved side	Horner's syndrome—enophthalmos (sinking eyeball), ptosis of upper eyelid, constriction of pupil, narrowed palpebral fissure, anhidrosis
Rib/vertebra erosion	Bone pain	Local pain on palpation
Hilar lymph node involvement	Usually asymptomatic	None
Mediastinal lymph node		
Recurrent laryngeal nerve involvement	Hoarseness with vocal cord paralysis, dysphagia	Paralyzed vocal cord on laryngoscopy
Phrenic nerve involvement	Shortness of breath	Decreased diaphragmatic excursion
Superior vena cava involvement	Swelling of face, neck, arms	Superior vena cava syndrome—venous stasis (secondary thrombus formation); distension of arm and neck veins; suffusion and/or edema of the face, neck, and arms; dilated tortuous collateral vessels (chest and back); elevated venous pressure in arms
Esophageal invasion	Dysphagia, fever, chills	Bronchoesophageal fistula, probably leading to aspiration pneumonia

(continued)

Assessment findings in lung cancer (continued)

Type of tumor, involved structures	History findings	Physical findings
Esophageal compression	Dysphagia	None
Mediastinal lymphatic obstruction	Dyspnea	Signs of pleural effusion—dullness on percussion, usually at lung base; breath sounds, tactile and vocal fremitus decreased below effusion, increased above

Specific metastatic sites

Central nervous system

Brain	Headache, nausea, vomiting, malaise, weakness, anorexia, alteration in mentation	Altered mental status, focal neurologic findings (including blindness, hemiparesis, aphasia), increased intracranial pressure
Meninges (carcinomatous meningitis)	Headache, nausea, vomiting, malaise, weakness, anorexia, alteration in mentation	Cranial nerve palsies, stiff neck, positive Kernig's and Brudzinski's signs
Spinal cord (vertebral involvement with collapse, extradural cord compression, spinal vascular occlusion)	Localized or radicular back pain; neurologic deficits—weakness, motor impairment, loss of sensation, incontinence, paralysis	Pain over affected vertebra, weakness and decreased sensation below compression

Bones

Destruction of weight-bearing bones	Bone pain, pathologic fractures	Local pain on palpation

Paraneoplastic syndromes

Skin

Acanthosis nigricans (adenocarcinoma)	Symmetric epidermoid thickening (hyperkeratosis, acanthosis); hyperpigmentation of axilla, flexural surfaces, palms, soles, oral membranes (not always linked with malignancy)	Thickening and blackish hyperpigmentation in skin folds, especially the axilla
Dermatomyositis	Muscle weakness, especially pelvic girdle; facial skin rash (erythematous butterfly distribution)	Weakness of pelvic and shoulder girdle muscles, facial skin rash in a butterfly distribution, violet coloration around eyes
Tylosis (squamous-cell)	Hyperkeratosis of palms and soles	Increased callus formation on palms and soles

Bones

Hypertrophic pulmonary osteoarthropathy (HPO)	Pain, swelling, tenderness over affected bones	Clubbing of fingers and toes, tenderness over distal portion of affected bones

Coagulation disorders

Hemorrhagic (common)

Disseminated intravascular coagulation (DIC)	Ecchymosis, hematoma	Ecchymoses, petechiae

Thrombotic (uncommon)

Nonbacterial thrombotic endocarditis (NBTE)	Emboli to brain: focal neurologic deficits, confusion, disorientation, seizures. Systemic emboli: usually to kidneys, spleen, or heart, with resulting disturbance in function	Altered mental status, increased intracranial pressure Signs of peripheral emboli (petechiae below nail beds, conjunctival hemorrhages)
Migratory venous thrombosis	Pain, swelling, tenderness over affected veins	Pain, swelling, tenderness over affected veins

Neuromuscular disorders

Cerebral encephalopathy	Dementia (varying degrees), psychosis	Altered mental status

(continued)

Assessment findings in lung cancer (continued)

Type of tumor, involved structures	History findings	Physical findings
Cerebellar degeneration	Bilateral weakness of arms or legs, intention tremors, dysarthria, vertigo	Nystagmus (seldom); difficulty in walking, standing, speaking, inability to coordinate movements
Peripheral nerve involvement	Pain, paresthesia, decreased deep tendon reflexes, sensory loss, ataxia, muscle weakness, wasting	Decreased deep tendon reflexes; decreased touch, vibration, and joint position sense; weakness
Myositis Degenerated muscle fibers (all cell types)	Proximal muscle weakness (thighs, pelvic girdle)	Tenderness and weakness of affected muscles
Myasthenia-like (Eaton-Lambert's syndrome) Defective neuromuscular transmission (small-cell)	Proximal muscle weakness (shoulder and pelvic girdle), paradoxic increase in muscle action potential after a few seconds of exercise	Weakness of affected muscles improves with repetitive contraction

Ectopic hormone production by cancer cells

Parathormone or parathormone-like	Alterations in mental status, constipation, urinary frequency	Altered mental status, decreased bowel sounds
Inappropriate antidiuretic hormone	Alterations in mental status	Hyponatremia-produced altered mental status
Gonadotropic hormone	Enlarged breasts	Unilateral or bilateral gynecomastia
Vasoactive peptide or serotonin	Facial flushing	Facial flushing, cardiac murmurs of aortic and/or mitral stenosis
Adrenocorticotropic hormone (ACTH)	Central obesity, round face, abdominal striae	Signs of Cushing's syndrome (central obesity, buffalo hump, loss of subcutaneous tissue, purple striae)
Adrenocorticotropic/melanocyte stimulating hormone (ACTH/MSH)	Hyperpigmentation of exposed areas of body, lips, nipples, mucous membranes, skin creases, recent scars	Hyperpigmentation of skin folds and mucous membranes

Points to remember

• Lung cancer is the leading cause of cancer death in American men and is rapidly assuming similar status in women.
• Cigarette smoking is lung cancer's chief cause.
• Doubling time, the time a tumor takes to double in size, determines the elapsed time before lung cancer becomes clinically apparent.
• Chest X-ray is the most important detection method, and surgical resection the preferred treatment.
• Prognosis is poor because the disease usually escapes detection until an advanced stage.
• Early nursing recognition of potentially avoidable mental, emotional, and physical complications can significantly improve the quality of life remaining to the patient.

Teach the patient to reduce exertion, and make any necessary arrangements for a wheelchair or walking aids.

You'll know you've succeeded when the patient's skin, nail beds, and mucous membranes regain their normal color; when he appears to be breathing comfortably and reports no problems with breathing; when his arterial blood gases show improved to normal oxygen, carbon dioxide, and pH values; and when tests show evidence of tumor shrinkage.

Alteration in comfort: Pain resulting from tumor involvement of the lung parenchyma, lung pleura, or bones. Your goals include relieving the pain and resulting dyspnea, preventing or treating pathologic fracture, and promoting tumor shrinkage.

To meet these goals, assess the type, amount, and location of pain; administer analgesic drugs as ordered; monitor the patient's response; and intervene with the doctor on the patient's behalf as needed. To prevent pathologic fracture in patients with long-bone involvement, support the long bones, take care in turning the patient, and make sure the patient avoids bearing weight until ortho-pedic procedures are completed to strengthen the involved area. Also, administer and monitor antineoplastic drugs as ordered.

You'll know you've succeeded when the patient reports pain relief, orthopedic procedures allow him to bear weight, and scans and X-rays indicate tumor shrinkage.

Your support can make the difference

As the person who sees the patient daily and intervenes with other health-care professionals on his behalf, you can have tremendous influence in improving the quality of medical and nursing care he receives. Through all the stages of this intractable disease—from initial treatment response to relapse, further treatment, and, finally, relapse into terminal stages—you can ensure the ever-increasing supportive care the patient needs so desperately. Through your daily involvement and your sensitivity, you can recognize the patient's subtle mental, emotional, and physical changes and react promptly to their implications. Thus, you can prevent potentially avoidable complications and may add comfortable, productive time to the patient's life.

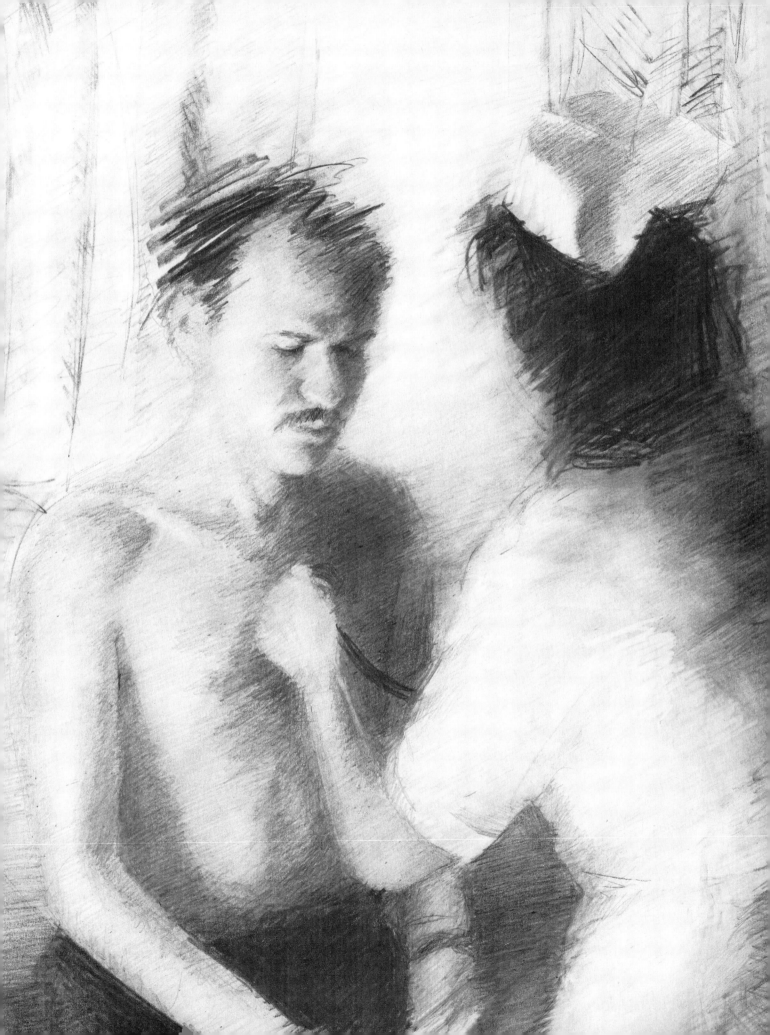

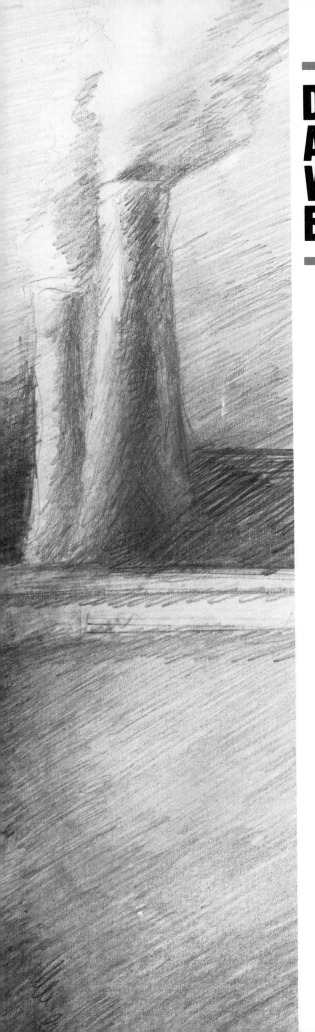

DISORDERS ASSOCIATED WITH THE ENVIRONMENT

12 CONTROLLING ENVIRONMENTAL DISEASE

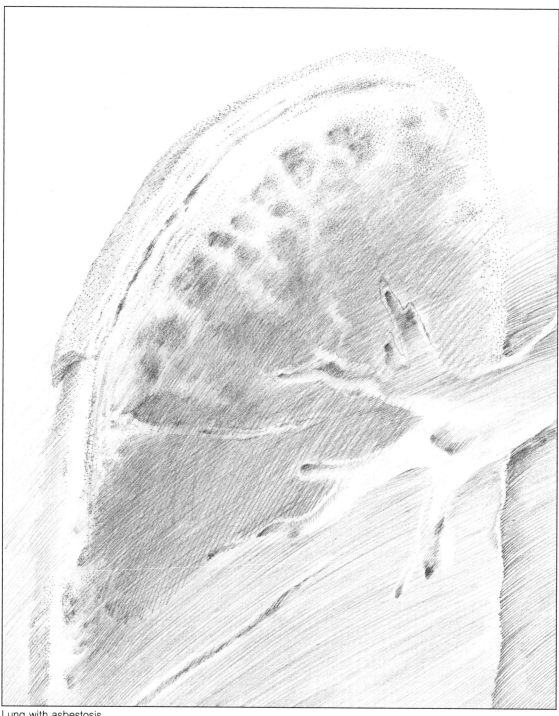

Lung with asbestosis

Occupational and environmental respiratory diseases have emerged recently as one of the most alarming of modern health problems. Traditionally, people have thought of their jobs and their homes in terms of security. Today, we know only too well that the kind of work a person does and where he lives can, in time, make him seriously ill and may even kill him.

Statistics tell only a part of the story: The U.S. Department of Labor estimates that 65,000 people develop occupational respiratory diseases each year, while another 25,000 people die from such diseases. Comparable statistics for the incidence of environmental respiratory diseases aren't available. But the hundreds of millions of dollars being spent to control industrial air pollution alone reflect widespread concern over environmental health hazards.

Both occupational and environmental respiratory diseases stem from some form of air pollution. Occupational respiratory diseases typically result from inhaling polluted air on the job. Three types of occupational respiratory diseases occur: *pneumoconiosis, hypersensitivity disease,* and *toxic lung injury.* Pneumoconiosis results from inhalation of inorganic dust, such as that produced during the manufacturing of asbestos materials or the mining of coal. Hypersensitivity disease results from inhalation of organic dust—for example, the dust found in farm crops or bird feathers. (See *Pneumoconioses* and *Hypersensitivity diseases,* pages 172 and 173.) Toxic lung injury results from inhalation of noxious chemicals contained in smoke and gases.

Environmental respiratory diseases usually result from inhaling polluted air in or around the home. This group of diseases can be classified according to its two most common causes—prevailing weather patterns and local industry. Respiratory disease resulting from prolonged inhalation of smog is an example of the first type; the second type can result from living near a factory that pollutes the air or disposes of its poisonous waste material improperly.

The distinction between occupational and environmental respiratory diseases can become blurred. For example, hypersensitivity disease can result from raising pigeons as a hobby. A fire at a chemical plant can cause toxic lung injury in nearby residents.

For health-care workers, the most important consideration is to identify patients at risk of developing these potentially life-threatening respiratory diseases—whatever their cause. That's where you come in. Nurses are in an ideal position to identify high-risk patients before the disease pursues its usual irreversible course. Mastering this skill will help you to prevent occupational and environmental respiratory diseases—the most effective form of treatment.

PATHOPHYSIOLOGY
To understand the pathophysiology of occupational and environmental respiratory diseases, you first have to be familiar with the lungs' *normal defense mechanisms* that protect the body from invasion. You also need to know the *predisposing factors* that make some people more likely to develop these diseases, as well as the characteristic *signs and symptoms* to look for in such patients.

Normal defense mechanisms
The lungs have three defense mechanisms to ward off invasion by harmful particles in polluted air. These mechanisms can be classified according to their functions: mechanical barriers, physical transport, and local detoxification.

Mechanical barriers. The anatomic structure of the respiratory system, with its progressively narrowing airways, prevents most harmful particles from reaching the lungs. Turbulent airflow through the larger upper airways brings most particles into contact with the mucosa, where they become trapped. Nasopharyngeal humidification of inhaled air also helps to trap particles. However, if a particle breaches this first line of defense and enters the trachea, it often triggers coughing, sneezing, or nose blowing and is forcefully expelled.

Physical transport. This second defense mechanism involves the so-called mucociliary escalator and possibly surfactant. The lining of the nose, trachea, bronchi, and large bronchioles consists of pseudostratified ciliated columnar epithelium. These epithelial cells are coated with a thin layer of watery mucus produced by goblet cells and serous glands. Very fine particles that pass through the hairs inside the nostrils may become trapped by this mucous layer and swept by ciliary action toward the pharynx to be swallowed or expectorated. Surfactant may assist in transporting particles toward the alveolar lumen, where they become exposed to the third defense mechanism.

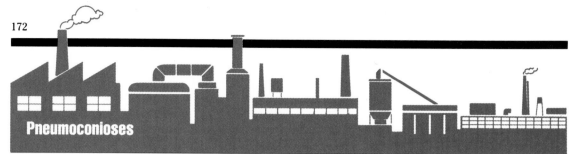

Pneumoconioses

Disease	Causative pollutant	High-risk occupations
Antimony pneumoconiosis	Antimony	• Mining and crushing antimony ore • Cleaning extraction chambers • Fumes from alloy production
Baritosis	Barium	• Mining crude barium ore • Drying and bagging ground ore
Carbon pneumoconioses	Carbon, carbon black	• Handling carbon black (used as a filler and coloring agent in rubber, plastics, printing inks, paints, or enamels) • Manufacturing carbon electrodes and carbon paper
	Graphite	• Mining and handling graphite • Manufacturing refractory ceramics and crucibles, pencils, lubricants, electrodes, and neutron moderators in atomic reactors
Anthracosilicosis	Coal	• Mining and handling coal
Siderosis	Iron	• Iron and steel rolling, steel grinding • Electric arc and steel welding • Silver and steel polishing with iron oxide • Scouring, chipping, and dressing castings in iron foundries • Boiler scaling (cleaning fireboxes) • Mining and crushing iron ores • Mining, milling, and mixing emery
Stannosis	Tin	• Milling, grinding, and handling tin ore • Tipping ore into and raking out refinery furnaces
Asbestosis	Asbestos	• Mining asbestos • Manufacturing asbestos-cement products (tiles and roofing) • Manufacturing and installing of insulating and fireproofing materials • Maintaining equipment in asbestos-processing factories
Diatomite silicosis	Diatomite	• Mining and processing of diatomite • Manufacturing of filters for inorganic and organic liquids • Manufacturing of bricks and cement used for heat and sound insulation • Handling diatomite (used as a filler for plastics, rubber, insecticides, paints, varnishes, floor coverings, or fertilizers)
Fuller's earth lung	Fuller's earth (type of clay)	• Mining and processing of fuller's earth • Clarifying of mineral, animal, or vegetable oils • Manufacturing herbicides, insecticides, paints, and cosmetics • Refining of mineral oils
Kaolin pneumoconiosis	Kaolin (china clay)	• Processing kaolin • Manufacturing paper, rubber, or plastics
Silicosis	Free silica	• Mining gold, tin, copper, platinum, and mica • Quarrying granite, slate, and pumice • Tunneling for sewers and roads; excavating sandstone • Stonecutting and polishing, cleaning, and carving of masonry • Manufacturing abrasives using crushed sand, sandstone, or quartzite; abrasive blasting • Manufacturing glass, enameling • Processing products that use rock-containing quartz • Working in iron and steel foundries • Manufacturing china, porcelain, stoneware, and earthenware • Building and dismantling kilns, steel furnaces, ovens in gas-making plants, and boiler houses • Cleaning and scaling boiler flues and fireboxes
Talc pneumoconiosis	Talc	• Mining and processing talc • Manufacturing cosmetic powders or paints

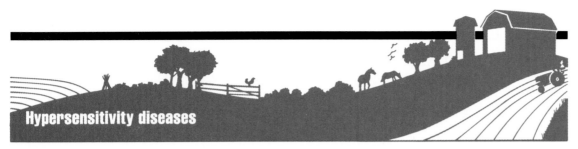

Disease	Pathogen	Environmental source
Bagassosis	*Thermoactinomyces sacharii*	Moldy sugarcane
Bird fancier's disease	Avian dust or serum	Birds
Byssinosis (brown lung)	Flax, hemp, or cotton dust	Textiles
Cheese washer's disease	*Penicillium, Aspergillus clavatus*	Cheese mold
Chicken handler's disease	Feathers, serum	Chickens
Coffee worker's lung	Unknown	Coffee dust
Coptic disease	Mold	Mummies
Duck fever	Serum	Ducks
Farmer's lung	*Micropolyspora faeni, Thermoactinomyces vulgaris, candidus,* and *virdis*	Moldy hay
Furrier's lung	Unknown	Hair dust
Humidifier or forced-air-system lung	*Thermoactinomyces candidus* and *vulgaris*	Fungal spores
Malt worker's disease	*Aspergillus clavatus* and *fumigatus*	Malt and barley dusts
Maple bark stripper's disease	*Cryptostroma corticale*	Moldy maple bark
Mushroom worker's disease	*Micropolyspora faeni, Thermoactinomyces vulgaris*	Mushroom compost
New Guinea lung	*Streptomyces olivaceous*	Thatched roof dust
Paprika splitter's lung	*Mucor stolonifer*	Moldy pods
Pituitary snuff taker's disease	Bovine and porcine proteins	Pituitary powder
Rodent worker's lung	Dried rat serum	Laboratory rats
Sauna taker's disease	*Pullaria* species	Moldy water and bucket
Sequoiosis	*Graphium aureobasidium pullulans*	Moldy redwood sawdust
Turkey handler's disease	Serum	Turkeys
Wheat weevil disease	*Sitophilus granarius*	Wheat flour
Wood dust disease	Unknown	Mahogany and oak dust
Wood pulp worker's disease	*Alternaria tenuis*	Moldy logs

Pathologic responses to smoke inhalation

Initial responses
• Constriction of bronchioles
• Increased carboxyhemoglobin saturation
• Laryngeal edema
• Signs and symptoms: cough, cherry-red mucosa, stridor

Delayed responses
• Increased pulmonary capillary permeability
• Destruction of lung parenchyma
• Signs and symptoms: dyspnea and rales, increased sputum production, hyperinflation of lungs, rhonchi

Local detoxification. Macrophages in the alveoli and the interstitium carry the primary responsibility for this last line of defense. These highly specialized, mobile cells can isolate and ingest a particle through phagocytosis. Macrophages can also detoxify certain particles and possibly transport others to the mucociliary escalator or lymphatic fluid for removal.

Pathologic responses
When the lungs' normal defense mechanisms become overwhelmed by the sheer number of invading particles or wear out from prolonged activity, pathologic responses develop. The nature of these responses depends on the chemical composition of the invading particles.

With inorganic dust particles, the initial pathologic response is usually *fibrosis,* which restricts lung movement and impairs ventilation. Fibrosis can occur after inorganic particles have been ingested by the interstitial macrophages. The macrophages then release various enzymes, which damage the alveolar walls and stimulate the deposition of fibrous tissue.

Organic dust particles typically produce an *antibody response,* which may be immediate or delayed, depending on where the particles lodge. Larger particles that lodge in the bronchi and bronchioles produce an immediate antibody response. This may lead to the condition known as occupational asthma. The characteristics of occupational asthma are: smooth muscle contractions, which cause bronchospasms; mucosal edema, which decreases the bronchial lumen and reduces airflow to the lungs; and stimulation of goblet cells, which increases mucus production.

A delayed antibody response occurs when smaller organic dust particles lodge in the alveoli, producing allergic alveolitis (or hypersensitivity pneumonitis). Allergic alveolitis is characterized by localized inflammation of the alveoli, with increased white blood cell (WBC) production and possible fluid accumulation within the alveoli. Long-term exposure to the harmful particles may cause chronic inflammation of the alveoli and surrounding tissue, eventually leading to fibrosis.

Fibrosis and antibody responses typify the pathologic responses that occur in pneumoconiosis and hypersensitivity disease as well as in environmental respiratory diseases caused by inorganic or organic dusts. However, in toxic lung injury the pathologic response depends on whether the noxious chemicals are inhaled in the form of smoke or gas (see *Pathologic responses to smoke inhalation* and *Pathologic responses to gas inhalation,* pages 174 and 175).

Effects of accompanying respiratory disorders
Chronic obstructive pulmonary disease (COPD) isn't usually considered an occupational or environmental respiratory disease. Nevertheless, its characteristic pathology—alveolar wall destruction, mucous gland hypertrophy, and ciliated epithelium damage—represents a generalized lung response to chronic irritation. The incidence of the disease is higher among workers exposed to air pollutants and among residents of industrialized areas.

Lung cancer also occurs more often among those two population groups. But many of these workers and residents smoke cigarettes, which contain known carcinogens. Fewer carcinogens have been identified in environmental and industrial air pollution. Therefore, the causative link between lung cancer and air pollution is weak, since it's not known whether the incidence of lung cancer would be as high in the absence of cigarette smoking.

Predisposing factors
In occupational and environmental respiratory diseases, the health of a person's lungs at the time of exposure is of paramount importance. Even normal lungs vary in the amount of mucus produced, the efficiency of the mucociliary escalator, and the extent of macrophagic activity. Predisposing factors in the development of occupational and environmental respiratory diseases, therefore, include the presence of preexisting lung disease, a history of cigarette smoking, the duration and concentration of exposure, and particle size.

Preexisting lung disease. Any preexisting disease that decreases airflow, disrupts cellular functions, or destroys lung tissue will have already compromised the lungs' normal defense mechanisms, increasing the risk of occupational and environmental respiratory diseases. One notable exception to this rule is preexisting pulmonary edema. The excess fluid produced in pulmonary edema may actually help minimize retention of harmful particles before they make contact with the alveolar wall.

Cigarette smoking. Like preexisting lung disease, cigarette smoking compromises the

Pathologic responses to gas inhalation

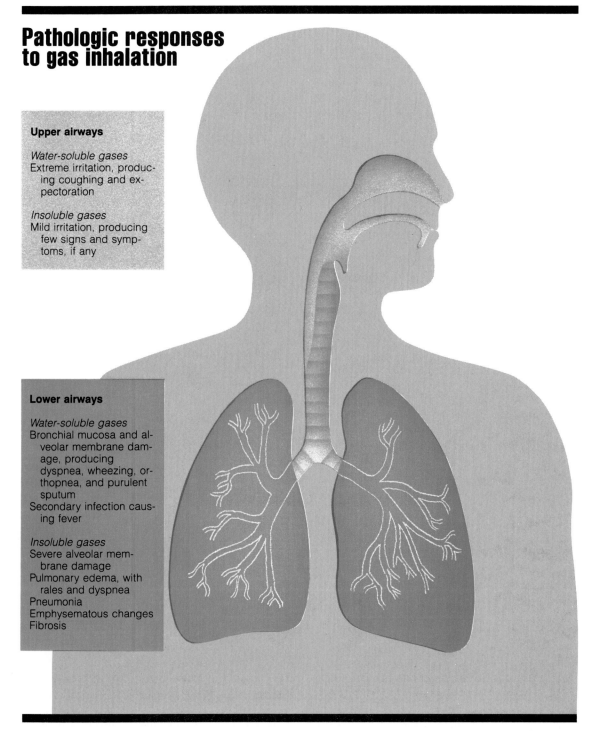

Upper airways

Water-soluble gases
Extreme irritation, producing coughing and expectoration

Insoluble gases
Mild irritation, producing few signs and symptoms, if any

Lower airways

Water-soluble gases
Bronchial mucosa and alveolar membrane damage, producing dyspnea, wheezing, orthopnea, and purulent sputum
Secondary infection causing fever

Insoluble gases
Severe alveolar membrane damage
Pulmonary edema, with rales and dyspnea
Pneumonia
Emphysematous changes
Fibrosis

Solubility factor

Solubility often determines how much of a gas is inhaled, thereby influencing the pathologic response. Water-soluble gases, such as ammonia and sulfur dioxide, cause extreme irritation of the upper airways. Typically, a person who inhales such a gas quickly flees the contaminated area, if he can, thereby minimizing lung damage. However, a person trapped in a contaminated area inhales a much greater volume of gas. As a result, the gas penetrates deeper into the respiratory system, usually causing acute respiratory dysfunction and possibly chronic disease.

Insoluble gases, such as nitrogen dioxide, cause only mild irritation of the upper airways. Consequently, a person is more likely to inhale a greater volume of such a gas—compared to a water-soluble gas—before fleeing. Lung damage at the alveolar level, therefore, is probably greater.

lungs' normal defense mechanisms. Besides known carcinogens, inhaled cigarette smoke contains many potent irritants that paralyze the mucociliary escalator, cause bronchoconstriction, and induce production of thick mucus. Such irritants also impair macrophagic activity.

Duration of exposure. With the exception of toxic lung injury, which can occur within minutes of exposure, occupational and environmental respiratory diseases typically require considerable time to develop. Black lung disease, for example, develops only after years of exposure to the toxic agent.

High-concentration exposure. The concentration of the inspired pollutant is as important as the duration of exposure. Inhaling excessively high concentrations of a pollutant may quickly overwhelm the lungs' defense mechanisms. On the other hand, decades of exposure to low concentrations may be insufficient to cause disease.

Particle size. The size of the harmful particles determines where they lodge in the lungs. This, in turn, affects the extent of the damage they cause. Usually, particles from 3 to 5 microns in diameter (such as bacteria, fly ash, and metallurgic dusts) are retained in the alveoli and cause the most damage. Many of these same particles, however, may be only 1 to 3 microns in diameter. In this case they'll usually reach the alveoli, but they won't adhere to the alveolar walls because they're so small. Particles less than 1 micron in diameter—aerosols, fumes, smoke, and viruses, for example—most often penetrate the alveolar walls and enter the interstitium. An exception to this last group of particles is filamentous particles (such as asbestos and talc), which don't penetrate the alveolar wall. Instead, they usually remain lodged in the alveolar wall, causing chronic inflammation that may extend to the adjacent alveolar ducts and bronchioles.

Signs and symptoms

Most pollutants capable of causing occupational and environmental respiratory diseases don't immediately produce a dramatic and unmistakable set of signs and symptoms. This fact, coupled with widespread ignorance of the many possible causes of air pollution, makes early diagnosis extremely difficult.

In the early stage of these diseases, patients usually complain of a chronic cough, but rarely do they suspect a specific occupational or environmental pollutant as the cause. Progressive dyspnea on exertion and increased susceptibility to respiratory infections are also common early signs. In some patients, wheezing may occur only in the presence of a cold; in other patients, only in the presence of the causative pollutant.

Because these early signs and symptoms tend to be nonspecific and fairly tolerable, many patients avoid seeking help until the advanced stage of the disease. By then, the signs and symptoms may indeed be quite dramatic, reflecting irreversible lung damage. The chronic cough may have become spasmodic, with copious sputum or mucus production. Dyspnea may now be limiting, at best, in terms of the patient's life-style; at worst, it may be disabling. Persistent hypoxemia and hypercapnia may produce cyanosis, headaches, insomnia or somnolence, and personality changes. The patient may also complain of weight loss. In very late stages of these diseases, you may detect signs and symptoms of right-sided heart failure, such as peripheral edema, jugular vein distention, and weight gain.

MEDICAL MANAGEMENT

A suspected occupational or environmental respiratory disease requires thorough diagnostic testing. If test results confirm disease, treatment begins at once with an attempt to end the patient's exposure to the causative agent. When this isn't possible, other forms of treatment—less assured of success than termination of exposure—may be pursued.

Radiologic findings in pulmonary disease

Characteristic patterns on the chest X-ray help detect pulmonary diseases. The three X-rays at right show linear, nodular, and reticular patterns.

Linear pattern

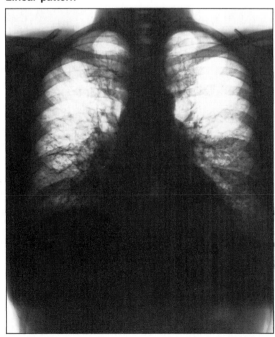

Nodular pattern

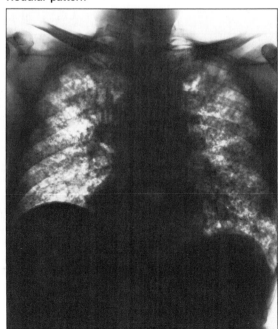

Diagnostic tests

In suspected occupational or environmental respiratory disease, diagnostic tests may reveal the functional status of the patient's lungs, provide objective evidence of various causes for respiratory signs and symptoms, and identify the causative pollutant. A typical diagnostic workup includes:

Chest X-rays. Routine posteroanterior and lateral chest X-rays may show anatomic changes in the lungs, such as nodules, fibrosis, and calcifications resulting from deposits of dust particles. Pneumoconiosis and hypersensitivity disease usually produce one of three distinctive radiographic patterns—nodular, reticular, and linear (see *Radiologic findings in pulmonary disease,* page 176). Hyperinflation of the lung fields may be seen in advanced stages of COPD. While a chest X-ray is the first and most important diagnostic test for a suspected occupational or environmental respiratory disease, negative findings don't necessarily exclude such a disease; neither do positive findings confirm it.

Lung scan. In this test, a radioactive substance is introduced into the pulmonary circulation and the airways. A gamma camera then takes pictures of the lungs at various angles, showing the distribution of the radioactive substance. Failure to detect the substance on the lung scan indicates a ventilation or perfusion defect. Ventilation defects may occur with fibrosis, emphysema, and chronic bronchitis; perfusion defects, with COPD. Lung

Reticular pattern

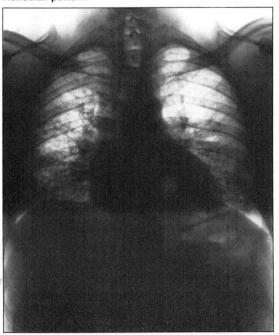

scanning can confirm clinical findings, evaluate the degree of functional impairment, and detect early changes in the lungs. The results, however, aren't specifically diagnostic for occupational and environmental respiratory diseases.

Sputum analysis. Under the microscope, sputum smears that have been properly stained may show a causative pollutant, such as *Aspergillus clavatus* or an asbestos fiber. The growth of fungi in characteristic patterns can also be evaluated microscopically to substantiate clinical findings.

Complete blood count with differential. The results of this test may show infection, inflammation, or allergic reactions in the body. An elevated WBC count indicates infection or inflammation; eosinophilia is associated with allergic reactions.

Pulmonary function tests. Functional impairment may be *restrictive* (interfering with lung expansion) or *obstructive* (interfering with airflow). Both types of impairment may result from occupational and environmental respiratory diseases. They produce different pulmonary function test results (see *Pulmonary function test results,* page 178).

Arterial blood gas analysis. As mentioned earlier, hypoxemia usually occurs in the late stages of an occupational or environmental respiratory disease. Usually, the lower the PaO_2 level, the more advanced the disease. Oxygen saturation percentage, which measures the degree to which the body's oxygen needs are being met, reflects pulmonary function even more accurately than the PaO_2 level. The percentage usually doesn't fall until PaO_2 decreases markedly, making it another common late-stage finding.

The $PaCO_2$ level reflects alveolar ventilation. Most patients with an occupational or environmental respiratory disease initially have a decreased $PaCO_2$ and an alkalotic pH level (above 7.45). These findings occur because the body initially compensates for impaired alveolar ventilation by increasing the respiratory rate and minute volume. Once the disease progresses and compensating mechanisms fail, $PaCO_2$ rises.

Skin testing and inhalation challenge. These tests may be indicated for patients with suspected hypersensitivity disease. A positive reaction to a test antigen administered by intradermal injection is demonstrated by erythema, tenderness, and induration at the site 4 to 6 hours after the test. Such a reaction, however, doesn't confirm the presence of the

Pulmonary function test results

Restrictive impairment
• Decreased total lung capacity, inspiratory capacity, and vital capacity
• Decreased or normal functional residual capacity, inspiratory reserve volume, expiratory reserve, residual volume, and tidal volume
• Normal flow rates
• Decreased lung compliance

Obstructive impairment
• Decreased expiratory flow rates (including forced expiratory volume in 1 second, maximal breathing capacity, forced expiratory flow rate, and maximal midexpiratory flow rate)
• Increased residual volume, functional residual capacity, and residual volume/total lung capacity ratio

disease. It may simply indicate previous exposure to the antigen. An inhalation challenge is more definitive. A positive reaction to inhalation of the suspected causative antigen will reproduce the respiratory signs and symptoms that occur during on-the-job exposure, including changes in the results of pulmonary function tests.

Treatment: Two major goals

Treatment for occupational and environmental respiratory diseases aims to prevent further lung damage and to relieve the patient's signs and symptoms. The best way to achieve the first goal is to end the patient's exposure to the causative pollutant. Unfortunately, this is often impossible. In many cases, the causative pollutant can't be identified; in other cases, the causative pollutant may be identified, but for personal or economic reasons the patient can't change jobs or move to a healthier environment. As a result, treatment usually must focus on achieving the second goal through one or more of the following measures.

Corticosteroids. Administering corticosteroids may slow the progression of an occupational or environmental respiratory disease. In fact, corticosteroid therapy has actually reversed some cases of pneumoconiosis and hypersensitivity disease. It may also benefit patients with toxic lung injury caused by gas inhalation. However, corticosteroid therapy is controversial in burn patients with toxic lung injury caused by smoke inhalation, because it promotes infection at burn sites.

Bronchodilators. These drugs help maintain airway patency by altering cellular levels of cyclic adenosine monophosphate, the cyclic nucleotide that relaxes bronchial smooth muscle. Bronchodilators may be administered intravenously, orally, or as an aerosol—alone or with other drugs. Intravenous theophylline, for example, may be administered alone or with a beta$_2$-adrenergic agonist (such as terbutaline sulfate) to achieve maximum relief. Aerosol preparations—administered by metered-dose, hand-held, or compressor-driven nebulizers or by positive pressure ventilation—can provide supplemental therapy. Oral bronchodilators may provide long-term relief.

Intermittent positive pressure ventilation (IPPB). Although its effectiveness has been questioned, this form of therapy may be used occasionally to deliver aerosolized bronchodilators. Its purpose is to help expand the airways and loosen secretions. IPPB treatments

also distend the tracheobronchial tree, reducing resistance to airflow and the work of breathing. In addition, they usually enhance the distribution of inspired oxygen and the flow of blood, which improves ventilation/perfusion ratios. These treatments are usually administered for 15 to 20 minutes several times a day.

Postural drainage. The simplest form of therapy for respiratory disease, postural drainage uses gravity to drain bronchial secretions toward the trachea. Percussion and vibration may help loosen secretions during the procedure. The patient can assume various positions for postural drainage several times a day, depending on the amount of secretions present. Recognize that postural drainage may be contraindicated in obese patients or those with severely compromised respiratory or cardiovascular status. Like IPPB, postural drainage is controversial, primarily because no evidence exists that it increases sputum production or improves ventilation.

Deep breathing and coughing. These traditional chest physiotherapy techniques may also help clear secretions from the airways. Deep breathing can be used during postural drainage; the patient breathes deeply with each change of position.

Oxygen therapy. The goal of oxygen therapy is to restore the patient's PaO$_2$ level to its baseline. However, if the baseline level is unknown, therapy aims to maintain oxygen saturation at 80% (normal is 94% to 100%). When administered for acute conditions, such as smoke inhalation or hypersensitivity reactions, oxygen therapy may be stopped once the condition is corrected. Patients with obstructive respiratory impairment, however, often need long-term low-flow oxygen therapy. Patients with diseases such as asbestosis or silicosis, where fibrosis and restrictive impairment progressively worsen, may also need long-term oxygen therapy, with the flow rate periodically increased. If the patient's resting PaO$_2$ level is more than 60 mm Hg but his oxygen saturation falls below 80% during exercise, oxygen therapy may be prescribed only during exercise.

NURSING MANAGEMENT

Nursing management of the patient with an occupational or environmental respiratory disease begins with a careful analysis of the *subjective data* gathered during history taking. The accuracy and completeness of such data

Classifying respiratory signs and symptoms

Classification	Dyspnea	Coughing	Sputum production
None	During strenuous exercise	Occasionally with colds	Only with colds
Slight or mild	While hurrying on a level surface or walking up a slight incline	Occasionally in morning	Occasionally in morning
Moderate	While walking for some time on a level surface	Four to six times daily	Twice daily, 4 or more days a week
Severe to very severe	After walking about 100 yards or a few minutes on a level surface. Very severe: breathlessness during routine activities	Throughout the day for at least 3 consecutive months	Throughout the day for at least 3 consecutive months

carry enormous significance with these patients. It usually raises the suspicion that the patient might have such a disease in the first place—a suspicion that may be strengthened by the *objective data* obtained during the physical examination. Working with these two types of data, you can then formulate *nursing diagnoses* that suggest realistic goals and effective interventions.

Subjective data

With suspected occupational or environmental respiratory diseases, the importance of a detailed patient history can't be overemphasized. The patient's occupational history should include a description of his current job, as well as any other jobs he has held, presented in chronologic order. Try to obtain exact dates of employment. They may be helpful in determining the risk of exposure to a harmful pollutant. Remember that because air quality regulations are constantly being revamped, occupations that were hazardous 10 years ago may be safe today. Or the opposite may be the case—the patient may work for a company that has recently relaxed its regulations, putting him at risk for exposure once again. Remember that small companies are less likely to have stringent environmental regulations than large companies.

Because job titles don't always reveal the actual nature of the work, make sure you find out exactly what the patient's job entails. Ask him to describe his workplace environment. What kinds of materials does he work with? Is he protected against harmful exposure? Does he wear a respirator, for example, or protective clothing? Are exhaust fans used? Do any of his co-workers have respiratory diseases that may be linked to the workplace? If so, do these diseases produce any signs and symptoms in common with the patient's?

For unemployed patients or white-collar workers, explore the possibility of an environmental cause for their respiratory complaints. Ask the patient about local industry. Are there any factories near the patient's house? If so, what do they manufacture or produce? Have these factories ever been charged with violating air pollution standards? Explore details of the patient's domestic life—hobbies, pets, cigarette smoking, hazardous dusts or fibers on the clothes of other family members, and so forth.

The onset and duration of the patient's signs and symptoms may also provide clues to a possible occupational or environmental cause. For example, signs and symptoms that occur mostly during the workweek obviously point to a possible occupational cause.

Establishing baseline levels of dyspnea, coughing, and sputum production (see *Classifying respiratory signs and symptoms*) helps you evaluate the progression of an occupational or environmental respiratory disease as well as the effectiveness of nursing and medical interventions. You may need to obtain more detailed descriptions from patients with advanced disease.

While patients are often quick to complain about cardinal signs and symptoms of these diseases—such as dyspnea, coughing, and sputum production—they frequently neglect to mention an increased susceptibility to upper respiratory tract infections and postnasal discharge. These are also important signs of respiratory irritation, so ask the patient about them.

Tripod position makes breathing easier

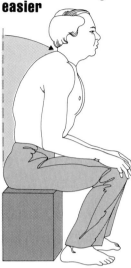

Assuming the tripod position makes breathing easier by allowing maximal excursion of the diaphragm, which promotes chest expansion. Have the patient sit and lean forward, as shown above, resting his hands on his knees to support the upper torso.

Objective data

Physical examination of the patient may provide important objective data to support your suspicion that an occupational or environmental respiratory disease exists. To begin with, you can form a general impression of the patient's respiratory status simply by noting his facial expression, positioning, and speech pattern. Chronic shortness of breath typically produces a pained facial expression. An obstructive impairment often causes the patient to instinctively lean forward to aid chest expansion. Decreased inspiratory capacity causes frequent interruptions of speech to allow breathing.

Any lung dysfunction causes an increased respiratory rate (normal is 12 to 16 respirations per minute). Shallow breathing and limited chest expansion occur in patients with severe restrictive impairment secondary to fibrosis. A barrel chest and the use of accessory muscles to breathe may indicate obstructive impairment.

On inspection, you may also find coal miner's tattoos—black marks that remain on exposed areas of the skin long after the person has stopped working in the mines. Note the color of the patient's sputum. Red sputum may result from siderosis, an occupational respiratory disease (usually benign) caused by exposure to iron dust.

Decreased chest expansion and increased vocal fremitus noted on palpation usually indicate fibrosis. If fibrosis is extensive, you'll detect dullness on percussion. With severe obstructive impairment, however, you'll find hyperresonance.

Auscultation can yield a wealth of clinical information. Extensive fibrosis decreases ventilation, producing diminished breath sounds. Obstructive impairment produces the same finding, but for a different reason—decreased airflow. Rales are audible when secretions or fluid clog the airways, as in allergic alveolitis, chronic bronchitis, and pulmonary edema. Rhonchi can be heard when air passes through constricted airways, as in occupational asthma and the bronchospasms that accompany chronic bronchitis.

You'll want to auscultate the patient's heart, too. Remember that cor pulmonale is associated with chronic respiratory disease. Listen for a ventricular gallop that intensifies during normal inspiration, which usually reflects right ventricular hypertrophy, the hallmark of cor pulmonale. Ankle edema and jugular vein distention usually precede this condition.

Nursing diagnoses

Occupational and environmental respiratory diseases impair not only the ability to breathe but also the ability to live a full, meaningful life. Your nursing diagnoses, therefore, can be divided into physiologic and psychological categories. Under physiologic effects, we'll discuss alterations in breathing patterns, airway clearance, and gas exchange; under psychological effects, disturbances in self-concept, body image, self-esteem, and role performance.

Your overall goal, of course, is to provide the patient and his family with the knowledge and skills they'll need to cope with the disease as comfortably as possible. Specific goals and interventions hinge on problems identified in the nursing diagnosis and on the patient's life-style priorities.

Let's consider the more obvious physiologic effects first:

Alteration in breathing patterns. This first physiologic nursing diagnosis may be related to structural or functional changes in the respiratory system caused by exposure to harmful pollutants. Your primary nursing goals are:
• to teach the patient to breathe more effectively by practicing various techniques, such as stabilization of the shoulders and abdomen during breathing, the use of accessory muscles of respiration, and pursed-lip breathing to prolong the expiratory phase.
• to promote chest expansion by having the patient assume positions that allow maximum excursion of the diaphragm, such as the tripod position (see *Tripod position makes breathing easier,* page 180), and by instructing him to wear supportive or nonrestrictive clothing.

Your nursing interventions include assessing the patient for dyspnea, increased respiratory rate, and hypoxemia (with or without hypercapnia), as well as shortness of breath, cyanosis, and coughing. Look, too, for nasal flaring during inspiration, changes in the depth of inspirations, and an increased anteroposterior chest diameter. These assessments allow you to evaluate the patient's breathing patterns accurately. You can then teach him the techniques and positions that'll help him breathe more effectively. Other appropriate interventions include administering oxygen, if necessary, and emphasizing the importance of avoiding smoking and other harmful pollutants.

Alterations in airway clearance. This second

physiologic nursing diagnosis may be related to airway infection, tracheobronchial secretions, ineffective coughing, or bronchoconstriction. Your primary nursing goals are:
• to help prevent airway infections by instructing the patient to avoid crowds and close contact with persons who are prone to such infections and by recommending annual vaccination for influenza or vaccination for pneumococcus (Pneumococcal vaccine guarantees immunity for 3 to 5 years, but recent studies indicate possible lifetime immunity from the vaccine.)
• to teach the patient the early signs and symptoms of airway infection, such as fever, increased shortness of breath, wheezing, and a change in sputum color, consistency, amount, or odor
• to teach the patient to clear his airways of tracheobronchial secretions by performing various maneuvers, such as deep breathing, controlled coughing, and postural drainage
• to minimize bronchoconstriction secondary to airway infections by teaching the patient to adjust dosages of bronchodilators and corticosteroids.

Your nursing interventions include assessing the patient for dyspnea, tracheobronchial congestion, rhonchi, wheezing, coughing, and sputum production. Also observe for fever, cyanosis, and hypoxemia (with or without hypercapnia). Evaluate sputum color, consistency, amount, and odor. To facilitate expectoration of sputum, ensure adequate hydration.

Have the patient perform airway clearance maneuvers, as necessary. For controlled coughing, teach the patient the "forceful" or "huff" technique. The forceful technique involves having the patient take a slow, deep breath, which he holds for the count of three. On the count of two, he contracts his abdominal muscles; on the count of three, he exhales forcefully and coughs at the same time. A patient who can't cough forcefully can try the huff technique: He inhales deeply, then exhales as rapidly as possible while repeatedly whispering the word "huff."

Alterations in gas exchange. This third physiologic nursing diagnosis may be related to a poor ventilation/perfusion ratio, bronchoconstriction, intrapulmonary shunting, or diffusion impairment. Your primary nursing goals are:
• to teach the patient the early signs and symptoms of hypoxemia and hypercapnia, such as headache, irritability, facial flushing, diaphoresis, confusion, and tachypnea

• to prevent or control hypoxemia and hypercapnia by teaching the patient relaxation and deep-breathing techniques
• to teach the patient to avoid drugs that depress the respiratory system, such as sedatives, analgesics, narcotics, tranquilizers, and alcohol
• to decrease oxygen consumption by advising appropriate modification of the patient's daily activities.

Your nursing interventions include assessing the patient for signs and symptoms of hypoxemia and hypercapnia. Besides those mentioned above, look for a decreased PaO_2 level (with or without an increased $PaCO_2$ level), dysrhythmias, polycythemia, and cyanosis. Recognize that cyanosis is a relatively late sign of hypoxemia. Administer oxygen therapy, if necessary.

Disturbances in self-concept, body image, self-esteem, and role performance. This key psychological nursing diagnosis may be related to changes in physical appearance or to increased physical or psychological dependence. Your primary nursing goals are:
• to teach the patient to avoid activities that require physical exertion and to explore alternative activities
• to promote the patient's sense of self-worth and independence and to encourage him to set realistic goals.

Your nursing interventions include assessing the patient for carelessness in dressing or grooming, difficulty in making decisions, withdrawal from family and social interactions, expressions of decreased self-worth, and increasingly dependent behavior. Try to determine the reasons for the patient's feelings by getting him to talk about them openly and honestly. Help him to identify and make the most of his physical and emotional strengths. Make sure you include the family in these discussions. If necessary, refer the patient for vocational rehabilitation.

A matter of skill—and compassion
Remember that occupational and environmental respiratory diseases often strike people with limited education and financial resources, to whom personal appearance and physical prowess are extremely important. If you keep this in mind, you'll be able to care for these patients as human beings—not statistics. As victims of one of the sorrier legacies of modern industrialization, they need your compassion and emotional support as much as your nursing knowledge and skills.

Points to remember

• All occupational and environmental respiratory diseases stem from some form of air pollution.
• Treatment for occupational and environmental respiratory diseases has two major goals: to prevent further lung damage and to relieve the patient's signs and symptoms.
• With these diseases, the importance of a *detailed* patient history can't be overemphasized.
• Your nursing diagnoses must consider the physical *and* psychological effects of these diseases on the patient.

APPENDIX

Respiratory drugs

Adrenergics

Drug, dose, and route	Interactions	Side effects	Special considerations
albuterol 1 or 2 inhalations q 4 to 6 hours; 2 to 4 mg P.O. t.i.d. or q.i.d.	*Beta-adrenergic blockers:* blocked bronchodilating effect. Monitor patient carefully.	Tremor, nervousness, insomnia, palpitations	Tablets and aerosol may be used concomitantly. Monitor the patient closely for toxicity. Note that elderly patients usually require a lower dose. To help prevent dry mouth and throat, have the patient rinse his mouth with water after each inhaled dose. Albuterol reportedly produces less cardiac stimulation than other sympathomimetics, especially isoproterenol. It's also known by the generic name of salbutomol.

ephedrine
12.5 to 50 mg P.O. b.i.d., t.i.d., or q.i.d.
	Beta-adrenergic blockers: blocked bronchodilating effect. Monitor patient carefully.
	Urinary alkalinizers: may increase ephedrine's toxic effects.
	MAO inhibitors, tricyclic antidepressants: may cause hypertension. Give cautiously with ephedrine.
	Guanethidine: antihypertensive action may be antagonized.
		Insomnia, nervousness, palpitations, tachycardia, urinary retention, hypertension	Warn the patient not to take over-the-counter drugs that contain ephedrine without informing the doctor.
			    To prevent insomnia, avoid giving this drug within 2 hours before bedtime.
			    Because effectiveness decreases after 2 to 3 weeks, the dosage may need to be increased. Although tolerance develops, ephedrine isn't known to cause addiction.

epinephrine 0.1 to 0.5 ml of 1:1,000 S.C. or I.M. Repeat dose q 10 to 15 minutes p.r.n.	*Beta-adrenergic blockers:* blocked bronchodilating effect. Monitor patient carefully. *Tricyclic antidepressants:* may cause hypertension. Give cautiously with epinephrine. *Guanethidine:* antihypertensive action may be antagonized.	Nervousness, headache, palpitations, tachycardia, cardiac dysrhythmias, hyperglycemia, hypertension	Use this drug cautiously in elderly patients and those with a history of heart disease, hyperthyroidism, angina, hypertension, or diabetes. After injection, observe the patient closely for side effects. Massage injection site to counteract possible vasoconstriction. Repeated local injection can cause necrosis at site due to vasoconstriction. In the event of a sharp blood pressure rise, rapid-acting vasodilators, such as the nitrites or alpha-adrenergic blocking agents, can be given to counteract the marked pressor effect of large doses of epinephrine.
isoetharine mesylate 1 to 2 inhalations q 4 hours.	*Beta-adrenergic blockers:* blocked bronchodilating effect. Monitor patient carefully.	Tremor, headache, palpitations	Recognize that some patients may require more inhalations or more frequent doses to achieve effectiveness. However, excessive use can decrease drug effectiveness. Monitor for severe paradoxical bronchoconstriction after excessive use. Discontinue the drug immediately if bronchoconstriction occurs.

isoproterenol
1 or 2 inhalations q.i.d.; 10 to 20 mg sublingually q 6 to 8 hours.
	Beta-adrenergic blockers: blocked bronchodilating effect. Monitor patient carefully.	Headache, palpitations, tremor, nervousness, insomnia, tachycardia, angina	Sublingual tablets are often poorly and erratically absorbed. Teach the patient how to take these tablets properly. Tell him to hold the tablet under his tongue until it dissolves and is absorbed and not to swallow saliva until that time.
			    Warn the patient using an oral inhalant that the drug may turn his sputum and saliva pink. Advise the patient not to take more than 2 inhalations at one time and to wait 2 minutes between inhalations.
			    Since the patient may develop a tolerance to this drug, warn against overuse.

metaproterenol
2 or 3 inhalations q 3 to 4 hours, not to exceed 12 inhalations daily; 20 mg P.O. q 6 to 8 hours.
	Beta-adrenergic blockers: blocked bronchodilating effect. Monitor patient carefully.	Tremor, nervousness, insomnia, palpitations	Tablets and aerosol may be used concomitantly. Monitor the patient closely for toxicity.
			    Tell the patient to notify doctor if no response to prescribed dosage. Warn against changing dose without calling doctor.
			    Metaproterenol reportedly produces less cardiac stimulation than other sympathomimetics, especially isoproterenol.

terbutaline 2.5 to 5 mg P.O. q 8 hours; 0.25 mg S.C. Repeat subcutaneous dose if no improvement occurs, but don't exceed more than 0.5 mg S.C. in a 4-hour period.	*Beta-adrenergic blockers:* blocked bronchodilating effect. Monitor patient carefully.	Tremor, nervousness, insomnia, palpitations	Protect the injection from light. Avoid using discolored injections. Give subcutaneous injections in the lateral deltoid area. Recognize that tolerance to this drug may develop with prolonged use.

Theophylline and derivatives

Drug, dose, and route	Interactions	Side effects	Special considerations
aminophylline (theophylline ethylene diamine) 5.6 mg/kg I.V. as a loading dose; 0.3 to 0.9 mg/kg hourly by I.V. infusion as a maintenance dose. Oral maintenance dose is 250 to 500 mg q 6 to 8 hours.	*Beta-adrenergic blockers:* may antagonize pharmacologic effect of aminophylline. May cause bronchospasm. Use together cautiously. *Erythromycin, cimetidine:* decreased hepatic clearance of aminophylline, causing elevated aminophylline levels. Monitor for toxicity. *Phenytoin:* increased pharmacologic effects of both drugs possible.	Restlessness, dizziness, insomnia, convulsions, palpitations, nausea, vomiting, anorexia	Before giving loading dose, check that patient hasn't had recent theophylline therapy. Warn elderly patients of dizziness, a common side effect at start of therapy. Individuals metabolize xanthines at different rates. Adjust dose by monitoring response, tolerance, pulmonary function, and aminophylline blood levels. Consider 10 to 20 mcg/ml a therapeutic aminophylline level. Levels more than 20 mcg/ml indicate toxicity. Monitor carefully for GI symptoms, which usually accompany toxicity. Note that plasma clearance may be decreased in patients with congestive heart failure, hepatic dysfunction, or pulmonary edema. Smokers show accelerated clearance. Adjust dose as necessary. Suppositories are unreliably absorbed. Avoid rectal administration or schedule after evacuations, if possible.
dyphylline 200 to 800 mg P.O. q 6 hours; 250 to 500 mg I.M. q 6 hours. Never administer drug intravenously.	*Beta-adrenergic blockers:* may antagonize pharmacologic effect of dyphylline. May cause bronchospasm. Use together cautiously. *Probenecid:* may decrease renal excretion of dyphylline. Monitor for dyphylline toxicity.	Restlessness, dizziness, insomnia, convulsions, palpitations, nausea, vomiting, anorexia	Question the patient closely about other drugs used. Warn that over-the-counter drugs may contain ephedrine in combination with theophylline salts. Concomitant use may cause excessive CNS stimulation. Tell the patient to check with the doctor before taking any other drugs. Warn elderly patients of dizziness, a common side effect. Also advise taking the oral dose after meals to help reduce gastric irritation. Discard dyphylline ampul if precipitate is present. Protect ampul from light. Note that dyphylline is a chemical derivative of theophylline, but is not a theophylline "salt" as are the other spasmolytics.
oxtriphylline 200 mg P.O. q 6 hours.	*Beta-adrenergic blockers:* may antagonize pharmacologic effects of oxtriphylline. Use together cautiously. *Erythromycin, cimetidine:* decreased hepatic clearance of oxtriphylline, causing elevated oxtriphylline levels. Monitor for toxicity. *Phenytoin:* increased pharmacologic effects of both drugs possible.	Restlessness, dizziness, insomnia, convulsions, palpitations, nausea, vomiting, anorexia	Question the patient closely about other drugs used. Warn that over-the-counter drugs may contain ephedrine in combination with theophylline salts. Concomitant use may cause excessive CNS stimulation. Tell the patient to check with the doctor before taking any other drugs. Advise the patient to report GI distress, palpitations, irritability, restlessness, nervousness, or insomnia; these signs may indicate excessive CNS stimulation. Store this drug at 15° to 30° C. (59° to 86° F.). Protect elixir from light, tablets from moisture.
theophylline 100 to 200 mg P.O. q 6 hours or q 8 to 12 hours for time-release form.	*Beta-adrenergic blockers:* may antagonize pharmacologic effects of theophylline. Use together cautiously. *Erythromycin, cimetidine:* decreased hepatic clearance of theophylline, causing elevated theophylline levels. Monitor for toxicity. *Phenytoin:* increased pharmacologic effects of both drugs possible.	Restlessness, dizziness, insomnia, convulsions, palpitations, nausea, vomiting, anorexia	Question the patient closely about other drugs used. Warn that over-the-counter drugs may contain ephedrine in combination with theophylline salts. Concomitant use may cause excessive CNS stimulation. Tell the patient to check with the doctor before taking any other drugs. Warn elderly patients of dizziness, a common side effect at start of therapy. Individuals metabolize xanthines at different rates. Adjust dose by monitoring response, tolerance, pulmonary function, and theophylline plasma levels. Consider 10 to 20 mcg/ml a therapeutic theophylline level. Be careful not to confuse sustained-release with standard-release dosage forms.

Antituberculars

Drug, dose, and route	Interactions	Side effects	Special considerations
ethambutol 15 mg/kg P.O. in a single daily dose.	None significant.	Optic neuritis with loss of color perception, hyperuricemia	Perform visual acuity and color discrimination tests before and during therapy. Also monitor serum uric acid; observe patient for symptoms of gout.
isoniazid 300 mg P.O. in a single daily dose.	*Disulfiram:* possible neurologic symptoms, including changes in behavior and coordination. *Phenytoin:* possible phenytoin toxicity. Use together cautiously.	Peripheral neuropathy, hepatitis (occasionally severe), allergic skin rashes	Monitor hepatic function during therapy. Tell the patient to notify doctor if symptoms of hepatic dysfunction (loss of appetite, fatigue, malaise, jaundice, dark urine) occur. Discourage use of alcohol, which may be associated with increased incidence of isoniazid-related hepatitis. Administer pyridoxine concomitantly to prevent peripheral neuropathy, especially in malnourished patients.

Antituberculars (continued)

Drug, dose, and route	Interactions	Side effects	Special considerations
rifampin 600 mg P.O. in a single daily dose.	*Corticosteroids:* decreased therapeutic effect of corticosteroids possible. *Oral contraceptives:* decreased pharmacologic effect of oral contraceptives. Suggest alternate form of birth control. *Oral anticoagulants:* decreased effectiveness of oral anticoagulants. Monitor prothrombin time. *Quinidine:* decreased levels of quinidine possible. Monitor blood levels and EKG.	Serious hepatotoxicity and transient abnormal liver function tests, drowsiness, mental confusion, thrombocytopenia, leukopenia, gastrointestinal irritation	Give this drug 1 hour before or 2 hours after meals for optimal absorption; however, if GI irritation occurs, patient may take rifampin with meals. Monitor hepatic function during therapy. Tell the patient to notify doctor of symptoms of hepatic dysfunction (loss of appetite, fatigue, malaise, jaundice, dark urine). Also monitor hematopoietic studies. Warn the patient about drowsiness and the possibility of red-orange discoloration of urine, feces, saliva, sweat, sputum, and tears. Soft contact lenses may be permanently stained.
streptomycin 1 g I.M. daily in a single dose, 2 to 3 times weekly.	*Ethacrynic acid, bumetanide, furosemide:* may increase streptomycin's ototoxic effects. Monitor patient carefully. *Dimenhydrinate:* may mask symptoms of ototoxicity. Use together cautiously.	Tinnitus and high frequency hearing loss, vertigo, nausea, vomiting, nephrotoxicity	Inject this drug deeply into upper outer quadrant of buttocks. Protect your hands when preparing drug, as it's very sensitizing topically. Test patient's hearing before, during, and 6 months after therapy. Notify doctor if patient complains of tinnitus, roaring noises, or fullness in his ears.

Antifungals

Drug, dose, and route	Interactions	Side effects	Special considerations
amphotericin B 0.25 mg/kg daily by slow I.V. infusion over 6 hours. Increase dose up to 1 mg/kg daily.	None significant.	Thrombophlebitis, pain at injection site, fever, chills, hypokalemia, nephrotoxicity, nausea, vomiting	Monitor potassium levels closely during therapy. Report any signs of hypokalemia. Check calcium and magnesium levels periodically. Obtain renal function studies weekly. If BUN exceeds 40 mg/100 ml, or if serum creatinine exceeds 3 mg/100 ml, doctor may reduce or stop this drug until renal function improves. Severity of some side effects can be reduced by premedication with aspirin, antihistamines, antiemetics, or small doses of corticosteroids.
flucytosine (5-FC) 50 to 150 mg/kg P.O. daily in divided doses q 6 hours.	None significant.	Nausea, vomiting, diarrhea, anorexia, leukopenia, thrombocytopenia	Obtain hematologic tests and renal and liver function studies before therapy, and repeat them frequently during therapy. Also perform susceptibility tests beforehand to establish that organism is flucytosine-sensitive. Repeat tests weekly. Give capsules over a 15-minute period to reduce nausea, vomiting, and stomach upset. Note that drug is often combined with amphotericin B; use may be synergistic.
ketoconazole 200 to 400 mg P.O. in a single daily dose.	*Antacids, anticholinergics, cimetidine, ranitidine:* decreased absorption of ketoconazole. Schedule these drugs at least 2 hours after administering the ketoconazole dose.	Nausea; vomiting; abdominal pain; serious, and possibly fatal, hepatotoxicity	Reassure patient that, although nausea is common early in therapy, it will subside. Monitor for elevated liver enzymes and persistent nausea, possible signs of hepatotoxicity.
miconazole 600 to 1,200 mg daily by I.V. infusion, divided over 3 infusions.	None significant.	Hyponatremia, nausea, vomiting, thrombophlebitis, pruritic rash	Inform patient that adequate response may take weeks or months. Monitor levels of hemoglobin, hematocrit, electrolytes, and lipids regularly. Recognize that pruritic rash may persist for weeks after drug is discontinued.

Broad-spectrum anti-infectives

Drug, dose, and route	Interactions	Side effects	Special considerations
ampicillin 250 mg to 1 g P.O., I.M., or I.V. q 6 hours.	*Tetracycline:* antibiotic antagonism. Give ampicillin at least 1 hour before tetracycline. *Aminoglycoside antibiotics:* separate ampicillin dose by at least 1 hour. Also, don't mix together in the same I.V. container.	Diarrhea, nausea, vomiting, maculopapular skin rash, hypersensitivity	When giving drug I.V., mix with dextrose 5% in water or a saline solution. Don't mix with other drugs or solutions; they might be incompatible. When given orally, drug may cause GI disturbances. Food may interfere with absorption, so give drug 1 to 2 hours before meals or 2 to 3 hours after.
cefazolin 500 mg to 1 g I.M. or I.V. q 6 to 8 hours.	*Probenecid:* may increase blood levels of cephalosporins. Use together cautiously.	Thrombophlebitis at I.V. injection site, maculopapular skin rash, diarrhea	Use cautiously in patients with impaired renal status and in those with history of sensitivity to penicillin. Avoid doses greater than 4 g daily in patients with severe renal impairment. Ask the patient if he's ever had any reaction to cephalosporin or penicillin therapy before administering first dose. Alternate injection sites if I.V. therapy lasts longer than 3 days. Use of small I.V. needles in the larger veins may also be preferable. About 40% to 75% of patients receiving cephalosporins show a false-positive direct Coombs' test; only a few of these indicate hemolytic anemia.

Broad-spectrum anti-infectives (continued)

Drug, dose, and route	Interactions	Side effects	Special considerations
cloxacillin 250 to 500 mg P.O. q 6 hours.	*Tetracycline:* antibiotic antagonism. Separate cloxacillin dose by at least 1 hour.	Nausea, vomiting, diarrhea, skin rash, hypersensitivity	Before giving cloxacillin, ask the patient if he's had any allergic reactions to penicillin. Be alert to cross allergenicity with cephalosporins. Food may interfere with absorption, so give this drug 1 to 2 hours before meals or 2 to 3 hours after.
erythromycin 500 mg to 1 g P.O. or I.V. q 6 hours.	*Digoxin:* increased digoxin blood levels and possibly toxicity. *Theophylline derivatives:* increased theophylline blood levels. Monitor for toxicity.	Abdominal pain and cramping, nausea, vomiting, diarrhea, thrombophlebitis at I.V. injection site	Erythromycin estolate may cause serious hepatotoxicity in adults (reversible cholestatic jaundice). Monitor hepatic function for increased levels of bilirubin, SGOT, SGPT, and alkaline phosphatase. Other erythromycin salts cause hepatotoxicity to a lesser degree. Report side effects, especially nausea, abdominal pain, or fever.
gentamicin 1.5 mg/kg I.V. or I.M. q 8 hours.	*Bumetanide, ethacrynic acid, furosemide:* increased ototoxicity. Use together cautiously. *I.V. penicillins:* separate gentamicin dose by at least 1 hour. Also, don't mix together in the same I.V. container. *Nondepolarizing muscle relaxants:* increased neuromuscular blocking effects of these drugs. Use together cautiously.	Nephrotoxicity (directly related to high blood levels), ototoxicity, skin rash	Weigh the patient and obtain baseline renal function studies (output, specific gravity, urinalysis, BUN, creatinine levels, and creatinine clearance) before therapy begins. Monitor renal function studies during therapy and notify the doctor of signs of renal impairment. Ensure that the patient is well hydrated while taking this drug to minimize chemical irritation of the renal tubules. Evaluate the patient's hearing before and during therapy. Notify the doctor if the patient complains of tinnitus, vertigo, or hearing loss. After completing I.V. infusion, flush the line with normal saline solution.
oxacillin 0.5 to 1 g P.O., I.M., or I.V. q 4 to 6 hours.	*Aminoglycoside antibiotics:* separate I.V. oxacillin dose by at least 1 hour. Also, don't mix together in the same I.V. container. *Tetracycline:* antibiotic antagonism. Give oxacillin at least 1 hour before tetracycline.	Nausea, vomiting, diarrhea, elevated liver enzymes, thrombophlebitis, skin rash, hypersensitivity	Before giving oxacillin, ask the patient if he's had any allergic reactions to penicillin. Be alert to cross allergenicity with the cephalosporins. When given orally, this drug may cause GI disturbances. Food may interfere with absorption, so give drug 1 to 2 hours before meals or 2 to 3 hours after. Obtain periodic liver function studies during therapy. Watch for elevated SGOT and SGPT.
penicillin G 1.6 to 3.2 million units P.O. daily in divided doses q 6 hours; 1.2 to 12 million units I.M. or I.V. daily in divided doses q 6 hours.	*Aminoglycoside antibiotics:* separate I.V. penicillin dose by at least 1 hour. Also, don't mix together in the same I.V. container. *Tetracycline:* antibiotic antagonism. Give penicillin at least 1 hour before tetracycline.	Hypersensitivity, skin rash, thrombophlebitis	Before giving penicillin, ask the patient if he's had any allergic reactions to this drug. Check the drug's expiration date. Warn the patient never to use leftover penicillin for a new illness or to share penicillin with family and friends. Tell the patient to call the doctor if rash, fever, or chills develop. A rash is the most common allergic reaction.
tobramycin 1.5 mg/kg I.V. or I.M. q 8 hours.	*Bumetanide, ethacrynic acid, furosemide:* increased ototoxicity. Use cautiously together. *I.V. penicillins:* separate tobramycin dose by at least 1 hour. Also, don't mix together in same I.V. container. *Nondepolarizing muscle relaxants:* increased neuromuscular blocking effects of these drugs. Use together cautiously.	Nephrotoxicity (directly related to high blood levels), ototoxicity, skin rash	Weigh the patient and obtain baseline renal function studies (output, specific gravity, urinalysis, BUN, creatinine levels, and creatinine clearance) before therapy begins. Monitor renal function during therapy. Notify the doctor of signs of renal impairment. Evaluate the patient's hearing before and during therapy. Notify doctor if the patient complains of tinnitus, vertigo, or hearing loss. After I.V. infusion, flush line with normal saline solution.

Miscellaneous respiratory drugs

Drug, dose, and route	Interactions	Side effects	Special considerations
acetylcysteine *For congestion:* 1 or 2 inhalations of a 10% to 20% solution by direct instillation into the trachea.	None significant.	Bronchospasm, stomatitis, rhinorrhea, hemoptysis	Monitor frequency and nature of the patient's cough. For maximum effect, instruct patient to clear his airway by coughing before aerosol administration. Use plastic, glass, stainless steel, or another nonreactive metal when administering drug by nebulization. After opening, solution color may change to light purple. This doesn't affect its safety or mucolytic activity. Store solution in refrigerator and use it within 96 hours.
cromolyn sodium *For asthma:* contents of 20 mg capsule inhaled q.i.d. at regular intervals.	None significant.	Bronchospasm following inhalation of dry powder, irritation of throat and trachea	Before cromolyn therapy, obtain pulmonary function tests to show significant bronchodilator-reversible component to patient's airway obstruction. Administer drug only when acute episode has been controlled, airway is cleared, and patient is able to inhale.

Miscellaneous respiratory drugs (continued)

Drug, dose, and route	Interactions	Side effects	Special considerations
heparin *For pulmonary embolism:* 7,500 to 10,000 units I.V. bolus, then 1,000 units hourly by I.V. infusion.	*Aspirin:* may increase bleeding risk. Don't use together.	Hemorrhage and excessive bleeding, thrombocytopenia	Measure partial thromboplastin time (PTT) carefully and regularly. Anticoagulation is present when PTT values are 1.5 to 2 times control values. When intermittent I.V. therapy is used, always draw blood ½ hour before next scheduled dose to avoid false-elevated PTT. 　Note that elderly patients typically start at lower doses. Avoid excessive I.M. injections of other drugs to prevent or minimize hematomas. If possible, don't give I.M. injections at all.
naloxone *For narcotic-induced respiratory depression:* 0.4 mg I.V., S.C., or I.M. May repeat dose q 2 to 3 minutes, p.r.n. for 3 doses.	None significant.	None significant	Use cautiously in patients with cardiac irritability and narcotic addiction. Monitor respiratory rate and rhythm. Be prepared to provide oxygen, ventilation, and other resuscitative measures. 　Naloxone is the safest drug to use when the cause of respiratory depression is uncertain. Because it's short-acting, be prepared to administer follow-up doses.
warfarin *For pulmonary embolism:* 2 to 10 mg daily P.O. is usual maintenance dose.	*Allopurinol, chloramphenicol, danazol, cloifibrate, diflunisal, dextrothyroxine, thyroid drugs, heparin, anabolic steroids, cimetidine, disulfiram, glucagon, inhalation anesthetics, metronidazole, quinidine, influenza vaccine, sulindac, sulfonamides:* increased prothrombin time. Monitor patient carefully for bleeding. Consider anticoagulant dose reduction. *Ethacrynic acid, indomethacin, mefenamic acid, oxyphenbutazone, phenylbutazone, salicylates:* increased prothrombin time; ulcerogenic effects. Don't use together. *Griseofulvin, haloperiodol, carbamazepine, paraldehyde, rifampin:* decreased prothrombin time with reduced anticoagulant effect. Monitor patient carefully. *Glutethimide, chloral hydrate, sulfinpyrazone, triclofos sodium:* increased or decreased prothrombin time. Avoid use if possible, or monitor patient carefully.	Hemorrhage and excessive bleeding, dermatitis, rash, fever	Recognize that PT determinations are essential to monitor anticoagulant effect. Doctors usually try to maintain PT at 1.5 to 2 times normal. A high incidence of bleeding occurs when PT exceeds 2.5 times control values. 　Give this drug at the same time daily. Stress importance of complying with recommended dosage and keeping follow-up appointments. Advise patient to carry a card that identifies him as a potential bleeder. Also suggest that he use an electric razor when shaving to avoid scratching skin and to brush his teeth with a soft toothbrush. Tell the female patient to notify the doctor if menses is heavier than usual. The dosage may need to be adjusted. Note that fever and skin rash signal severe complications. Elderly patients and patients with renal or hepatic failure are especially sensitive to warfarin effect.
hydrocortisone *For inflammation:* 50 to 250 mg I.M. or I.V. q 6 hours. **prednisone** *For inflammation:* 2.5 to 15 mg P.O. b.i.d., t.i.d., or q.i.d.	*Barbiturates, phenytoin, rifampin:* decreased corticosteroid effect. Corticosteroid dose may need to be increased. *Indomethacin, aspirin:* increased risk of GI distress and bleeding. Give together cautiously.	Hypokalemia, hyperglycemia, peptic ulcer, euphoria, insomnia, hypertension, edema and fluid retention	Give I.M. injection deep into gluteal muscle. Avoid subcutaneous injection, as atrophy and sterile abscesses may occur. Give P.O. dose with food when possible. 　Unless contraindicated, give salt-restricted diet rich in potassium and protein. Potassium supplement may be needed. Watch for additional potassium depletion from diuretics and amphotericin B. 　Warn patients on long-term therapy about cushingoid symptoms. Gradually reduce drug dosage after long-term therapy. Tell the patient not to discontinue the drug abruptly or without doctor's consent.
streptokinase *For pulmonary embolism:* 250,000 IU by I.V. infusion over 30 minutes, then 100,000 IU hourly by I.V. infusion for 24 to 72 hours. **urokinase** *For pulmonary embolism:* 4,400 IU/kg by I.V. infusion over 10 minutes, then 4,400 IU/kg hourly by I.V. infusion for 12 to 24 hours.	*Anticoagulants:* concurrent use of anticoagulants is not recommended. Reversing the effects of oral anticoagulants must be considered before beginning therapy, and heparin must be stopped and its effects allowed to diminish. *Aspirin, indomethacin, phenylbutazone, drugs affecting platelet activity:* increased risk of bleeding. Don't use together.	Severe bleeding, decreased hematocrit, thrombophlebitis, anaphylaxis (especially with streptokinase)	These drugs should be used only by doctors with wide experience in thrombotic disease management in a setting where clinical and laboratory monitoring can be performed. Before therapy, draw blood to determine PTT and PT. Monitor patient for excessive bleeding during therapy; if evident, discontinue drug. Pretreatment with heparin or drugs affecting platelets increases risk of bleeding. Have typed and crossmatched packed red cells and whole blood available to treat possible hemorrhage. Also keep aminocaproic acid available to treat bleeding. Keep venipuncture sites to a minimum; use pressure dressing on puncture sites for at least 15 minutes. Monitor vital signs frequently. Watch for signs of hypersensitivity. Notify the doctor immediately if these signs occur. Corticosteroids are used to treat allergic reactions.

Selected References and Acknowledgments

Selected References

Anderson, Sandra V., and Eleanor E. Bauwens. *Chronic Health Problems: Concepts and Applications.* St. Louis: C.V. Mosby Co., 1981.

◆

Bates, Barbara. *A Guide to Physical Examination,* 2d ed. New York: Harper & Row, 1979.

◆

Beamis, J.F., A. Stein, and J.L. Andrews. *Changing Epidemiology of Lung Cancer: Increasing Incidence in Women.* Medical Clinics of North America, vol. 33, no. 1. Philadelphia: W.B. Saunders Co., 1983.

◆

Bone, R.C., ed. *Respiratory Failure.* Medical Clinics of North America, vol. 67, no. 3. Philadelphia: W.B. Saunders Co., 1983.

◆

Borrie, John. *Management of Thoracic Emergencies,* 3d ed. New York: Appleton-Century-Crofts, 1980.

◆

Brunner, Lillian S. *The Lippincott Manual of Nursing Practice,* 3d ed. Philadelphia: J.B. Lippincott Co., 1982.

◆

Cameron, Terrie J. "Fiberoptic Bronchoscopy." *American Journal of Nursing,* August 1981.

◆

Campbell, Claire. *Nursing Diagnosis and Intervention in Nursing Practice.* New York: John Wiley & Sons, 1978.

◆

Chaffee, Ellen E., et al. *Basic Physiology and Anatomy,* 4th ed. Philadelphia: J.B. Lippincott Co., 1980.

◆

Chronic Obstructive Pulmonary Disease. New York: American Lung Association, 1981.

◆

Cline, Barbara A., and Mary L. Fisher. "A.R.D.S. Means Emergency." *Nursing82* 12 (February 1982): 62-67.

◆

Eighth Report of the Director, National Heart, Lung and Blood Institute, Bethesda, Md.: National Institutes of Health.

◆

Erickson, Roberta. "Chest Tubes: They're Really Not That Complicated." *Nursing81* 11 (May 1981).

◆

Facts in Brief About Lung Disease. New York: American Lung Association, 1982.

Glezen, W.P., et al. "Mortality and Influenza." *Journal of Infectious Diseases* 146:3 (September 1982): 313-321.

◆

Griffin, Joyce P. "Acquired Immune Deficiency Syndrome: A New Epidemic." *Critical Care Nurse* 3:2 (March-April 1983).

◆

Guenter, Clarence A., and Martin H. Welch, eds. *Pulmonary Medicine,* 2d ed. Philadelphia: J.B. Lippincott Co., 1982.

◆

Guyton, Arthur C. *Textbook of Medical Physiology,* 6th ed. Philadelphia: W.B. Saunders Co., 1981.

◆

Harper, R.W. *A Guide to Respiratory Care: Physiology and Clinical Application.* Philadelphia: J.B. Lippincott Co., 1981.

◆

Kaye, Donald, and Louis F. Rose. *Fundamentals of Internal Medicine.* St. Louis: C.V. Mosby Co., 1983.

◆

Kenner, Cornelia V., et al. *Critical Care Nursing: Body—Mind—Spirit.* Boston: Little, Brown, 1981.

◆

Kinney, Marguerite, et al. *AACN's Reference for Critical Care Nursing.* New York: McGraw-Hill Book Co., 1981.

◆

Light, R.W. *Pleural Effusions.* Medical Clinics of North America, vol. 61. Philadelphia: W.B. Saunders Co., 1977.

◆

Luckmann, Joan, and Karen C. Sorenson. *Medical-Surgical Nursing: A Psychophysiologic Approach,* 2d ed. Philadelphia: W.B. Saunders Co., 1980.

◆

Meador, Billie. "Pneumothorax: Providing Emergency and Long-Term Care." *Nursing78* 8 (May 1978).

◆

Melan, E.D., et al. "Detection of True Pathologic Stage I Lung Cancer in a Screening Program and the Effect on Survival." *Cancer* 47 (1981): 1182-1187.

◆

Miller, Martha J. *Pathophysiology: Principles of Disease.* Philadelphia: W.B. Saunders Co., 1983.

◆

Moser, Kenneth M., and Roger G. Spragg. *Respiratory Emergencies,* 2d ed. St. Louis: C.V. Mosby Co., 1982.

◆

Netter, Frank H. *The CIBA Collection of Medical Illustrations.* Summit, N.J.: Ciba-Geigy Corp., 1974.

Parkes, W. Raymond. *Occupational Lung Disorders,* 2d ed. Boston: Butterworth, 1982.

◆

Sana, Josephine M., and Richard P. Judge. *Physical Assessment Skills for Nursing Practice,* 2d ed. Boston: Little, Brown, 1982.

◆

Shapiro, Barry A., et al. *Clinical Application of Respiratory Care,* 2d ed. Chicago: Yearbook Medical Pub., 1979.

◆

Sjoberg Eileen. "Nursing Diagnosis and the COPD Patient." *American Journal of Nursing,* February 1983.

◆

Snider, Gordon L. *Clinical Pulmonary Medicine.* Boston: Little, Brown, 1981.

◆

Traver, Gayle A. *Respiratory Nursing: The Science and the Art.* New York: John Wiley & Sons, 1982.

◆

Trichopoulos, D., et al. "Lung Cancer and Passive Smoking." *International Journal of Cancer* 27 (1981): 1-4.

◆

Tucker, Susan M., et al. *Patient Care Standards,* 2d ed. St. Louis: C.V. Mosby Co., 1980.

◆

Weaver, Terri E. "Bronchoscopy, Laryngoscopy, and Their Potential Complications." *RN,* December 1982.

◆

Weaver, Terri E. "Getting the Most from Chest X-rays and Lung Scans." *RN,* November 1982.

◆

West, John B. *Respiratory Physiology: The Essentials,* 2d ed. Baltimore, Md.: Williams & Wilkins, 1979.

◆

Woodin, Linda M. "Your Patient with a Pneumothorax—A Patient in Distress." *Nursing82,* November 1982.

◆

Youtsey, John W., and Kanube P. Rarey. *Respiratory Patient Care.* Englewood Cliffs, N.J.: Prentice-Hall, 1981.

Acknowledgments

◆ pp.46, 49, 62, 120 (X-ray upper right) Photo courtesy: Marc S. Lapayowker, MD, Chairman, Department of Radiology, Abington Memorial Hospital, Abington, Pa.

◆ p.161 Adapted with permission from *Manual for Staging of Cancer,* 2nd ed. (Philadelphia: J.B. Lippincott, 1983).

INDEX

i = illustration; t = table

i = illustration; t = table

i = illustration; t = table

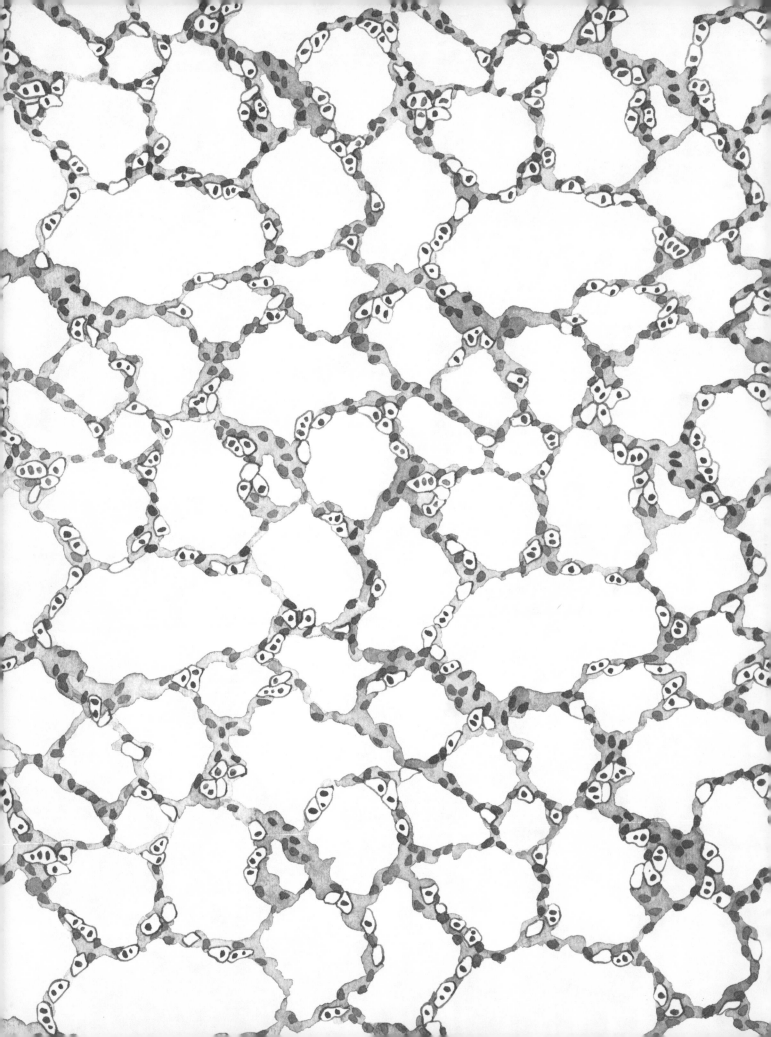